Prescribing Health

Prescribing Health

Transcendental Meditation in Contemporary Medical Care

Edited by David F. O'Connell
and Deborah L. Bevvino

ROWMAN & LITTLEFIELD
Lanham • Boulder • New York • London

Published by Rowman & Littlefield
A wholly owned subsidiary of The Rowman & Littlefield Publishing Group, Inc.
4501 Forbes Boulevard, Suite 200, Lanham, Maryland 20706
www.rowman.com

Unit A, Whitacre Mews, 26-34 Stannary Street, London SE11 4AB

Copyright © 2015 by Rowman & Littlefield

British Library Cataloguing in Publication Information Available

Library of Congress Cataloging-in-Publication Data

Prescribing health : transcendental meditation in contemporary medical care / edited by David F. O'Connell and Deborah L. Bevvino.
    p. ; cm.
  Includes bibliographical references and index.
  ISBN 978-1-4422-2626-5 (cloth : alk. paper) — ISBN 978-1-4422-2627-2 (electronic) 1. Meditation—Health aspects. 2. Meditation—Therapeutic use. 3. Transcendental meditation—Health aspects. 4. Transcendental meditation—Therapeutic use. I. O'Connell, David F., editor. II. Bevvino, Deborah, editor.
  [DNLM: 1. Meditation. 2. Mind-Body Relations, Metaphysical—physiology. BF 637.T68]
  RC489.M43P74 2015
  158.1'28—dc23   2014047418

∞™ The paper used in this publication meets the minimum requirements of American National Standard for Information Sciences—Permanence of Paper for Printed Library Materials, ANSI/NISO Z39.48-1992.

Printed in the United States of America

Contents

Foreword   vii
  Norman Rosenthal, M.D.

Preface   ix
  David F. O'Connell, Ph.D., and Deborah L. Bevvino, Ph.D., NP

SECTION I: THEORY

1 Transcendental Meditation: What, How, and Why   3
   Robert W. Boyer, Ph.D.

2 How Meditation Heals: The Brain and Higher States
   of Consciousness   25
   Fred Travis, Ph.D.

3 Stress, Illness, and Transcendental Meditation: A Triad
   Worth Re-exploring   47
   Deborah L. Bevvino, Ph.D., NP

SECTION II: RESEARCH

Medical Disorders

4 Transcendental Meditation and Cardiovascular Health   69
   Vernon A. Barnes, Ph.D.

5 Transcendental Meditation and the Prevention of Diabetes Mellitus
   and Other Disorders   87
   David Lovell-Smith, Ph.D., M.B., CH.B. FRNZCGP

Mental Health Disorders

6 Transcendental Meditation Research on Anxiety and
   Anxiety Disorders   121
   Sarina Grosswald, Ed.D., David F. O'Connell, Ph.D., M.S.,
   CFC, DABPS, and James Krag, M.D.

7 Transcendental Meditation in the Treatment of Depression   137
   James S. Brooks, M.D.

8 The Use of Transcendental Meditation Practice
   in Promoting Recovery and Preventing Relapse
   for Addictive Diseases   157
   David F. O'Connell, Ph.D., M.S., CFC, DABPS,
   and Alarik Arenander, Ph.D.

9 Transcendental Meditation and the Treatment of
   Childhood Disorders   177
   William R. Stixrud, Ph.D., and Sarina Grosswald, Ed.D.

SECTION III: APPLICATIONS

10 Transcendental Meditation as a Preventative Approach for
    Improving Healthcare Outcomes   205
    Maxwell V. Rainforth, Ph.D., M.S., M.A., B.Sc (Hons),
    and Robert E. Herron, Ph.D., M.B.A., M.S.C.I., B.A.

11 Addressing Societal Problems through Transcendental
    Meditation: Aging, Prison Rehabilitation, and
    Collective Health   243
    David W. Orme-Johnson, Ph.D., and David F. O'Connell,
    Ph.D., M.S., CFC, DABPS

Index   285

The Editors   299

Contributors   301

Foreword

In the nearly forty years since Transcendental Meditation (TM®) was introduced into the United States and the rest of the world by Maharishi Mahesh Yogi, millions of people have learned the simple yet powerful practice. TM has been thoroughly studied scientifically, resulting in over 330 peer-reviewed publications.

Many medical and psychological benefits of TM have been documented. TM has been shown convincingly to reduce blood pressure, reduce cardiovascular disease, and increase longevity. Psychological benefits include reduced anxiety, depression, and addictions. In addition, TM can improve functioning in a variety of stressful circumstances, such as inner-city schools and prisons. The power of TM, however, is not confined to helping heal disease and alleviating situations of dire stress. Happily, the practice also helps to optimize brain function.

Anecdotes of psychological and physical relief thanks to TM abound. Although fascinating in their own right, they are powerfully buttressed by numerous research studies in all the areas of interest mentioned above. What a delight it is to find the most important of these studies described, distilled, and analyzed by leading figures in the field and then brought together and beautifully edited by Drs. O'Connell and Bevvino, who are themselves meditation experts. The resulting volume, *Prescribing Health: Transcendental Meditation in Contemporary Medical Care*, will be a valuable resource for all who seek to understand the potential benefits of TM.

It is my sincere desire and hope that publication of *Prescribing Health* will stimulate serious efforts by the medical and scientific communities to make TM widely available to patients, to implement evidence-based TM programs for a broad range of health disorders, and to vigorously promote and conduct continuing research on TM to address the many ills of society.

Norman E. Rosenthal, M.D., author of *Transcendence: Healing and Transformation through Transcendental Meditation,* and clinical professor of psychiatry, Georgetown University School of Medicine

Preface

Prescribing Health: Transcendental Meditation in Contemporary Medical Care was inspired by a recent huge surge of impressive research on the effects of Transcendental Meditation (TM®) on mental and physical disorders. This increase in research studies, most of it initiated, supported, and funded by the David Lynch Foundation, builds on and extends over four decades of scientific inquiry into the beneficial impact of this ancient meditation technique. The goal of this book is simple and straightforward: to make healthcare professionals—physicians, nurse practitioners, nurses, psychiatrists, psychologists and counselors, and other allied health professionals—aware of the vital contributions the practice of TM can offer in relieving the pain and suffering of a range of disorders and diseases. TM has emerged as a powerful approach to healing many types of health disorders worldwide with over 30 countries carrying out research on its impact and 150 countries offering TM instruction. TM research is increasingly socially conscious and is being utilized in treating many of the most vulnerable, underserved patient populations, including African American children, abused women, young girls forced into prostitution, U.S. combat veterans, Native Americans, inner-city residents, underprivileged minority students, and prison inmates as well as Congolese war refugees and impoverished Latin American children. TM has been deployed to war-torn countries to assist in easing suffering through the positive effects that large groups of meditators can exert on the collective consciousness of a society. TM programs have been introduced into the prison system, resulting in dramatic drops in criminal recidivism and much-improved inmate rehabilitation. The elderly have enjoyed greater longevity, decreased morbidity, and better

overall health, happiness, and wellbeing as measured by the effects of
TM with nursing home and assisted living patients.

The wide-ranging effects of TM extend well beyond health, and research has solidly established its positive effects in many domains of
human functioning including increased intelligence, creativity, cognitive
flexibility, personality and moral development, academic achievement,
organizational effectiveness, job satisfaction and performance, and overall stability and quality of life.

TM research is at the forefront of neuroscientific investigation into the
nature, function, and expression of consciousness, an area that has mysti-
fied and perplexed scientists and philosophers for centuries. The brain
changes associated with the long-term effects of TM on the development
of higher states of consciousness are being mapped, and the phenomenon
of enlightenment itself is increasingly becoming more clearly understood
and appreciated. The implications of this research are enormous as the
highest levels of human development are recognized and harnessed.

In the final analysis, the practice and experience of TM is designed for
and has as its goal the development of a permanent, stable, irreversible,
and unbounded style of human functioning known traditionally as *enlightenment*, the highest state of consciousness. Indeed, all of the wonderful health benefits described in this text can be conceived as really only
fortuitous side effects of this process. Following the beautiful expressions
of the eminent Vedic scholar Dr. Vernon Katz, through TM, the state of
transcendental, pure awareness is first located in the depths of meditation then found to be persisting during daily life until finally, like a river
devouring its banks, it cannot be contained and spills over and flows into
more and more of the domains of life until all objects of awareness reflect
this glorious state. TM purifies and clarifies the senses and perceptions
so we move from an incomplete, concrete, filtered, distorted appreciation
of life to an experience of subtler and subtler and more abstract universal
levels of objects of the senses. As concentration becomes more diffused
through continued meditation, the senses are cleansed and reset. The
awareness of the boundaries of objects becomes so refined and delicate
so as to not disturb the awareness of the less bounded, more universal
aspects of objects until eventually the very boundaries of life become concrete expressions of the radiating and reflecting of complete unboundedness: the true nature of consciousness itself. This unbounded inner awareness becomes complete so that the wholeness of life can be lived within
the boundaries of space and time. The local and the universal aspects of
life interfuse and a gradual, orderly process of transformation takes place,
culminating in the state of Unity of life. Growth continues even more until
the entirety of life, from the nearest to the farthest unperceivable ranges
of reality, are cognized and appreciated in terms of the pure being of the

Self. This is the ultimate state of the human condition, known in Vedic knowledge as *Brahman*, or the full expression of Unity Consciousness.

Prescribing Health is interdisciplinary in scope, and the esteemed contributors to this volume, all prolific researchers and clinicians and many at the vanguard of research on consciousness and health, come from many disciplines, including education, medicine, pediatric neuropsychology, psychiatry, and neuroscience. The editors, and the reader, are fortunate to have the benefit of their knowledge and experience, and the culmination of their efforts has produced what we believe to be a highly useful, enlightening text for those interested in creating, maintaining, and recovering health for patients and themselves.

We sincerely hope this volume will stimulate further interest and scientific inquiry into the role of TM in the treatment of disease and will result in the implementation of TM–based treatment programs for increased quality of care for all who need help in reestablishing true health and happiness in their lives.

The editors would like to express their appreciation to the David Lynch Foundation and the Maharishi Foundation, in particular Mario Orsatti, for ideas and encouragement for this project and for promoting TM research and programs worldwide.

Transcendental Meditation and TM® are trademarks registered in the U.S. Patent and Trademark Office, licensed to Maharishi Vedic Education Development Corporation and are used with permission.

David F. O'Connell, Ph.D., M.S., CFC, DABPS
Deborah L. Bevvino, Ph.D., NP
September 2014, Reading, Pennsylvania

SECTION I

THEORY

ONE

Transcendental Meditation: What, How, and Why

Robert W. Boyer, Ph.D.

This introductory chapter summarizes the Transcendental Meditation (TM®) technique, explains how to learn and practice it, and shows why it is uniquely effective as an approach to healing and personal development. Although TM is systematic and does not require any belief system or lifestyle, its origin is in the ancient knowledge approach to consciousness of *Veda* (total knowledge).[1] Principles of this approach of *Consciousness-Based*® Education are also overviewed, including related principles of natural medicine in *Ayurveda* (knowledge of the lifespan).

In this consciousness-based approach, transcending mental activity to *pure consciousness*—the simplest state of awareness—is considered the *holistic active ingredient* to promote physical and mental wellbeing and complete awakening to the highest state of human consciousness. Historically, this highest state has been characterized by direct experience of the seamless unity of everything in nature. Subsequent chapters discuss this highest state in detail with regard to applications and supporting research for psychiatric and medical disorders, and societal ills generally.

WHAT IS TM?

TM is a simple mental procedure practiced while sitting comfortably with eyes closed. It is distinct from contemplation, concentration, chanting, and other practices that frequently are associated with meditation. In TM, mental activity naturally settles to softer, less-excited states and is transcended to inner, silent wakefulness. Historically, this state has been referred to as *samadhi* or *turiya*, a fourth natural state

3

of *pure consciousness* in addition to and underlying the ordinary three states of sleep, dreaming, and waking. It is also called *transcendental consciousness* because it transcends ordinary perception, thinking, and feeling. However, it is transcending deeper inside, not to something outside—similar to an individual, bounded wave that naturally settles back to its source in the unbounded ocean. This completely holistic experience has the most profound implications for healing and development of full potential.

HOW IS TM TAUGHT AND PRACTICED?

TM is taught only by certified TM teachers who have completed extensive training. Because instructions are personalized depending on *in vivo* experiences, including questions and answers to guide the delicate experiences, it cannot be learned from a book or recording. Personal instruction is standardized worldwide in a series of seven steps that includes introductory lectures, a personal interview with a TM teacher, private instruction, and follow-up sessions. Private, individual instruction includes guidance through verbal instructions and immediate feedback about experiences to ensure correct practice. There is assignment of a sound, or a *mantra*, in this case a sound with no meaning attached to it, and guidance in its use as a vehicle for natural transcending.

Instruction is preceded by a simple ceremony that is an established cultural tradition for beginning a knowledge program, which the student is asked to witness. It sets the stage for the teacher to teach the technique correctly by recognizing the ancient Vedic tradition of teachers and the importance of maintaining its time-tested effectiveness.

Because TM is simple to learn and effortless to do, in the first session the new practitioner enjoys deep relaxation and expansion of conscious experience. It is practiced twice daily, once in the morning and once in the afternoon, for 15–20 minutes each time, while sitting comfortably.

The next three days after instruction include follow-up sessions to ensure correct practice and provide further training in the principles of transcending, normalization, and natural development. Typically there is a 10-day follow-up, as well as periodic meetings available for group practice, questions and answers, and additional knowledge, including deeper understanding of higher stages of development resulting from regular, long-term TM practice.

Importantly, there is also a systematic procedure to ensure correctness of the practice, called *checking*, an essential part of the regular, life-long follow-up program. It is recommended that checking be done each month for the first few months then periodically thereafter.

The TM technique is a systematic procedure that does not require any particular belief system or lifestyle to learn and practice correctly. In order to foster clear experiences at the initial instruction, however, students are required to attend all four consecutive days of instruction and to not use psychoactive drugs for at least fifteen days prior to instruction.

Effortlessness of TM

In ordinary waking, mental attention is directed outward toward the objects of sense. This can be viewed as the opposite of attention naturally turning inward and the mind settling to less-excited states. As a simple comparison, included in the ability to run is the ability to run slower and to walk; and included in the ability to walk is the ability to stand still. Included in the ability to talk is the ability to talk softly, or to be silent. Likewise, included in the ability to think is the ability to settle mental activity and transcend to the least excited ground state of the mind. Revived from ancient Vedic science by Maharishi Mahesh Yogi and systematized as the Transcendental Meditation technique, this effortless mental process is so simple, natural, and subtle that it was overlooked for millennia.

When we attempt to control the mind and settle it down, a typical experience is that the mind is fickle and shifts from one object of experience to another. Many traditions have concluded that the mind then must be actively controlled in order to be resolute and to attain inner stillness.

Methods of mental control apply forms of contemplation and concentration. Contemplation has come to mean thoughtful reflection on concepts such as peace, quietude, or the grace of God. Because the mind tends to wander, contemplation is frequently modified to include some form of concentration on a particular object such as an idea, an image, or breathing. These practices can be difficult to do and have led to the conclusion that an austere, reclusive lifestyle may be necessary to minimize distractions in the hope of practicing them well. Unfortunately, this has contributed to the view that meditation is not for the general population—which has marginalized the practice in active mainstream society.

In contrast, transcending to pure consciousness through TM takes place *effortlessly* based on the natural tendency of the mind, and, practically speaking, it can be enjoyed by anyone. Emphasizing the effortlessness of TM is not a promotional tool such as advertising; it is essential for correct practice and the full benefits of meditation. This technology has been trademarked in order to distinguish and maintain recognition of its uniqueness and the importance of its proper instruction. There are numerous other practices available that miss the essential nature and subtlety of TM and that unfortunately do not produce the desired results that naturally come from systematic, effortless transcending of mental activity.

When Maharishi began teaching meditation, he first called it "a simple system of deep meditation." However, as he saw that the term "meditation" was commonly understood to involve active, effortful thinking as in contemplation and concentration, he added "transcendental" to clarify that it involves a natural transcending of all mental activity. The TM technique avoids active sensory, intellectual, or emotional processing, which can interfere with the natural transcending process. It is based on two empirical principles: the natural tendency of the mind to go to a field of greater happiness, and that more-refined levels of experience are inherently more enjoyable. Based on these principles, the mind automatically settles down under appropriate conditions.

The contrast between pure, transcendental consciousness and active mental states of thinking and feeling is now being documented in direct experimental comparisons. Some mental practices from other traditions quite different from TM and its effects, such as "mindfulness," correlate with increased EEG gamma synchrony, proposed as the best measurable neural correlate of consciousness.[2,3] This view is consistent with the active waking state experience of being *conscious of* an object. This particular EEG pattern is not correlated with reported experiences of the fourth state, transcendental consciousness unmixed with thoughts and feelings, which is described in ancient Vedic literature and commonly reported by TM practitioners.[4,5,6,7]

Transcendental consciousness during TM is correlated with peak alpha power and frontal alpha coherence. EEG coherence is positively correlated with neural integration, indicating improved mental health, such as emotional stability, self or ego development, and normalization of mood and affect, as well as moral maturity.[8,9,10] These empirical findings clearly identify transcendental consciousness during TM as distinct from other mental practices.

Extensive research also has accumulated on additional benefits of TM. The research covers areas such as the neuroendocrinology of stress, stress reactivity, cardiovascular health, rehabilitation, substance abuse, academic performance, IQ, cognitive efficiency, ADHD, PTSD, and self-actualization, as well as reduced anxiety and depression.[11,12,13,14,15,16,17,18]

The Process of Normalization in Natural Healing

A key principle relating to TM is that *rest is the basis of activity*. Rest is a natural antidote to stress and disease, and it is typically the first commonsense recommendation for healing. Generally the deeper the rest, the deeper the healing. Deep rest in the mind is correlated with deep rest in the body. The deepest rest is said to be gained when mental activity settles to the fourth state, transcendental consciousness. In this context, transcendental consciousness can be thought of as the essential *holistic active ingredient* for healing and human development.

The transcending process is frequently described as a deeply relaxing, enjoyable, and—at times—quite blissful experience in which the individual naturally wants to remain. If the mind-body system contains deep-rooted imbalances, however, its functioning is not refined enough to maintain the inner silence of the state of transcendental consciousness, except for brief episodes. From the deeply restful ground state of the mind, healing mechanisms that dissolve obstacles to healthy functioning are naturally induced in a manner similar to the way in which sleep and dreaming rejuvenate from fatigue, only it is much deeper due to deeper rest.

Sub-periods of reported transcendental consciousness during TM are positively correlated with breath quiescence or virtual breath suspension suggestive of profound physiological rest.[19,20,21] Transcendental consciousness also is positively correlated with increases in skin conductance—a measure of autonomic arousal—and alpha-band EEG patterns indicative of *restful alertness*.[22,23,24]

As the mind-body system is purified of deep-rooted stress and naturally reflects a more refined style of functioning, the individual is able to sustain deeply settled states for more than brief episodes. Eventually an unbounded, inner, wakeful background to the ordinary three states of waking, dreaming, and sleep is said to be enlivened, becoming permanent in higher states of consciousness that define enlightenment. Higher states are *spontaneously* lived as the natural result of refinement and integration and not by intentionally holding a mood in the mind or heart, which can interfere with transcending and natural growth to higher states.

With sufficient degrees of deep rest, biochemical and structural imbalances in the body are naturally dissolved and eliminated—this is called the *process of normalization*. The activity of dissolving imbalances in the body increases mental activity, bringing the mind outward to feeling and thinking. Mental activity arising in this way results from dissolving imbalances in the body due to deep rest.

Typically the mental activity resulting from this process reflects a mixture of levels and types of imbalance released at the moment and doesn't correspond directly to the nature of imbalances eliminated. A subtle but important point is that because this type of mental activity occurs as a result of, and subsequent to, the release of stress, it is a by-product of the purification and normalization that has already taken place. Thus attention is not placed on the contents of these thoughts or emotions, and they are not examined or analyzed. At times during regular practice, some of the thoughts resulting as a by-product of the normalization process can be somewhat distressing or uncomfortable. Mental alertness is held to be expanded and stronger when experiencing refined, deeply relaxed states, and it is the strongest when mental activity is transcended. It strengthens and protects the mind during these natural normalizing processes.

It is important to understand these processes accurately and not to get confused or distracted by them. Cases in which individuals report experiences such as depersonalization or emotional release are understood in the context of normalization. The checking procedure, which reestablishes and ensures correct practice, also helps to strengthen correct understanding and to smooth out normalizing processes.

TM has been taught to individuals with different levels of education and from a wide range of cultural and religious backgrounds. It also has been applied in diverse conditions including maximum security prisons, psychiatric wards, substance-abuse treatment programs, nursing homes, and discipline-challenged school settings plagued by despondency and violence. Insurance statistics indicate that utilization rates for many chronic medical and psychiatric conditions are lower in TM practitioners compared to matched samples drawn from the general population. These outcomes support the safety and wide applicability of this practical mental technology.[25,26,27,28,29,30,31]

Eliminating accumulated stress, strain, and fatigue is an important result of this technology. To keep the practice itself simple and to avoid straining or interfering expectations, however, the emphasis is on cumulative benefits outside of the practice and natural integration of expanded awareness into daily activity toward permanent higher states of consciousness.

TM involves neither intellectual analysis of what is occurring during the practice nor focusing on problems or disease. It does not bring pathogenic beliefs or repressed material into conscious attention to analyze them. Such problem-focused approaches attempt to draw traumatic memories outward, toward more expressed levels of experience. Whether biobehavioral or psychological, this can foster analytic habits with iatrogenic effects, such as retraumatization, that can stir up past emotions and over time increase negative mental sets and depressive affect.[32]

In distinct contrast, the TM program involves gentle progress to refine and integrate consciousness, mind, and body by appreciating and utilizing the subtle mechanics of how the mind naturally functions. It does not apply methods to draw out and consciously work through past accumulated stresses or traumatic memories. Maharishi[33] has indicated that problem-focused methods develop in the absence of knowledge of the natural tendency of the mind and the subtle dynamics of healing. He makes a strong point about iatrogenic effects of these types of therapeutic interventions.

Analyzing an individual's way of thinking and bringing to the conscious level the buried misery of the past, even for the purpose of enabling him to see the cause of the stress and suffering, is highly deplorable; for it helps to strengthen directly the impressions of the miserable past and serves to suppress his consciousness in the present.

A key principle in this Vedic approach is that "what you put your attention on grows in your life."[34] For example, putting attention on music, politics, gardening, or a sport tends to increase its prominence in one's life—consistent with research on long-term memory. Putting attention on negative events from past experience tends to increase negativity in patterns of thinking, emotions, and memory. This can subtly train the mind to focus on problems and inadequacies in cognitive schemas (such as diagnostic labels), which can complicate the mind, rather than support positive solutions to current challenges. This does not prevent discussion of past traumatic experiences such as in psychotherapy, but it does not include trying to draw them out, dwelling on them, and interpreting them in a manner that can complicate the mind—which are common practices in many traditional psychotherapeutic approaches based on completely different models of the mind and its functioning.

Again, in the approach associated with TM, the underlying level of the mind is *consciousness itself*, not the *unconscious*. It does not bring repressed traumatic or unconscious material to ordinary awareness. It is a much subtler, simpler, and more positive healing technology that is based on a profound understanding of the natural tendency of the mind.

To summarize, the overall approach to natural healing and higher development in the TM program is to calm the mind to its ground state in the inner silence of transcendental consciousness, a restfully alert state of unbounded inner wakefulness correlated with EEG alpha coherence and physiological indicators of deep rest. This natural transcending process brings the body into a state of deep, rejuvenating rest, which purifies the system from accumulated imbalances and increases coherence in consciousness, mind, and body.

After practice, the emphasis shifts to integrating expanded awareness through enhanced conscious experiences and the vigorous pursuit of personal goals in daily living. This is said to result eventually in permanent actualization of full human potential through a sequence of higher states of consciousness, described in detail by Maharishi according to the ancient Vedic tradition and outlined later in this chapter.

THE ADVANCED TM-SIDHI® PROGRAM

Once effortless transcending has been established as a daily routine in TM, additional technologies are available. These additional technologies, taught by extensively trained advanced-technique instructors, are to further accelerate the progress of development. They also are associated with *sadhana*, the transcending practice in the yoga aspect of the Vedic tradition.

The word *yoga* has become increasingly popular in recent decades with growing interest in healthier lifestyles and appreciation of the interconnectedness of mind and body in holistic health, as well as in preventive and integrative medicine. Frequently the emphasis is on the aspect of yoga associated with light physical exercise and body postures, *hatha yoga*, which is a beneficial physical approach. Less emphasized is the deeper aspect of yoga as a systematic mental technology for knowledge and experience of full human development.

The mental technology of transcending associated with yoga is described in the *Yoga Sutras of Patanjali*, an important aspect of Vedic knowledge. "Yoga" refers to *union*, and "Sutra" to *stitch* or *thread*. The Yoga Sutras detail knowledge and experience that stitch or thread together individual being with the unbounded universal Being. They describe subtle experiences to unify the consciousness-mind-body connection, called *sidhis*, also revived by Maharishi from ancient Vedic science into a systematic developmental technology called the *TM-Sidhi Program*.

In a scientific context, the Yoga Sutras can be understood to serve as a description of the results of practical means to develop higher states of consciousness through regular transcending. They also can be understood as constituting *empirical tests* of the degree to which higher states of consciousness have been stabilized in the individual.

SEVEN STATES OF HUMAN CONSCIOUSNESS

In the Vedic approach, as revived by Maharishi Mahesh Yogi, the natural desire to "know thyself" impels each individual to progress through distinguishable stages of self-knowledge. The full range of human development is described in terms of a developmental sequence of seven states of consciousness, each state with its own phenomenal reality.[35] This sequence includes four higher states in addition to ordinary waking, dreaming, and sleep. Maharishi's model of the developmental sequence of states of consciousness provides milestones to help clarify descriptions of peak experiences and higher states.

Respecting religious, cultural, and language differences, most historical and contemporary descriptions of higher state experiences can be placed in this developmental sequence. Briefly, the seven states of consciousness are distinguishable by the experience of *self and environment* (subject/object, self/other) on a continuum from virtually no wakefulness to full wakefulness.[36]

Sleep—(*Sushupti Chetana*) virtually no experience of self or environment
Dreaming—(*Swapn Chetana*) imaginary individual self and environment
Waking—(*Jagaret Chetana*) individual self and relative environment
Transcendental consciousness—(*Turiya Chetana*) pure wakefulness, universal Self only
Cosmic consciousness—(*Turyatit Chetana*) universal Self and relative environment
Refined cosmic consciousness—(*Bhagavad Chetana*) universal Self and maximum value of relative environment
Unity consciousness—(*Brahma Chetana*) self and environment are one; all is universal Self.

ORIGIN OF THE TM AND TM-SIDHI PROGRAM

The TM and TM-Sidhi program are based on principles of the subtle natural functioning of the mind in the *Veda*, the oldest continuous tradition of knowledge. This tradition of knowledge has been revived and extensively explained in the language of modern science by Maharishi as *Maharishi Vedic Science and Technology*.

In this perennial tradition, about 2,500 years ago the celebrated sage Shankara established four *Maths*, or centers of learning, in India (North, East, South, West). From time to time, great teachers represent the Vedic tradition as the head, or *Shankaracharya*, of one of these centers of learning. The seat of the Shankaracharya of the North at Jyotir Math, Himalayas, had been vacant for over 100 years until 1940, when the revered Vedic sage Brahmananda Saraswati consented to fill the seat.[37]

Upon becoming a student of Brahmananda Saraswati, Shankaracharya of Jyotir Math, Maharishi followed his teacher's direction to finish studies in physics at Allahabad University. Maharishi then worked closely with the Shankaracharya as administrative secretary, learning from him and experiencing the integration of life that is the essence of Veda, including the Vedic principles from which the TM program was drawn.

In 1955 Maharishi came out of the Himalayas and began teaching this revival of Vedic technology throughout India, eventually traveling around the world several times to fill the need of making it available to as many individuals as possible. He established TM centers and formal educational institutions worldwide, including Maharishi Vedic University (MVU) in Vlodrop, Holland, and, perhaps the most publicly recognized, Maharishi University of Management (MUM) in Fairfield, Iowa. These schools teach traditional academic disciplines in the context of holistic Vedic knowledge and development of higher states of consciousness through the TM technique and related technologies, called consciousness-based education. Accredited at the doctoral level, the currently most popular undergraduate degrees at MUM are in business, sustainability, and Maharishi Vedic Science.[38]

The TM Program and Vedic Science Are Not a Religion

It is important to clarify that the TM program and Maharishi Vedic Science and Technology do not constitute a faith-based approach and are not a religion. The programs and courses certainly have practical significance as a systematic means of living the essence of spirituality in higher states of consciousness. However, Maharishi has consistently emphasized gaining fulfillment in the context of one's own religion or belief system. The essential truth of the programs and courses is universal. He also has emphasized that the TM program fosters deeper appreciation of the essential knowledge in one's own secular or non-secular belief system.

Maharishi has further pointed out that science is the language of our times, and he has emphasized Vedic knowledge in the modern scientific context of systematic understanding and empirical validation, both experimentally and experientially. This is consistent with the historical understanding that Vedic knowledge is a holistic system of understanding and practical experience—a comprehensive, integrated science and technology for daily living.

This ancient, integrated knowledge system did not reflect the current sociopolitical distinction of secular and non-secular areas of societal life, which separates science and government from religion. This view of social structure has its roots in the experience associated with the ordinary waking state of consciousness that separates object from subject, and it overlooks the underlying unity. The differences in this fragmented view were emphasized during the British colonial occupation of India, in part to contrast Christianity and Hinduism in efforts to evangelize Indian society.

The general academic understanding has been that Vedic records originated about 5,000 to 1,500 years ago and reflect pre-scientific thought. However, this is now under revision as a longer time frame and deeper understanding of Vedic records are unfolding. Various philosophical and religious traditions emerged over the centuries from different interpretations of Vedic literature, including Hinduism and Buddhism. Because it has been extensively drawn on by these religions, Vedic knowledge as a systematic means of gaining knowledge, or *science*, rather than as a philosophy or a faith-based religion, was not appreciated.

This distinction also was more difficult to make due to the loss of an essential, holistic understanding of Vedic developmental technologies. Without systematic applications to verify its knowledge as a science, thus making this knowledge seemingly unverifiable, Vedic science was not clearly distinguished from philosophy or faith-based traditions. And its practical benefits to human life were rendered unavailable. Maharishi's re-clarification of the essential holistic value of Vedic science and reestablishment of its systematic technologies—especially meditation as an *effortless* natural process of transcending mental activity—is a crucial contribution to healing and full human development.

In Maharishi Vedic Science and Technology, the standard for validation is not only through indirect objective experimental means; it also goes deeper to include direct experiential validation emphasizing the practical principle of "knowing by being." Knowledge has to be validated by direct experience, not just intellectual understanding.

This integration of theoretical knowledge and practical empirical experience promotes further progress beyond the Age of Reason that established modern science in the eighteenth and nineteenth centuries, also sometimes referred to as the Enlightenment. By applying completely holistic knowledge to develop higher states of consciousness, an era worthy of the name *Age of Enlightenment* is fortunately emerging. An essential point which now makes this possible is reflected in Maharishi's statement emphasizing the value of regular transcending of even the discriminating intellect as practical means for establishing permanent enlightenment:[39] "Transcending thought is infinitely more valuable than thinking."

WHAT DOES "CONSCIOUSNESS-BASED" MEAN?

To appreciate the unique contribution of Maharishi Vedic Science and Technology, it is helpful to clarify what is meant by "consciousness-based education." Consciousness has been the constitutive issue for psychology.[40] It also is now a core issue in diverse fields from quantum physics to evolutionary biology and cognitive neuroscience.[41] The mainstream view of consciousness in psychology—and also modern science generally—is based on the reductive physicalist worldview that the only real level of nature is the physical.

In this view, consciousness is commonly defined as the ability to be *aware of* an object of experience, attributed a functional role in attention, intention, and the sense of self. It is further characterized as fading out during sleep and coma, restricted by brain malfunctioning, and ceasing when the body no longer sustains life. Consciousness is held to be an emergent property of neural and biophysical processes in the brain. But despite massive efforts to locate consciousness in the brain, it is increasingly recognized that only its physiological correlates have been found.

Fundamental challenges to the reductive physicalist worldview and its understanding of consciousness are emerging in nonlocal quantum and information field theories, in consideration of the relationship between consciousness and a theorized unified field. As modern science has advanced to the stage where it is seriously considering the most fundamental level of nature in unified field theories, the relevance of ancient Vedic science to cutting-edge issues in modern science is beginning to be appreciated. Here are a few statements from scientists who have recognized the fundamental role of consciousness in nature:

"I consider consciousness as primary. I consider matter as derivative from consciousness." Nobel Laureate physicist Max Planck[42]

"All through the physical world runs that unknown content, which must surely be the stuff of our consciousness." Astrophysicist Sir Arthur Eddington[43]

"It will remain remarkable, in whatever way our future concepts may develop, that the very study of the external world led to the conclusion that the content of the consciousness is an ultimate reality." Physicist Eugene Wigner[44]

The Unified Field as a Field of Consciousness

An analysis of the overall trend in scientific theories in the past century toward deeper and more integrated levels of nature reveals that modern science has been converging on the model of the relationship of objective nature, subjective mind, and the underlying unified field that is described extensively in ancient Vedic records.[45,46,47] Unified field theories in physics now posit a single, abstract, infinite field as the ultimate source and container of everything in existence, logically including all the laws of nature that structure the universe.

In the ancient Vedic tradition, as well as other ancient traditions, albeit with various cultural and language differences, there is purported to be a transcendent universal essence of nature. This universal essence has an obvious correspondence to developing unified field theory. Previously thought to contrast with modern scientific accounts, ancient Vedic views correspond with recent descriptions of an infinitely dynamic, self-interacting unified field.[48,49,50] The most parsimonious explanation for the correspondence is that these knowledge traditions converge on the same unified field from their respective vantage points.[51,52] Logically, there is only one completely unified field.

Ancient knowledge traditions further hold that direct experience of the transcendent universal essence of nature is possible because it is the essence of one's own consciousness—*universal Being* as the basis of *individual being*. Consistent with these views, Maharishi Vedic Science and Technology describes the universal essence of nature as consciousness itself—universal Being.[53,54,55,56,57,58]

The reductive physicalist account in modern science can be character-ized as an *unconscious-based* matter → mind → consciousness model in which the conscious mind emerges and is entirely dependent on uncon-scious processes in the physical brain. The ancient Vedic account can be viewed in the reverse way as a consciousness → mind → matter model in which the unified field of consciousness is the basis of mind and matter. In this holistic view of subjective and objective levels, the brain mediates conscious experience in the physical level of nature but does not cause or create consciousness. Maharishi explains,

> Underneath the subtlest layer of all that exists in the relative field is the ab-stract, absolute field of pure Being which is unmanifested and transcendental . . . Experience shows that Being is the essential, basic nature of the mind; but, since It commonly remains in tune with the senses projecting outwards toward the manifested realms of creation, the mind misses or fails to appreciate its own essential nature, just as the eyes are unable to see themselves. Everything but the eyes themselves can be seen through the eyes. Similarly, everything is based on the essential nature of the mind . . . and yet, while the mind is en-gaged in the projected field of manifested diversity, Being is not appreciated by the mind, although It is the very basis and essential constituent.[59]

In the physicalist approach, consciousness is underpinned by uncon-scious biophysical processes and inert elemental, atomic and subatomic processes and quantum fields that are fundamentally random, valueless, and meaningless. Thus it is an unconscious-based approach. In contrast, in consciousness-based education, the individual body and mind are ulti-mately based on the unified field of nature. In this Vedic approach, heal-ing and personal development are facilitated holistically through direct experience of pure consciousness itself.

Eventually this state of pure consciousness itself is said to stabilize as the non-changing platform of unbounded awareness in permanent indi-vidual enlightenment, the building block for an enlightened society. Each individual is inherently capable of fully unfolding the universal value of life, reflected in Maharishi's holistic principle that *the individual is cosmic*. This means that the individual is composed of all levels of nature. This fundamental holistic principle reflects the highest respect for each indi-vidual and his or her highest potential contribution to the world by living in full enlightenment.[60,61,62]

WHAT DOES "COMPLETELY HOLISTIC" MEAN?

Maharishi Vedic Technologies represent a *completely holistic* approach to healing and health promotion, according to the principle that *the*

individual is cosmic.[63,64,65] Individual body, mind, and consciousness are
ultimately connected to the totality of the unified field of universal Being, and individuals can directly access that universal level through the
effortless process of transcending. Transcending is possible by virtue
of the total holistic structure of nature that comprises each individual
human being. Each healing and developmental technology in this completely holistic approach—whether emphasizing outer environmental,
interpersonal, behavioral, physical, or inner psychological levels—is
drawn from the integrated totality.

In other words, the parts come from the whole, and the wholeness is not
lost in the parts. Each part or specific aspect is connected to the totality. That
is the *completely holistic* approach. It is in direct contrast to the fragmented,
reductive physicalist view that the whole emerges from the parts.

The numerous approaches to healing developed in recent years are
based on insights and sometimes evidence-based theories not established
in the understanding and experience of the wholeness or ultimate unity
of nature. Such non-integrated healing approaches can produce some
limited benefit in one area or system of the body, or symptom complex,
but they do not act in an integrated fashion with the total physiology,
which can result in unintended and often serious and unwanted side effects. Though certainly an important contribution to healthcare, a prime
example is pharmacotherapy, in which active ingredients are extracted
from basic elements and natural organisms and then administered with
little regard for the larger context of holistic mind-body functioning and
the inherent balance in "nature's intelligence."

Natural vs. Artificial Means for Healing and Personal Development

In mainstream modern science, nature is viewed as fundamentally
random, valueless, and devoid of inherent order and meaning. Although
modern technology is making major contributions to health and healing,
for the most part its mainstream worldview is frozen in reductive physicalism, which is now becoming recognized as untenable. Well-intentioned
scientists and entrepreneurs are forging ahead with fragmenting technologies without understanding the subtle and unified levels of nature. This
could actually hinder the progress of more integrated natural approaches
to solving long-standing societal ills.

A defining crisis is on the horizon. Fragmented technological innovations
such as in biotechnology, genomics, and cyborg nano-technologies based
on reductive physicalism are rapidly leading to a *post-human era* that could
seriously distort or even end human nature and the human species. Because it is not *completely holistic*, modern science in its current state is powerful enough to *disintegrate* us, but not powerful enough to *integrate* us.[66]

On the other hand, unified field theory, which is developing in modern science, is consistent with fundamental order, not fundamental randomness. Maharishi Vedic Science and Technology applies the principle of fundamental order to all of nature—including subjective and objective, mind and matter. It emphasizes natural *alignment with* the underlying totality of nature to develop the full potential inherent in each individual as the basis for a healthy, enlightened society. Hopefully, completely holistic technologies, especially the TM technique, will soon be applied to reverse the disintegrating influence of fragmenting technologies based on reductive views limited to the material surface of nature, including only the surface levels of our own nature as human beings.

MAHARISHI AYURVEDA AND NATURAL MEDICINE

The ancient Vedic approach as revived by Maharishi Mahesh Yogi and described here includes extensive therapeutic strategies to reestablish and maintain balance in mind and body. In addition to the TM and TM-Sidhi program, there is a wide range of technologies in *Maharishi Ayurveda*. Emphasizing primary prevention, it sets forth the consciousness-mind-body connection and how to optimize health. Most fundamentally, it views disease as lack of alignment of individual consciousness with universal consciousness.

Maharishi Ayurveda is an extensive body of natural medicine with specificity and detail. It includes dietetics and natural organic foods, herbal therapies, body purification therapies (*panchakarma*), gentle exercise routines (*asanas*), simple breathing exercises (*pranayama*), music therapy (*gandharvaveda*), aromatherapies, Vedic sound vibration therapy, Vedic light therapy, and specific daily and seasonal routines (*behavioral rasayanas*), as well as many other approaches for the promotion of health, vitality, mental clarity, muscle tone, digestion, skin condition, immune system strength, and longevity. Although supported by extensive clinical practice and observation, these technologies did not originate from experimental laboratory findings or theoretical insights based on fragmented understanding in disease-oriented medicine.

Another interesting and related technology concerns structural features of living environments based on principles of Maharishi *Sthapatya-Veda*. This aspect includes construction of ecologically sustainable buildings and community environments that promote individual and societal health.[67,68,69,70]

In Maharishi Ayurveda, the five senses have direct correspondence with the natural elements—which can be related to fundamental particle-forces in modern physics. Experiencing different sensory objects affects the consciousness-mind-body system. Experiences of smell, taste, sight, touch, and sound are directly related to their objects, and each has specific effects that promote or disturb natural psychophysiological balance. When we disregard these natural relationships, mind and body can become less refined, eventually resulting in disorder and disease. Countering these results involves establishing an integrated balance based on a holistic understanding of objects of sense and their natural effects.

An important corresponding feature is classification into *mind-body types*, the inherited genetic constitution of the individual as manifested physically and behaviorally. In addition to reactions to specific sensory inputs, mind-body types react differentially to basic cycles in nature, such as diurnal and seasonal cycles. Each mind-body type has strengths as well as vulnerabilities. Illness and disease are understood to be the consequences of behavior that is not in tune with the natural balance for the individual mind-body type in the time and place in which the individual is living.

Maharishi Ayurveda is a profound integration of natural cause-effect relationships between the individual and his or her environment. It provides subtle assessments of the relationships between individual mind-body types and the influences of sensory objects in the environment in order to apply more refined and integrated means to promote optimal health.

CONCLUSION

Maharishi Vedic Science and Technology and Maharishi Ayurveda, including the TM and TM-Sidhi program, have revolutionary implications for contemporary healthcare. They represent a practical integration of holistic knowledge into modern science, crucially needed in our highly stressed and crisis-laden civilization. These approaches emphasize the deep rest of inner silence, along with biobehavioral therapies and balanced daily routines, to refine the consciousness-mind-body connection toward optimal health and higher human development. Each technology is directly linked to its source in the unified field of consciousness, universal Being.

The above description is included to provide information on the origins of the TM technique. It may be important, however, to restate that TM's benefits are automatic outcomes of effortless TM and not due to acceptance of or adherence to any particular system of beliefs or lifestyle.

To summarize this chapter, my key points include the following.

- The unified field of all the laws of nature is the field of consciousness itself.
- Consciousness is the basis of individual mind/body.

- Transcending to pure consciousness is an effortless process.
- Deep rest is the basis of activity.
- The deepest rest is gained by transcending all mental activity.
- Deep rest activates natural healing mechanisms that prevent and reduce imbalances.
- The individual is cosmic.

The next chapters examine in detail published research on TM and related programs across a broad spectrum of psychological, behavioral, social, and sociological measures. This research further corroborates Maharishi Vedic Science and Technology and Maharishi Ayurveda for natural healing and personal development toward full realization of the cosmic nature of each individual in the highest state of unity consciousness.

NOTES

1. *Maharishi Vedic University: Introduction* (Vlodrop, The Netherlands: Maharishi Vedic University Press, 1994).

2. S. R. Hameroff, "The 'Conscious Pilot': Synchronized Dendritic Webs Move through the Brain Neurocomputational Networks to Mediate Consciousness," paper presented at the bi-annual conference *Toward a Science of Consciousness*, Tucson, Arizona, April 8–12, 2008.

3. H. P. Stapp, *Mindful Universe: Quantum Mechanics and the Participating Observer* (New York: Springer-Verlag, 2007).

4. *Scientific Research on Maharishi's Transcendental Meditation and TM-Sidhi Programme—Collected Papers*, vols. 1–5 (Fairfield, IA: Maharishi University of Management *Press*, 1977–1990).

5. M. C. Dillbeck, ed., *Scientific Research on Maharishi's Transcendental Meditation and TM-Sidhi Programme—Collected Papers*, vol. 6 (Vlodrop, The Netherlands: Maharishi Vedic University Press, 2011).

6. F. Travis and A. Arenander, "Cross-sectional and Longitudinal Study of Effects of Transcendental Meditation Practice on Interhemispheric Frontal Asymmetry and Frontal Coherence," *International Journal of Neuroscience* 116 (2006): 1519–38. D. W. Orme-Johnson, "Commentary of the AHRQ Report on Research on Meditation Practices in Health," *Journal of Alternative and Complementary Medicine* 14, no. 10 (2008): 1215–21.

7. J. Hebert, D. Lehmann, G. Tan, F. Travis, and A. Arenander, "Enhanced EEG Alpha Time-Domain Phase Synchrony during Transcendental Meditation: Implications for Cortical Integration Theory," *Signal Processing* 85, no. 11 (2005): 2213–32.

8. P. Sauseng and W. Klimesch, "What Does Phase Information of Oscillatory Brain Activity Tell Us about Cognitive Processes?" *Neuroscience Biobehavioral Review* 32, no. 5 (2008): 1001–13.

9. Travis and Arenander, "Cross-sectional and Longitudinal Study."

10. Dillbeck, *Scientific Research on Maharishi's Transcendental Meditation*.

11. C. N. Alexander, P. Robinson, and Maxwell V. Rainforth, "Treating and Preventing Alcohol, Nicotine, and Drug Abuse through Transcendental Meditation: A Review and Statistical Meta-analysis," *Alcoholism Treatment Quarterly* 11, nos. 1 and 2 (1994): 13–87.

12. A. Deans. *A Record of Excellence* (Fairfield, IA: Maharishi University of Management Press, 2005).

13. R. H. Schneider and Jeremy Z. Fields, *Total Heart Health* (Laguna Beach, CA: Basic Health Publications, 2006).

14. V. A. Barnes and D. W. Orme-Johnson, "Prevention and Treatment of Cardiovascular Disease in Adolescents and Adults through the Transcendental Meditation® Program: A Research Update," *Current Hypertension Reviews* 8, no. 3 (2012): 227–42.

15. D. W. Orme-Johnson and V. A. Barnes, "Effects of TM Practice on Trait Anxiety: A Meta-analysis of Randomized Control Trials," *Journal of Alternative and Complementary Medicine* 19, no. 10 (2013): 1–12.

16. D. F. O'Connell and C. N. Alexander, eds., *Self-Recovery: Treating Addictions Using Transcendental Meditation and Maharishi Ayur-Veda* (Binghamton, NY: Haworth Press, 1994).

17. D. L. Bevvino, this volume.

18. J. T. Farrow and J. Russell Hebert, "Breath Suspension During the Transcendental Meditation Technique," *Psychosomatic Medicine* 44, no. 2 (1982): 133–53.

19. K. Badawi, R. K. Wallace, D. W. Orme-Johnson, and A. M. Rouzere, "Electrophysiologic Characteristics of Respiratory Suspension Periods Occurring During the Practice of the Transcendental Meditation Technique," *Psychosomatic Medicine* 46, no. 3 (1984): 267–76.

20. F. Travis and R. K. Wallace, "Autonomic Patterns During Respiratory Suspension: Possible Markers of Transcendental Consciousness," *Psychophysiology* 34, no. 1 (1997): 39–46.

21. Travis and Arenander, "Cross-sectional and Longitudinal Study."

22. Orme-Johnson, "Commentary of the AHRQ Report."

23. D. W. Orme-Johnson, www.truthabouttm.com.

24. Orme-Johnson and Barnes, "Effects of TM Practice on Trait Anxiety."

25. Barnes and Orme-Johnson, "Prevention and Treatment of Cardiovascular Disease."

26. Orme-Johnson, www. truthabouttm.com.

27. D. W. Orme-Johnson, "Commentary of the AHRQ Report."

28. D. W. Orme-Johnson, "Medical Care Utilization and the Transcendental Meditation Program, *Psychosomatic Medicine* 49, no. 1 (1997): 493–507.

29. D. W. Orme-Johnson and Robert E. Herron, "An Innovative Approach to Reducing Medical Care Utilization," *American Journal of Managed Care* 3, no. 1 (1987): 135–44.

30. www.tm.org/research-on-meditation.

31. R. Boyer, *Vedic Principles of Therapy* (Malibu, CA: Institute for Advanced Research, 2012).

32. M. M. Yogi, *Science of Being and Art of Living* (Washington, DC: Age of Enlightenment Publications, 1963), 258–59.

33. M. M. Yogi, *Science of Being.*

34. B. Morris, *Maharishi's Global News Conference*, May 5, 2004.

35. R. W. Boyer, *Bridge to Unity: Unified Field-Based Science & Spirituality* (Malibu, CA: Institute for Advanced Research, 2008).

36. M. M. Yogi, *Maharishi Mahesh Yogi on the Bhagavad-Gita: A New Translation and Commentary* (London: Penguin Books, 1967).

37. www.mum.edu.

38. M. M. Yogi, *Maharishi Mahesh Yogi on the Bhagavad-Gita.*

39. G. A. Miller, "Trends and Debates in Cognitive Psychology," *Cognition* 10 (1981): 215–25.

40. Boyer, *Bridge to Unity.*

41. M. Planck, *Observer*, January 31, 1931.

42. A. Eddington, *The Nature of the Physical World* (Ann Arbor: University of Michigan Press, 1974), 276.

43. E. Wigner, quoted in Nick Hebert, *Quantum Reality: Beyond the New Physics* (New York: Anchor Books, 1985), 26.

44. M. M. Yogi, *Science of Being.*

45. M. M. Yogi, *Maharishi Mahesh Yogi on the Bhagavad-Gita.*

46. M. M. Yogi, *Maharishi's Absolute Theory of Defence: Sovereignty in Invincibility* (India: Age of Enlightenment Publications, 1996).

47. M. M. Yogi, *Science of Being.*

48. J. S. Hagelin, "Is Consciousness the Unified Field? A Field Theorist's Perspective," *Modern Science and Vedic Science* 1 (1987): 29–87.

49. J. S. Hagelin, "Restructuring Physics from Its Foundation in Light of Maharishi's Vedic Science," *Modern Science and Vedic Science* 3, no. 1 (1989): 3–72.

50. Hagelin, "Is Consciousness the Unified Field?"

51. Hagelin, "Restructuring Physics."

52. M. M. Yogi, *Science of Being.*

53. M. M. Yogi, *Maharishi Mahesh Yogi on the Bhagavad-Gita.*

54. J. Shear, *The Experience of Meditation* (London: Paragon Press, 2006).

55. Boyer, *Bridge to Unity.*

56. R. W. Boyer, *Linking Mind and Matter: A New Scientific Model That Unifies Nonlocal Mind and Local Matter* (Malibu, CA: Institute for Advanced Research, 2012b).

57. R. W. Boyer, "A Critique of Scientific Realism Based in Vedic Principles," *NeuroQuantology* (September 2013): 477–502.

58. M. M. Yogi, *Science of Being.*

59. M. M. Yogi, Maharishi's Global News Conference, December 12, 2003.

60. T. Nader, *Human Physiology: Expression of the Veda and Vedic Literature* (Vlodrop, Holland: Maharishi Vedic University, 2000).

61. T. Nader, *Ramayan in Human Physiology: Discovery of the Eternal Reality of the Ramayan in the Structure and Function of Human Physiology* (Fairfield, IA: Maharishi University of Management Press, 2011).

62. Morris, *Maharishi's Global News Conference.*

63. Nader, *Human Physiology.*

64. Nader, *Ramayan in Human Physiology.*

65. Boyer, *Bridge to Unity.*

66. M. M. Yogi, *Maharishi's Absolute Theory*.
67. J. Lipman and A. Arenander, *Maharishi Vedic Architecture: Background and Summary of Scientific Research*, www.maharishivastu.org.
68. F. Travis, A. Bonshek, V. Butler, M. Rainforth, C. N. Alexander, and J. Lipman, "Can a Building's Orientation Affect the Quality of Life of the People Within? Testing Principles of Maharishi Sthapatya Veda," *Journal of Social Behavior and Personality* 17 (2005): 553–64.
69. A. Geller, "Smart Growth: A Prescription for Livable Cities," *American Journal of Public* Health (September 2003): 1410–15.
70. *Washington Post*, "Sprawl May Harm Health, Study Finds," September 27, 2004, A3.

BIBLIOGRAPHY

Alexander, C. N., Robinson P., and Rainforth, M. V. "Treating and Preventing Alcohol, Nicotine, and Drug Abuse through Transcendental Meditation: A Review and Statistical Meta-analysis." *Alcoholism Treatment Quarterly* 11, nos. 1 and 2 (1994): 13–87.
Badawi, K., Wallace, R. K., Orme-Johnson, D. W., and Rouzere, A. M. "Electrophysiologic Characteristics of Respiratory Suspension Periods Occurring During the Practice of the Transcendental Meditation Technique." *Psychosomatic Medicine* 46 no. 3 (1984): 267–76.
Barnes, V. A., and Orme-Johnson, D. W. "Prevention and Treatment of Cardiovascular Disease in Adolescents and Adults through the Transcendental Meditation®Program: A Research Update." *Current Hypertension Reviews* 8, no. 3 (2012): 227–42.
Bevvino, D. L. This volume.
Boyer, R. W. "A Critique of Scientific Realism Based in Vedic Principles." *NeuroQuantology* (September 2013): 477–502.
———. *Bridge to Unity: Unified Field-Based Science and Spirituality*. Malibu, CA: Institute for Advanced Research, 2008.
———. *Linking Mind and Matter: A New Scientific Model That Unifies Nonlocal Mind and Local Matter*. Malibu, CA: Institute for Advanced Research, 2012.
———. *Vedic Principles of Therapy*. Malibu, CA: Institute for Advanced Research, 2012.
Deans, A. *A Record of Excellence*. Fairfield, IA: Maharishi University of Management Press, 2005.
Dillbeck, M. C., ed. *Scientific Research on Maharishi's Transcendental Meditation and TM-Sidhi Programme—Collected Papers*, vol. 6. Vlodrop, The Netherlands: Maharishi Vedic University Press, 2011.
Eddington, A. *The Nature of the Physical World*. Ann Arbor: University of Michigan Press, 1974.
Farrow, J. T., and Hebert, J. R. "Breath Suspension During the Transcendental Meditation Technique." *Psychosomatic Medicine* 44, no. 2 (1982): 133–53.
Geller, A. "Smart Growth: A Prescription for Livable Cities." *American Journal of Public Health* (September 2003): 1410–15.

Hagelin, J. S. "Is Consciousness the Unified Field? A Field Theorist's Perspective." *Modern Science and Vedic Science* 1 (1987): 29–87.

———. "Restructuring Physics from Its Foundation in Light of Maharishi's Vedic Science." *Modern Science and Vedic Science* 3, no. 1 (1989): 3–72.

Hameroff, S. R. "The 'Conscious Pilot': Synchronized Dendritic Webs Move through the Brain Neurocomputational Networks to Mediate Consciousness." Paper presented at the bi-annual conference *Toward a Science of Consciousness*, Tucson, Arizona, April 8–12, 2008.

Hebert, J. R., Lehmann, D., Tan, G., Travis, F., and Arenander, A. "Enhanced EEG Alpha Time-Domain Phase Synchrony During Transcendental Meditation: Implications for Cortical Integration Theory." *Signal Processing* 85, no. 11 (2005); 2213–32.

Lipman, J., and Arenander, A. *Maharishi Vedic Architecture: Background and Summary of Scientific Research*, www.maharishivastu.org.

Maharishi Foundation. www.tm.org/research-on-meditation.

Maharishi Mahesh Yogi. *Maharishi Mahesh Yogi on the Bhagavad-Gita: A New Translation and Commentary*, chs. 1–6. London: Penguin Books, 1967.

———. *Maharishi's Absolute Theory of Defence: Sovereignty in Invincibility*. India: Age of Enlightenment Publications, 1996.

———. *Maharishi's Global News Conference*. December 12, 2003.

———. *Science of Being and Art of Living*. Washington, DC: Age of Enlightenment Publications, 1963, 258–59.

Maharishi University of Management, www.mum.edu.

Maharishi Vedic University: Introduction. Vlodrop, The Netherlands: Maharishi Vedic University Press, 1994.

Miller, G. A. "Trends and Debates in Cognitive Psychology." *Cognition* 10 (1981): 215–25.

Morris, B. *Maharishi's Global News Conference*. May 5, 2004.

Nader, T. *Human Physiology: Expression of the Veda and Vedic Literature*. Vlodrop, Holland: Maharishi Vedic University, 2000.

———. *Ramayan in Human Physiology: Discovery of the Eternal Reality of the Ramayan in the Structure and Function of Human Physiology*. Fairfield, IA: Maharishi University of Management Press, 2011.

O'Connell, D. F., and Alexander, C. N., eds. *Self-Recovery: Treating Addictions Using Transcendental Meditation and Maharishi Ayur-Veda*. Binghamton, NY: Haworth Press, 1994.

Orme-Johnson, D. W. www.truthabouttm.com.

———. "Commentary of the AHRQ Report on Research on Meditation Practices in Health." *Journal of Alternative and Complementary Medicine* 14, no. 10 (2008): 1215–21.

———. "Medical Care Utilization and the Transcendental Meditation Program." *Psychosomatic Medicine* 49, no. 1 (1997): 493–507.

Orme-Johnson, D. W., and Barnes, V. A. "Effects of TM Practice on Trait Anxiety: A Meta-analysis of Randomized Control Trials." *Journal of Alternative and Complementary Medicine* 19, no. 10 (2013): 1–12.

Orme-Johnson, D. W., and Herron, R. E. "An Innovative Approach to Reducing Medical Care Utilization." *American Journal of Managed Care* 3, no. 1 (1987): 135–44.

Planck, M. *Observer.* January 31, 1931.

Sauseng, P., and Klimesch, W. "What Does Phase Information of Oscillatory Brain Activity Tell Us About Cognitive Processes?" *Neuroscience Biobehavioral Review* 32, no. 5 (2008): 1001–13.

Schneider, R. H., and Fields, J. Z. *Total Heart Health.* Laguna Beach, CA: Basic Health Publications, 2006.

Scientific Research on Maharishi's Transcendental Meditation and TM-Sidhi Programme—Collected Papers. Vols. 1–5. Fairfield, IA: Maharishi University of Management Press, 1977–1990.

Shear, J. *The Experience of Meditation.* London: Paragon Press, 2006.

Stapp, P. *Mindful Universe: Quantum Mechanics and the Participating Observer.* New York: Springer-Verlag, 2007.

Travis, F., and Arenander, A. "Cross-sectional and Longitudinal Study of Effects of Transcendental Meditation Practice on Interhemispheric Frontal Asymmetry and Frontal Coherence." *International Journal of Neuroscience* 116 (2006): 1519–38.

Travis, F., Bonshek, A., Butler, V., Rainforth, M., Alexander, C. N., and Lipman, J. "Can a Building's Orientation Affect the Quality of Life of the People Within? Testing Principles of Maharishi Sthapatya Veda." *Journal of Social Behavior and Personality* 17 (2005): 553–64.

Travis, F., and Wallace, R. K. "Autonomic Patterns During Respiratory Suspension: Possible Markers of Transcendental Consciousness." *Psychophysiology* 34, no. 1 (1997): 39–46.

Washington Post. "Sprawl May Harm Health, Study Finds." September 27, 2004, A3.

Wigner, E. quoted in Herbert, N. *Quantum Reality: Beyond the New Physics.* New York: Anchor Books, 1985.

Two

How Meditation Heals: The Brain and Higher States of Consciousness

Fred Travis, Ph.D.

The brain is a living organ that adapts to every experience we have. Meditation practice heals the mind and body by providing fundamentally different kinds of experiences that re-shape brain connections. Every experience creates a wave of electrical activity over the brain that brings awareness of the world around us. At the same time, the brain connections activated by that experience become enhanced (long-term potentiation) or dampened (long-term depression) to more easily facilitate processing the same experience in the future.[1] Changes in brain connections lead to changes in larger cortical patterns. For instance, experienced London taxi-cab drivers, compared to novice drivers, have more richly connected circuits in those brain areas involved in planning a route through city traffic, time estimation of alternative routes, and dealing with unexpected delays.[2] The ongoing modification of brain circuits with experience is known as *neuroplasticity*.[3]

NEUROPLASTICITY—A DOUBLE-EDGED SWORD

Neuroplasticity is expressed on all levels of the individual from genetic expression to psychological states and to physical states, such as brain circuits. Neuroplasticity is value neutral; it reflects the frequency and intensity of whatever experience you are having. Trauma and stress produce dysfunctional circuits; positive, nurturing experiences produce functional circuits.

Effect of Stress, Abuse, and Trauma on Brain Circuits

On the level of the DNA, stress and trauma decrease the expression of synapse-related genes in the developing brain of a fetus, causing loss of dendritic spines and dendrites. This in turn leads to smaller memory centers (hippocampus), smaller executive brain areas (frontal areas), and reduced working memory.[4,5] Early childhood stress disrupts regulation of the immune response contributing to autoimmune diseases in genetically predisposed individuals and differences in immune response and degree of neural plasticity throughout life.[6,7]

Effects of maternal stress on brain functioning have been demonstrated by an elegant field study in Quebec, where in one severe winter, there was a month-long power outage. Researchers identified pregnant women who were affected or were not affected by the power outage. Stress and trauma are reported to decrease connections between the limbic system and the frontal executive system, and increases connections between the limbic system and the brainstem.[8] The child whose mother was caught in the power outage exhibited (1) significantly lower mental and motor development, (2) lower levels of receptive and productive language development, and (3) stereotypical rather than functional play.[9,10] Another study has reported that high levels of stress in early childhood predict lower reading scores and IQ scores in first-grade students.[11]

Traumatic experiences cause dysfunctional brain circuits in which limbic reactivity dominates responses in all situations.[12] The question naturally arises: Can positive, nurturing experiences buffer the effects of current stress and stimulate different circuits that will neutralize past trauma? The answer to both of these questions is yes.

Effect of Positive and Nurturing Experiences on Brain Circuits

Maternal care can buffer the effects of stress on brain structure and functioning. Luby and colleagues compared the size of the hippocampus—the memory centers in the brain—in school-age children who had been diagnosed with low or high levels of depression. Depression is associated with smaller hippocampus volumes. The researchers also measured the level of maternal support during a "waiting task," which requires the child to wait for eight minutes before opening a brightly wrapped gift which is sitting within their reach. In this study, higher levels of parental support during the "waiting task," which were assumed to reflect maternal support throughout the day, were associated with larger hippocampal volumes in both low and high depressive subjects.[13] Another buffer for effects of stress is leisure-time exercise. College students who reported higher levels of leisure activity reported lower levels of physical and psychological symptoms of stress.[14]

This line of discussion has practical implications for the healthcare professional. The level of safety, empathy, and unconditional regard in a therapeutic relationship is reported to predict treatment outcomes.[15] Thus the success of a patient's recovery in therapy stems not only from what the therapist does, but also from the character of the relationship that the therapist sets up. The supporting environment is a potent mechanism for healing of both mental and physical disorders.

Habits and Brain Functioning

We are guided by habit. One hundred years ago, William James, the father of American psychology observed,

> Could the young but realize how soon they will become mere walking bundles of habits. We are spinning our own fates, good or evil. Every smallest stroke of virtue or of vice leaves its ever so small scar . . . down amongst the nerve cells and fibers; the molecules are counting it, registering and storing it up to be used against him when the temptation occurs. Nothing we ever do is, in strict scientific literalness, wiped out.[16]

Our habits color how we see the world. We revolve every day through a *perception-choice-experience cycle*. Current brain circuits determine how we perceive a situation and, in turn, the choices we make. Those choices lead to specific experiences, which then reinforce the brain circuits used. This is the basis of learning—the basis of conditioning.

This means that a person can get into a rut. We continue to see the world in the same way, make the same choices, and reinforce the same brain circuits. Because the brain functions in this perception-choice-experience cycle, an individual can become trapped in a bad habit and not see the way out. They "want" to change, but they are "driven" to act in the same way. On the other hand, good habits can support continued growth in life. As Aristotle famously proclaimed, *"We are what we repeatedly do . . . Excellence, then, is not an act, but a habit."*

EXPERIENCES DURING MEDITATION PRACTICES

Typical experiences throughout the day involve the subject experiencing changing sensory, mental, or emotional states. The perception-choice-experience cycle biases our thoughts and actions. If we remain within the field of changing sensory, mental, or emotional states, then we remain in the sphere of the influence of the past.

Meditation practices give rise to different kinds of experiences. The degree to which meditation experiences differ from day-to-day experiences is the degree to which they can structure new circuits to support new ways to see and respond to the world.

Meditations Have Different Procedures

Various meditation practices all have one thing in common: they investigate inner subjectivity or inner awareness. However, they explore inner subjectivity from different angles and are associated with different brain activation patterns and lead to different benefits.[17] The common practice of grouping different types of meditation together ignores the inherent differences between meditation practices.

Three categories of meditation have been delineated based on procedures used during the meditation practice and the reported EEG signatures. These three categories are *focused attention, open monitoring,* and *automatic self-transcending.*[18] Meditations in the focused attention category keep the mind focused on one object of experience—a thought, an emotional state, a part of the body. Meditations in the open monitoring category allow experiences to pass through attention without manipulation, control, or rumination, which is termed "dispassionate observation." Meditations in the automatic self-transcending category transcend the steps of practice—they start from the thinking level and end up with silence, the level of being or inner wakefulness. Meditations in the first two categories keep you involved in subject/object relationships. Meditations in the last category transcend the subject/object relationship, resulting in pure self-awareness.

Meditations in the first two categories develop cognitive and affective skills during the meditation session that are then available to deal with challenges in daily life.[19] For instance, compassion meditation, which is in the focused attention category, leads to higher gamma (20–50 Hz) EEGs and activation of limbic brain circuits, including the insula and amygdala during the practice.[20] This meditation practice is reported to result in more compassionate behavior after the practice.[21]

Mindfulness meditation, which is in the open monitoring category, leads to increases in bilateral frontal theta2 (6–8 Hz) EEGs[22] and activation of anterior cingulate cortices during the practice.[23] Developing mindfulness during meditation practice helps one to be more mindful—more present-centered—during stressful experiences. Mindfulness is reported to decrease the impact of stress on one's mind and body.[24]

Meditation practices in the automatic self-transcending category transcend cognitive and affective processes to reveal a state of pure self-awareness—a state of *being* rather than a state of thinking or doing—called pure consciousness.[25] Pure consciousness is "pure" in that it is free from changing mental content. Transcendental Meditation (TM®), which is in this category, is marked by frontal alpha1 power and coherence[26] and elevated frontal blood flow and reduced brain-stem blood flow.[27] The word "automatic" is important in this category. Transcending is a delicate process that needs to go by itself. Any attentional control or manipulation leads to activity in localized brain areas that impede the process of transcending.

Meditations Have Different Effects on Mind and Body

Meditations use different procedures that produce different brain patterns and consequently have different effects. The more specific the meditation procedure, the more specific the effects will be. Sedlmeier compared effect sizes reported in 165 studies of effects of mindfulness meditation, TM, and "other meditations" on 22 psychological variables.[28] Transcending led to substantially greater decreases in negative psychological traits, such as depression and anxiety, and to significantly greater increases in positive psychological traits, such as self-esteem and self-actualization, than other meditations or mindfulness practice (effect sizes: TM = 0.34; other meditations = 0.27; mindfulness = 0.24).

A similar comparison among meditation practices has been conducted on studies of hypertension. After comparing all studies on meditation and hypertension, the American Heart Association supported physicians recommending TM to their patients, based on the strength of the research. They observed that all other meditation techniques (including mindfulness) received a "Class III, no benefit, Level of Evidence C" recommendation and were not recommended in clinical practice to lower blood pressure.[29] A similar finding was recently reported from a large random assignment study in Toronto of 101 subjects with stage-1 hypertension. Eight-weeks of mindfulness practice did not lead to significant decreases in hypertension.[30]

A comparison of meditation practices on decreases in posttraumatic stress disorder (PTSD) symptoms also yielded different effects with different meditation practices. Effect sizes from five published studies on meditation and PTSD are presented in figure 2.1. The first three studies investigated the effects of TM on PTSD symptoms; the fourth reported effects of loving-kindness; the last reported effects of mindfulness practice. All studies used the PTSD Checklist to assess post-traumatic stress symptoms. Effect sizes for reduction in PTSD symptoms were 2 to 4 times larger with transcending during TM compared to other meditation practices.

The three TM studies included a random assignment test of Vietnam veterans by Brooks (three months TM practice), a single-group design of Iraqi veterans by Rosenthal (3 months TM practice), and a random assignment test of refugees in Uganda by Rees (1 month and 4.5 months TM

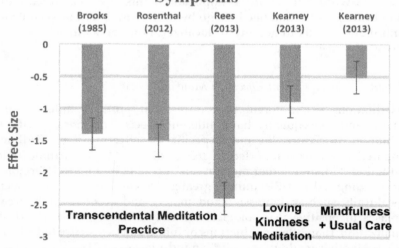

Figure 2.1.   Impact of different meditation practices on reducing posttraumatic stress symptoms.

practice).[31,32,33] The fourth study, with loving-kindness, was a pilot study with a single-group design by Kearney (3 months, and 6 months loving-kindness practice).[34] The fifth study was a random assignment study of treatment-as-usual or treatment-as-usual-plus-mindfulness-meditation, also by Kearney (2 months, and 4 months mindfulness practice).[35] In this study, the treatment-as-usual-plus-mindfulness-meditation group experienced reduced PTSD symptoms as much as the treatment-as-usual group. Mindfulness did not contribute to further reductions in PTSD symptoms.

Healing through Meditation Practice: State Effects Become Trait Effects

This brings us to the core of our discussion. Meditations heal by providing new experiences—*state* effects—that with regular practice over time change brain functioning and become *trait* effects. By our consciously adopting a meditation practice, brain structure and functioning can be systematically shaped.

Focused attention and open monitoring meditations have been discussed as a "family of complex emotional and attentional regulatory strategies developed for various ends, including the cultivation of well-being and emotional balance."[36] Research on these meditations has focused on developing cognitive and affective skills that can help patients cope with the effects of past stress and current challenges. However, the possible drawback of working on a single skill is that it could lead to unbalanced development and mental instability.[37]

Meditations in the automatic self-transcending category, such as TM, transcend the usual subject/object relationship; they lead to the experience of pure self-awareness without changing sensory, mental, or emotional content.[38,39] Pure self-awareness means that all mental structures, including categories, concepts, and memories, are transcended. In the experience of pure consciousness, even traumas are transcended, allowing the brain to begin to develop new connections to process experience in a different way.[40,41] Transcending changes the subject that identifies with changing objects. This provides a new basis for perceiving the world and making decisions, and so individuals begin to grow out of their situation. Establishing a new "ground" to process experience could explain the substantial benefits reported from TM. The next sections explore in detail the nature of pure consciousness.

What Is the Nature of Pure Consciousness?

The sense of self in waking state is called the "lower self" in Vedic science, and it includes that "aspect of the personality which deals only with the relative aspect of existence. It comprises the mind that thinks, the intellect that decides, and the ego that experiences."[42] Meditation practices that involve focused attention or open monitoring train the practitioner to use aspects of the lower self in different ways, such as by controlling one's attention or emotional state.

Pure consciousness, the "higher self," is that "aspect of the personality which never changes, absolute Being, which is the very basis of the entire field of relativity, including the lower self."[43] The Katha Upanishad, which explores the nature of pure consciousness, describes pure consciousness in this way: "The Self is without sound, without touch and without form . . . You will know the Self when your senses are still, your mind is at peace, and your heart is pure."[44] The word "self" is capitalized in this quotation to distinguish the higher Self from the lower self.

Pure consciousness is qualitatively distinct from waking, sleeping, and dreaming. Figure 2.2 presents a 2 × 2 grid with the presence/absence of thoughts, i.e., sensory, mental, or affective content (object) on the y-axis, and the presence/absence of self-awareness (subject) on the x-axis. Notice that the subject-object relation during pure consciousness is completely different from that during waking, sleeping, or dreaming. In sleeping, there is no sense of self and no content. In dreaming, an illusory sense of self is caught up with vivid, quickly changing dream images. In waking, there is a sense of self—the lower self—and there is changing content. That leaves the bottom-right cell—no sense of individual self or objects of

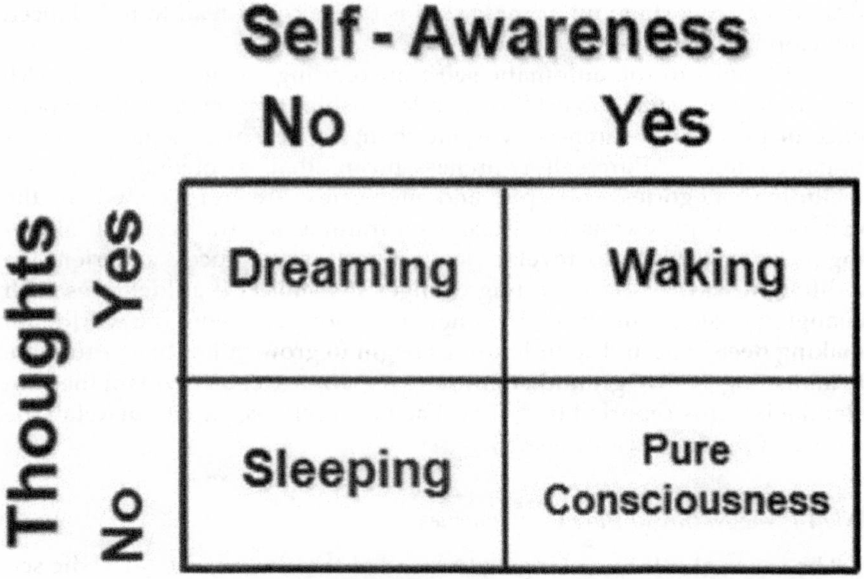

Self - Awareness

	No	Yes
Thoughts Yes	Dreaming	Waking
No	Sleeping	Pure Consciousness

Figure 2.2.　2×2 grid with the presence/absence of object on the y-axis, and the subject on the x-axis.

Note: Waking, dreaming, sleeping, and pure consciousness have different values of subject and object.

perception, which is the experience of pure consciousness, the higher Self, where the subject/object dichotomy is united in pure subjectivity.

Some scientists might comment that the bottom-right cell—pure consciousness—is not possible. How can you be aware of yourself without also being aware of your body, or your feelings, or your thoughts, or the fact you are thinking?[45] William James, in his *Principles of Psychology*, observed,[46]

> It is difficult for me to detect in [mental] activity any purely spiritual element at all. Whenever my introspective glance succeeds in turning round quickly enough to catch one of those manifestations of spontaneity in the act, all it can ever feel distinctly is some bodily process, for the most part taking place within the head.

This conclusion is a valid conclusion in discussions of the lower self in the waking state, which always includes a sense of (small) self with changing mental content. However, meditations such as TM lead to the experience of pure consciousness, in which consciousness is conscious of its own nature.

TM is a process of transcending perception of a mantra, a sound without meaning. During transcending, the mantra becomes increasingly secondary in experience, ultimately disappearing, and self-awareness becomes primary. Maharishi Mahesh Yogi, who brought TM to the West, described pure consciousness in this way:[47]

> The state of Being is one of pure consciousness, completely out of the field of relativity; there is no world of the senses or of objects, no trace of sensory activity, no trace of mental activity. There is no trinity of thinker, thinking process and thought, doer, process of doing and action; experiencer, process of experiencing and object of experience. The state of transcendental Unity of life, or pure consciousness, is completely free from all trace of duality.

On one hand, you can say there is no content in pure consciousness. On the other, you could say the content is wakefulness itself,[48] or consciousness itself.[49] A content analysis of thirty-five descriptions of pure consciousness yielded three common themes used to describe the experience: absence of time, absence of space, and absence of body sense.[50] Time, space, and body sense are the framework that gives meaning to waking experience. Notice that pure consciousness is not characterized by distorted sensory or body sensations but by the absence of the very framework that gives meaning to waking experience. This supports the Vedic tradition calling the experience of pure consciousness a fourth major state of consciousness, or *turiya chetanā*.[51]

PHYSIOLOGICAL PATTERNS OF PURE CONSCIOUSNESS

Changes in breath rate, skin conductance, and EEG patterns have been reported during the experience of pure consciousness. Farrow and Hebert[52] and later Badawi and colleagues[53] observed suspension of normal respiration for 10–40 seconds during the experience of pure consciousness. This type of breathing, while initially termed "respiratory suspension," is very often an example of *apneustic* breathing—slow, prolonged inspiration.[54] Apneustic breathing is supported by different respiratory drive centers in the brain stem than those that mediate breathing during waking.[55]

A second marker of this state is skin conductance responses, reflecting sympathetic nervous system activation at the onset of breath changes.[56] These autonomic responses are similar to those seen during *orienting*—attention switching to environmental stimuli that are novel or significant.[57] These autonomic responses could mark the transition of awareness from active thinking processes to the mental silence of pure consciousness.

A third marker of the experience of pure consciousness is increased frontal alpha1 (8–10 Hz) coherence as reported in two random assignment studies comparing TM to eyes-closed rest—one a random assignment within-subject study of 24 subjects,[58] the other a random assignment between-subject study of 50 subjects.[59]

It is important to note that frontal alpha1 (8–10 Hz) brain waves are most often seen during TM rather than alpha2 (10–12 Hz) brain waves. The alpha2 frequency is associated with lower thalamic activity and lower cerebral metabolic rate in sensory and motor areas.[60] This has been termed *cortical idling* since brain areas used in processing are inhibited.[61]

In contrast, alpha1 activity in frontal association cortices is correlated with higher cerebral metabolic rate. It is reported during tasks involving internally directed attention,[62] such as imagining a tune compared to listening to a tune.[63] Bursts of alpha1 EEG are also seen when the subject is solving a problem by intuition or insight.[64]

Thus pure consciousness is subjectively distinct from waking, sleeping, and dreaming and is marked by distinct physiological patterns. Discrete subjective and objective patterns support calling pure consciousness a *fourth* state of consciousness. Regular experience of pure consciousness transforms one's inner nature and leads to higher states of consciousness.

HIGHER STATES OF CONSCIOUSNESS: THE STATE OF ENLIGHTENMENT

Enlightenment in Buddhist Traditions

States beyond waking—dreaming and sleeping—are understandably hard to define. They represent types of experiences that do not readily fit into the categories of usual waking experience. Davis and Vago[65] summarized the discussion of enlightenment in the Buddhist traditions in this way:

> There are deep disagreements over the nature of the goal between and even within various Buddhist schools. Scientific investigations cannot assume that there is any commonality among the transformative changes referred to as "kensho," "stream entry," "realizing the nature of mind," and so on, that various Buddhist traditions take as various stages of awakening.

In contrast, the Vedic tradition clearly defines different levels or stages of enlightenment.

Enlightenment in the Vedic Tradition

Maharishi Mahesh Yogi has delineated milestones of four higher states of consciousness.[66] Pure consciousness, a fourth state of consciousness, is the first stage of enlightenment. It is transitory. However, by taking the mind to pure consciousness and back to waking activity, the *state* of pure consciousness becomes a permanent *trait*.[67] Pure consciousness becomes a continuous inner experience that forms a silent core of inner subjectivity that is independent from but supports processing of changing sensory, mental, and emotional states.

Cosmic Consciousness: The First Stabilized State of Enlightenment

The integration of pure consciousness with the other three states is the first stabilized state of enlightenment in the Vedic tradition and is called *Turyatit Chetana*, or Cosmic Consciousness.[68] In Cosmic Consciousness, perception, thinking, and feeling are on the surface of life; deep within is immovable silence, uninvolved with ongoing experience. Maharishi Mahesh Yogi describes Cosmic Consciousness in this way:[69]

> [In Cosmic Consciousness] Being is permanently lived as separate from activity. Then a man realizes that his Self is different from the mind which is engaged with thoughts and desires. It is now his experience that the mind, which had been identified with desires, is mainly identified with the Self. He experiences the desires of the mind as lying outside himself, whereas he used to experience himself as completely involved with desires. On the surface of the mind desires certainly continue, but deep within the mind they no longer exist, for the depths of the mind are transformed into the nature of the Self. All the desires which were present in the mind have been thrown upward, as it were, they have gone to the surface, and within the mind the finest intellect gains an unshakeable, immovable status. This is the "steady intellect" in the state of nitya-samadhi, Cosmic Consciousness.

In Cosmic Consciousness, the immovability of inner silence becomes the predominant element of experience because it does not change. Outer activity is constantly changing. Outer change is experienced, but it does not leave a strong impression to color future action. During sleep, this state is described by one meditator as

> a continuum there. It's not like I go away and come back. It's a subtle thing. It's not like I'm awake waiting for the body to wake-up or whatever. It's me there. I don't feel like I'm lost in the experience. That's what I mean by a continuum. You know, it's like the fizzing on top of a soda when you've poured it. It's there and becomes active so there's something to identify with. When I'm sleeping, it's like the fizzing goes down. (65-year-old male; 39 years of TM practice)

EEG patterns have been identified during the experience of inner wakefulness coexisting with the body while sleeping deeply. Individuals reporting this experience exhibit the brain-wave pattern of transcending (alpha) coexisting with the brain patterns of deep sleep (delta).[70]

Inner wakefulness during sleep cannot be feigned. The body is asleep, the senses are shut down, and the thinking mind is quiet, all while a continuum of self-awareness persists from falling asleep to waking up. The quote above uses an analogy: during sleep, the "fizzing," or stream of conscious experiences, goes down to reveal the underlying "soda," or pure self-awareness, that continues throughout the night. When one wakes up, the fizzing simply begins again.

PHYSIOLOGICAL PATTERNS DURING ACTIVITY IN SUBJECTS
REPORTING COSMIC CONSCIOUSNESS

Brain patterns were compared in three groups: 17 meditation-naive subjects; 17 subjects with 7 years TM experience (approximately 4,900 hours); and 17 subjects with 24 years TM experience (approximately 18,000 hours) who reported the experience of Cosmic Consciousness—inner self-awareness throughout sleep.[71] One person reported experiences that fit descriptions of the third state of enlightenment (sixth state of consciousness) delineated in the Vedic tradition, called *Bhagavad Chetanā*; another reported experiences of *Brahmi Chetanā*, or Unity consciousness, the fourth state of enlightenment (seventh state of consciousness). These last two higher states will not be discussed in detail because we do not have sufficient people in those states to discuss their subjective experiences and objective parameters.

EEGs were recorded in these subjects during simple and choice paired reaction-time tasks. The simple reaction task included an asterisk as a warning stimuli followed by a tone 1.5 seconds later. Subjects stopped the tone with a button press. The choice reaction task included a one- or two-digit number as a warning stimuli followed by a second one- or two-digit number 1.5 seconds later. Subjects indicated which number was larger with a button press. The EEG in the gap between the two stimuli captured how the brain was preparing to respond. The brain preparatory response as well as the EEG power and coherence were calculated during the reaction-time tasks.

During these computer tasks, the subjects reporting Cosmic Consciousness, in comparison to subjects in the other two control groups, exhibited higher levels of broad-band frontal EEG coherence, higher frontal and central alpha relative power, and a better match in brain preparatory response to task demands. These brain measures were transformed to z-scores and added together to yield a composite measure, called the Brain Integration Scale.[72]

BRAIN INTEGRATION AS A BIOMARKER OF GROWING ENLIGHTENMENT

Enlightenment is a very abstract state defined in terms that go beyond everyday experiences. The Brain Integration Scale could provide an objective means to bring enlightenment into the scientific dialogue. Scores on the Brain Integration Scale increase with three months of TM practice, suggesting that regular transcending may be the engine that drives growth of enlightenment. In a random assignment study with college students, Brain Integration Scale scores significantly increased over three months of TM practice compared to controls.[73]

A series of studies have taken the Brain Integration Scale out of the meditation setting. A canonical correlation analysis investigated the relation of Brain Integration Scale scores to measures of creativity, executive functioning, brain processing speed, and moral reasoning in a group of product development engineers. Scores on the Brain Integration Scale corresponded to faster speed of brain processing on a task, faster resolution of response conflict, higher moral reasoning, and higher manageability. As a set, these correlated with higher figural and verbal flexibility and originality scores on Torrance tests of creativity.[74] Flexibility and originality both represent the ability to change and adapt to new situations. Thus these data suggest that people with higher Brain Integration Scale scores should be better able to deal with uncertainty, generate novel solutions, and so be successful in different professions.

This prediction was tested with three groups of professionals: athletes, managers, and musicians. Thirty-three athletes who finished in the top ten for three consecutive years in Olympic and national games were compared to thirty-three control athletes who competed but did not consistently place. The top athletes had higher levels of brain integration.[75] A similar pattern was seen with twenty top-level managers, who had higher levels of brain integration than twenty middle-level managers.[76] A slightly different picture emerged for classical musicians. Both professional and amateur musicians had high levels of brain integration—higher than the other top professionals.[77] Amateur musicians are not less-successful musicians; they just do not make their living playing music. The amateur musicians were successful in other careers, such as education, business, IT, and healthcare.

Implications of Higher Consciousness for Better Health

Experience changes the brain. As we move through our daily activities, we are continually strengthening some circuits and dampening others. In this way, our lifestyle becomes imprinted in the structure and functioning of the brain. We create our reality in a real, physical sense. The brain we have today is the concrete expression of our thoughts and experiences of yesterday. The brain we have tomorrow is the concrete expression of our thoughts and experiences today.

Meditative practices that lead to transcending, such as TM, add a new engine to our growth. Rather than simply developing individual skills or changing our orientation for food, music, or activity, transcending gives the experience of who we are when we stop all skill development, all thinking, all evaluation, all decision making and all attempts to please others. That state of pure consciousness we experience to be outside of time and space. It is our universal Self.

Pure consciousness does not remain isolated to the periods of TM, but rather it begins to influence the depth of our sleep, the vitality of our waking, and the breadth of our vision. As we become more stable inside, our changing circumstances have less of an impact on us. Those things that were oppressive before become mere challenges now. We steadily move beyond "not being sick" to being healthy, whole, vibrant, and growing.

CONCLUSION

Meditation practices could be the core of the art of healing in the twenty-first century. Medications and medical interventions will still be needed to address emergency situations and to stabilize some disease conditions. However, psychotherapists and other healthcare professionals could prescribe behavioral recommendations that will give new experiences to their clients, leading to the development of new brain circuits. As the brain is transformed, clients can take control of their lives. By receiving the chance to transcend, they can discover the part of themselves that is outside change. That is the real foundation for breaking dysfunctional habits of thinking and acting. That is the real foundation to move from deficiency thinking and deficiency motivation to growth motivation. That is the foundation for the enjoyment of a healthy and happy life.

NOTES

1. D. Buonomano and M. Merzenich, "Cortical Plasticity: From Synapses to Maps," *Annual Review of Neuroscience* 21 (1998): 149.

2. E. Maguire, K. Woollett, and H. Spiers, "London Taxi Drivers and Bus Drivers: A Structural MRI and Neuropsychological Analysis," *Hippocampus* 16, no. 12 (2006): 1093.

3. M. Butz, F. Worgotter, and A. van Ooyen, "Activity-Dependent Structural Plasticity," *Brain Research Review* 60, no. 2 (2009): 293.

4. H. J. Kang, B. Voleti, T. Hajszan, G. Rajkowska, C. Stockmeier, P. Licznerski, A. Lepack, M. Majik, L. S. Jeong, M. Banasr, H. Son, and R. Duman, "Decreased Expression of Synapse-Related Genes and Loss of Synapses in Major Depressive Disorder," *Natural Medicine* 18, no. 9 (2012): 1416.

5. G. Evans and M. Schamberg, "Childhood Poverty, Chronic Stress, and Adult Working Memory," *Proceedings of the National Academy of Science USA* 106, no. 16 (2009): 6548.

6. F. Strickland and B. Richardson, "Epigenetics in Human Autoimmunity—DNA Methylation in Systemic Lupus Erythematosus and Beyond," *Autoimmunity* 41, no. 4 (2008): 282.

7. B. Keverne and J. Curley, "Epigenetics, Brain Evolution, and Behaviour," *Frontiers in Neuroendocrinology* 29, no. 3 (2008): 408.

8. J. Lauter, *How Is Your Brain Like a Zebra?* (New York: Xlibris Corporation, 2008), 78.

9. X. Cao, D. P. Laplante, A. Brunet, A. Ciampi, and S. King, "Prenatal Maternal Stress Affects Motor Function in 5 1/2-Year-Old Children: Project Ice Storm," *Developmental Psychobiology* 56, no. 1 (2014): 122.

10. S. King and D. P. Laplante, "The Effects of Prenatal Maternal Stress on Children's Cognitive Development: Project Ice Storm," *Stress* 8, no. 1 (2005): 41.

11. V. Delaney-Black., C. Covington, S. J. Ondersma, B. Nordstrom-Klee, T. Templin, J. Ager, J. Janisse, and R. J. Sokol, "Violence Exposure, Trauma, and IQ and/or Reading Deficits among Urban Children," *Archives of Pediatric and Adolescent Medicine* 156, no. 3 (2002): 284.

12. Lauter, *How Is Your Brain Like a Zebra?* 101.

13. J. Luby, D. Barch, A. Belden, M. Gaffrey, R. Tillman, C. Babb, T. Nishino, H. Suzuki, and K. Botteron, "Maternal Support in Early Childhood Predicts Larger Hippocampal Volumes at School Age," *Proceedings of the National Academy of Sciences USA* 109, no. 8 (2011): 2856.

14. C. L. Carmack, E. Boudreaux, M. Amaral-Melendez, P. Brantley, and C. de Moor, "Aerobic Fitness and Leisure Physical Activity as Moderators of the Stress-Illness Relation," *Annals of Behavioral Medicine* 21, no. 3 (1999): 254.

15. D. Murphy and D. Cramer, "Mutuality of Rogers's Therapeutic Conditions and Treatment Progress in the First Three Psychotherapy Sessions," *Psychotherapy Research* 27 (2014): 356.

16. W. James, *Principles of Psychology* (New York: Dover Books, 1951), 127.

17. F. T. Travis and Jonathan Shear, "Focused Attention, Open Monitoring and Automatic Self-Transcending: Categories to Organize Meditations from Vedic, Buddhist and Chinese Traditions," *Consciousness and Cognition* 19, no. 4 (2010): 1118.

18. Ibid., 1112.

19. P. Sedlmeier, J. Eberth, M. Schwarz, D. Zimmermann, F. Haarig, S. Jaeger, and S. Kunze, "The Psychological Effects of Meditation: A Meta-analysis," *Psychological Bulletin* 138, no. 6 (2012): 1147.

20. A. Lutz, H. Slagter, J. Dunne, and R. Davidson, "Attention Regulation and Monitoring in Meditation," *Trends in Cognitive Science* 12, no. 4 (2008): 166.

21. D. DeSteno, D. Condon, G. Desbordes, and W. Miller, "Can Meditation Make You a More Compassionate Person?" *Psychological Science* 24, no. 10 (2013): 2126.

22. J. F. Tsai, S. Hou Jou, W. Chun Cho, and C. M. Lin, "Electroencephalography When Meditation Advances: A Case-Based Time-Series Analysis," *Cognitive Processing* 14, no. 4 (2013): 375.

23. A. Chiesa and A. Serretti, "A Systematic Review of Neurobiological and Clinical Features of Mindfulness Meditations," *Psychological Medicine* 40, no. 8 (2010): 1245.

40   *Fred Travis*

24. F. Zeidan, K. Martucci, R. Kraft, J. McHaffie, and R. Coghill, "Neural Correlates of Mindfulness Meditation-Related Anxiety Relief," *Social Cognitive and Affective Neuroscience* 23 (2013): 9.

25. M. M. Yogi, *Maharishi Mahesh Yogi on the Bhagavad Gita* (New York: Penguin, 1969), 269.

26. F. Travis, D. Haaga, J. Hagelin, M. Tanner, A. Arenander, S. Nidich, C. Gaylord-King, S. Grosswald, M. Rainforth, and R. Schneider, "A Self-Referential Default Brain State: Patterns of Coherence, Power, and ELORETA Sources During Eyes-Closed Rest and Transcendental Meditation Practice," *Cognitive Processing* 11, no. 1 (2010): 28.

27. M. Ludwig, "Brain Activation in Experienced Meditators," doctoral dissertation, 2011, UMI no. 3114720, 246.

28. Sedlmeier, *Psychological Effects of Meditation*, 1168.

29. R. Brook, L. Appel, M. Rubenfire, G. Ogedegbe, J. Bisognano, W. Elliott, F. Fuchs, J. Hughes, D. Lackland, B. Staffileno, R. Townsend, and S. Rajagopalan, "Beyond Medications and Diet: Alternative Approaches to Lowering Blood Pressure, A Scientific Statement from the American Heart Association," *Hypertension* 61, no. 6 (2013): 1379.

30. K. Blom, B. Baker, M. How, M. Dai, J. Irvine, S. Abbey, B. Abramson, M. Myers, A. Kiss, N. Perkins, and S. Tobe, "Hypertension Analysis of Stress Reduction Using Mindfulness Meditation and Yoga: Results from the Harmony Randomized Controlled Trial," *American Journal of Hypertension* 27, no. 1 (2014): 127.

31. J. Brooks and T. Scarano, "Transcendental Meditation in the Treatment of Post-Vietnam Adjustment," *Journal of Counseling and Development* 64 (1985): 214.

32. J. Rosenthal, S. Grosswald, R. Ross, and N. Rosenthal, "Effects of Transcendental Meditation in Veterans of Operation Enduring Freedom and Operation Iraqi Freedom with Posttraumatic Stress Disorder: A Pilot Study," *Military Medicine* 176, no. 6 (2011): 628.

33. B. Rees, F. Travis, D. Shapiro, and R. Chant, "Reduction in Posttraumatic Stress Symptoms in Congolese Refugees Practicing Transcendental Meditation," *Journal of Traumatic Stress* 26, no. 2 (2013): 297.

34. D. Kearney, C. Malte, C. McManus, M. Martinez, B. Fellman, and T. Simpson, "Loving-Kindness Meditation for Posttraumatic Stress Disorder: A Pilot Study," *Journal of Trauma Stress* 4 (2013): 432.

35. D. Kearney, K. McDermott, C. Malte, M. Martinez, and T. Simpson, "Effects of Participation in a Mindfulness Program for Veterans with Posttraumatic Stress Disorder: A Randomized Controlled Pilot Study," *Journal of Clinical Psychology* 69, no. 1 (2013): 18.

36. Lutz et al., "Attention Regulation and Monitoring," 164.

37. L. J. Williamson, "Willoughby Britton at the Buddhist Geeks Conference, on the Problem with Meditation," *LA Weekly*, 2011.

38. F. Travis and C. Pearson, "Pure Consciousness: Distinct Phenomenological and Physiological Correlates of 'Consciousness Itself,'" *International Journal of Neuroscience* 100, nos. 1–4 (2000): 83.

39. F. Travis, "Transcendental Experiences During Meditation Practice," *Annals of the New York Academy of Sciences: Advances in Meditation Research: Neuroscience and Clinical Applications* 1307 (2014): 29.

40. F. Travis, "Core and Matrix Thalamic Nuclei: Parallel Circuits Involved in Content of Experience and General Wakefulness," *NeuroQuantology* 12, no. 2 (2012): 5.

41. Ibid., 31.

42. M. M. Yogi, *Maharishi Mahesh Yogi on the Bhagavad Gita*, 184.

43. Ibid.

44. K. Reddy, T. Egenes, and L. Egenes, *All Love Flows to the Self* (Schenectady, NY: Samhita Productions, 1999), 31.

45. T. Natsoulas, "The Concept of Consciousness," *Journal of Theory and Social Behavior* 29 (1999): 78.

46. James, *Principles of Psychology*, 300.

47. M. M. Yogi, *Maharishi Mahesh Yogi on the Bhagavad Gita*, 222.

48. Travis, *Core and Matrix Thalamic Nuclei*, 6.

49. M. M. Yogi, *Celebrating Perfection in Education* (Vlodrop, The Netherlands: Maharishi Vedic University Press, 1994): 10.

50. Travis and Pearson, "Distinct Phenomenological and Physiological Correlates," 83.

51. Ibid., 72.

52. J. Farrow and J. Hebert, "Breath Suspension During the Transcendental Meditation Technique," *Psychosomatic Medicine* 44 (1982): 148.

53. K. Badawi, R. K. Wallace, D. W. Orme-Johnson, and A. M. Rouzere, "Electrophysiological Characteristics of Respiratory Suspension Periods Occurring During Practice of the Transcendental Meditation Program," *Psychosomatic Medicine* 46 (1984): 272.

54. J. Kesterson and N. Clinch, "Metabolic Rate, Respiratory Exchange Ratio, and Apneas During Meditation," *American Journal of Physiology* 89 (1989): R636.

55. F. Plum and J. Posner, *The Diagnosis of Stupor and Coma* (Philadelphia, PA: F. A. Davis, 1980), 78.

56. F. Travis and R. K. Wallace, "Autonomic Patterns During Respiratory Suspensions: Possible Markers of Transcendental Consciousness," *Psychophysiology* 34, no. 1 (1997): 42.

57. J. A. Spinks, G. Blowers, and D. Shek, "The Role of the Orienting Response in the Anticipation of Information: A Skin Conductance Response Study," *Psychophysiology* 22 (1985): 388.

58. F. Travis and R. K. Wallace, "Autonomic and EEG Patterns During Eyes-Closed Rest and Transcendental Meditation (TM) Practice: The Basis for a Neural Model of TM Practice," *Consciousness and Cognition* 8, no. 3 (1999): 312.

59. Travis et al., "A Self-Referential Default Brain State," 25.

60. T. Oakes, D. Pizzagalli, A. Hendrick, K. Horras, C. Larson, H. Abercrombie, S. Schaefer, J. Koger, and R. Davidson, "Functional Coupling of Simultaneous Electrical and Metabolic Activity in the Human Brain," *Human Brain Mapping* 21, no. 4 (2004): 277.

61. G. Pfurtscheller, A. Stancak, and C. Neuper, "Event-Related Synchronization (ERS) in the Alpha Band—An Electrophysiological Correlate of Cortical Idling: A Review," *International Journal of Psychophysiology* 24 (1996): 42.

62. J. C. Shaw, "Intention as a Component of the Alpha-Rhythm Response to Mental Activity," *International Journal of Psychophysiology* 24 (1996): 19.

63. N. Cooper, A. Burgess, R. Croft, and J. Gruzelier, "Investigating Evoked and Induced Electroencephalogram Activity in Task-Related Alpha Power Increases During an Internally Directed Attention Task," *NeuroReport* 17 (2006): 207.

64. J. Kounios and M. Beeman, "The Aha! Moment: The Cognitive Neuroscience of Insight," *Current Directions in Psychological Science* 18 (2009): 215.

65. J. Davis and D. Vago, "Can Enlightenment Be Traced to Specific Neural Correlates, Cognition, or Behavior? No, and (a Qualified) Yes," *Frontiers in Psychology* 4 (2013): 870.

66. M. M. Yogi, *Celebrating Perfection in Education*, 10.

67. M. M. Yogi, *Maharishi Mahesh Yogi on the Bhagavad Gita*, 174.

68. Ibid.

69. M. M. Yogi, *Maharishi Mahesh Yogi on the Bhagavad Gita*, 85.

70. L. Mason, C. Alexander, F. Travis, G. Marsh, D. Orme-Johnson, J. Gackenbach, D. Mason, M Rainforth, and K. Walton, "Electrophysiological Correlates of Higher States of Consciousness During Sleep in Long-Term Practitioners of the Transcendental Meditation Program," *Sleep* 20, no. 2 (1997): 109.

71. F. Travis, J. Tecce, A. Arenander, and R. K. Wallace, "Patterns of EEG Coherence, Power, and Contingent Negative Variation Characterize the Integration of Transcendental and Waking States," *Biological Psychology* 61 (2002): 298.

72. Ibid., 300.

73. F. Travis, D. A. F. Haaga, J. Hagelin, M. Tanner, A. Arenander, S. Nidich, C. Gaylord-King, S. Grosswald, M. Rainforth, and R. H. Schneider, "A Self-Referential Default Brain State: Patterns of Coherence, Power, and eLORETA Sources During Eyes-Closed Rest and Transcendental Meditation Practice," *Cognitive Processing* 11, no. 1 (2010): 28.

74. F. Travis and Y. Lagrosen, "Creativity and Brain-Functioning in Product Development Engineers: A Canonical Correlation Analysis," *Creativity Research Journal* 1040 (2014): 423.

75. H. Harung, F. Travis, A. M. Pensgaard, R. Boes, S. Cook-Greuter, and K. Daley, "High Levels of Brain Integration in World-Class Norwegian Athletes: Towards a Brain Measure of Performance Capacity in Sports," *Scandinavian Journal of Medicine and Science in Sports* 21 (2011): 39.

76. H. Harung and F. Travis, "Higher Mind-Brain Development in Successful Leaders: Testing a Unified Theory of Performance," *Cognitive Processing* 13 (2012): 179.

77. F. Travis, H. Harung, and Y. Lagrosen, "Moral Development, Peak Experiences and Brain Patterns in Professional and Amateur Classical Musicians: Support for a Unified Theory of Performance," *Consciousness and Cognition* 20 (2011): 1262.

BIBLIOGRAPHY

Badawi, K., R. K. Wallace, D. W. Orme-Johnson, and A. M. Rouzere. "Electrophysiological Characteristics of Respiratory Suspension Periods Occurring During Practice of the Transcendental Meditation Program." *Psychosomatic Medicine* 46 (1984): 267–76.

Blom, K., B. Baker, M. How, M. Dai, J. Irvine, S. Abbey, B. L. Abramson, M. G. Myers, A. Kiss, N. J. Perkins, and S. W. Tobe. "Hypertension Analysis of Stress Reduction Using Mindfulness Meditation and Yoga: Results from the Harmony Randomized Controlled Trial." *American Journal of Hypertension* 27, no. 1 (2014): 122–29.

Brook, R. D., L. J. Appel, M. Rubenfire, G. Ogedegbe, J. D. Bisognano, W. J. Elliott, F. D. Fuchs, J. W. Hughes, D. T. Lackland, B. A. Staffileno, R. R. Townsend, and S. Rajagopalan. "Beyond Medications and Diet: Alternative Approaches to Lowering Blood Pressure: A Scientific Statement from the American Heart Association." *Hypertension* 61, no. 6 (2013): 1360–83.

Brooks, J. S. and T. Scarano. "Transcendental Meditation in the Treatment of Post-Vietnam Adjustment." *Journal of Counseling and Development* 64 (1985): 212–15.

Buonomano, D. V. and M. M. Merzenich. "Cortical Plasticity: From Synapses to Maps." *Annual Review of Neuroscience* 21 (1998): 149–86.

Butz, M., F. Worgotter and A. van Ooyen. "Activity-Dependent Structural Plasticity." *Brain Research Review* 60, no. 2 (2009): 287–305.

Cao, X., D. P. Laplante, A. Brunet, A. Ciampi, and S. King. "Prenatal Maternal Stress Affects Motor Function in 5 1/2-Year-Old Children: Project Ice Storm." *Developmental Psychobiology* 56, no. 1 (2014): 117–25.

Carmack, C. L., E. Boudreaux, M. Amaral-Melendez, P. J. Brantley, and C. de Moor. "Aerobic Fitness and Leisure Physical Activity as Moderators of the Stress-Illness Relation." *Annuals of Behavioral Medicine* 21, no. 3 (1999): 251–57.

Chiesa, A. and A. Serretti. "A Systematic Review of Neurobiological and Clinical Features of Mindfulness Meditations." *Psychological Medicine* 40, no. 8 (2010): 1239–52.

Cooper, N. R., A. P. Burgess, R. J. Croft, and J. H. Gruzelier. "Investigating Evoked and Induced Electroencephalogram Activity in Task-Related Alpha Power Increases During an Internally Directed Attention Task." *NeuroReport* 17 (2006): 205–8.

Davis, J. H. and D. R. Vago. "Can Enlightenment Be Traced to Specific Neural Correlates, Cognition, or Behavior? No, and (a Qualified) Yes." *Frontiers in Psychology* 4 (2013): 870.

Delaney-Black, V., C. Covington, S. J. Ondersma, B. Nordstrom-Klee, T. Templin, J. Ager, J. Janisse, and R. J. Sokol. "Violence Exposure, Trauma, and IQ and/or Reading Deficits among Urban Children." *Archives of Pediatric and Adolescent Medicine* 156, no. 3 (2002): 280–85.

DeSteno, D., P. Condon, G. Desbordes, and W. Miller. "Can Meditation Make You a More Compassionate Person?" *Psychological Science* 24, no. 10 (2013): 2125–27.

Evans, G. W. and M. A. Schamberg. "Childhood Poverty, Chronic Stress, and Adult Working Memory." *Proceedings of the National Academy of Science USA* 106, no. 16 (2009): 6545–49.

Farrow, J. T. and J. R. Hebert. "Breath Suspension During the Transcendental Meditation Technique." *Psychosomatic Medicine* 44 (1982): 133–53.

Harung, H. S. and F. Travis. "Higher Mind-Brain Development in Successful Leaders: Testing a Unified Theory of Performance." *Cognitive Processing* 13 (2012): 171–81.

Harung, H. S., F. Travis, A. M. Pensgaard, R. Boes, S. Cook-Greuter, and K. Daley. "High Levels of Brain Integration in World-Class Norwegian Athletes: Towards a Brain Measure of Performance Capacity in Sports." *Scandinavian Journal of Medicine and Science in Sports* 21 (2011): 32–41.

James, W. *Principles of Psychology*. New York: Dover Books, 1951.

Kang, H. J., B. Voleti, T. Hajszan, G. Rajkowska, C. A. Stockmeier, P. Licznerski, A. Lepack, M. S. Majik, L. S. Jeong, M. Banasr, H. Son, and R. S. Duman. "Decreased Expression of Synapse-Related Genes and Loss of Synapses in Major Depressive Disorder." *Natural Medicine* 18, no. 9 (2012): 1413–17.

Kearney, D. J., K. McDermott, C. Malte, M. Martinez, and T. L. Simpson. "Effects of Participation in a Mindfulness Program for Veterans with Posttraumatic Stress Disorder: A Randomized Controlled Pilot Study." *Journal of Clinical Psychology* 69, no. 1 (2013): 14–27.

Kearney, D. J., C. A. Malte, C. McManus, M. E. Martinez, B. Fellman, and T. L. Simpson. "Loving-Kindness Meditation for Posttraumatic Stress Disorder: A Pilot Study." *Journal of Trauma Stress* 4 (2013): 426–34.

Kesterson, J. and N. Clinch. "Metabolic Rate, Respiratory Exchange Ratio, and Apneas During Meditation." *American Journal of Physiology* 89 (1989): R632–R638.

Keverne, E. B. and J. P. Curley." Epigenetics, Brain Evolution and Behaviour." *Frontiers in Neuroendocrinology* 29, no. 3 (2008): 398–412.

King, S. and D. P. Laplante. "The Effects of Prenatal Maternal Stress on Children's Cognitive Development: Project Ice Storm." *Stress* 8, no. 1 (2005): 35–45.

Kounios, J. and M. Beeman. "The Aha! Moment: The Cognitive Neuroscience of Insight." *Current Directions in Psychological Science* 18 (2009): 210–16.

Lauter, J. L. *How Is Your Brain Like a Zebra?* New York: Xlibris Corporation, 2008.

Luby, J. L., D. M. Barch, A. Belden, M. S. Gaffrey, R. Tillman, C. Babb, T. Nishino, H. Suzuki, and K. N. Botteron. "Maternal Support in Early Childhood Predicts Larger Hippocampal Volumes at School Age." *Proceedings of the National Academy of Sciences USA* 109, no. 8 (2011): 2854–59.

Ludwig, M. "Brain Activation in Experienced Meditators." Doctoral Dissertation. Dissertations and Theses Database, UMI no. 3114720, 2011.

Lutz, A, H Slagter, J. D. Dunne, and R. J. Davidson. "Attention Regulation and Monitoring in Meditation." *Trends in Cognitive Science* 12, no. 4 (2008): 163–69.

Maguire, E. A., K. Woollett, and H. J. Spiers. "London Taxi Drivers and Bus Drivers: A Structural MRI and Neuropsychological Analysis." *Hippocampus* 16, no. 12 (2006): 1091–101.

Maharishi Mahesh Yogi. *Celebrating Perfection in Education*. Vlodrop: Maharishi Vedic University Press, 1994.

Maharishi Mahesh Yogi. *Maharishi Mahesh Yogi on the Bhagavad Gita*. New York: Penguin, 1969.

Mason, L. I., C. N. Alexander, F. T. Travis, G. Marsh, D. W. Orme-Johnson, J. Gackenbach, D. C. Mason, M. Rainforth, and K. G. Walton. "Electrophysiological Correlates of Higher States of Consciousness During Sleep in Long-Term Practitioners of the Transcendental Meditation Program." *Sleep* 20, no. 2 (1997): 102–10.

Murphy, D. and D. Cramer. "Mutuality of Rogers's Therapeutic Conditions and Treatment Progress in the First Three Psychotherapy Sessions." *Psychotherapy Research* 27 (2014).

Natsoulas, T. "The Concept of Consciousness." *Journal of Theory and Social Behavior* 29 (1999): 59–87.

Oakes, T. R., D. A. Pizzagalli, A. M. Hendrick, K. A. Horras, C. L. Larson, H. C. Abercrombie, S. M. Schaefer, J. V. Koger, and R. J. Davidson. "Functional Coupling of Simultaneous Electrical and Metabolic Activity in the Human Brain." *Human Brain Mapping* 21, no. 4 (2004): 257–70.

Pfurtscheller, G., A. Stancak, and C. Neuper. "Event-Related Synchronization (ERS) in the Alpha Band—An Electrophysiological Correlate of Cortical Idling: A Review." *International Journal of Psychophysiology* 24 (1996): 39–46.

Plum, F. and J. B. Posner. *The Diagnosis of Stupor and Coma*. Philadelphia, PA: F. A. Davis, 1980.

Reddy, K., T Egenes, and L Egenes. *All Love Flows to the Self*. Schenectady, NY: Samhita Productions, 1999.

Rees, B., F. Travis, D. Shapiro, and R. Chant. "Reduction in Posttraumatic Stress Symptoms in Congolese Refugees Practicing Transcendental Meditation." *Journal of Traumatic Stress* 26, no. 2 (2013): 295–98.

Rosenthal, J. Z., S. Grosswald, R. Ross, and N. Rosenthal. "Effects of Transcendental Meditation in Veterans of Operation Enduring Freedom and Operation Iraqi Freedom with Posttraumatic Stress Disorder: A Pilot Study." *Military Medicine* 176, no. 6 (2011): 626–30.

Sedlmeier, P., J. Eberth, M. Schwarz, D. Zimmermann, F. Haarig, S. Jaeger, and S. Kunze. "The Psychological Effects of Meditation: A Meta-analysis." *Psychological Bulletin* 138, no. 6 (2012): 1139–71.

Shaw, J. C. "Intention as a Component of the Alpha-Rhythm Response to Mental Activity." *International Journal of Psychophysiology* 24 (1996): 7–23.

Sokolov, E. N. *Perception and the Conditioned Reflex*. Oxford: Pergamon, 1963.

Spinks, J. A., G. H. Blowers, and D. T. L. Shek. "The Role of the Orienting Response in the Anticipation of Information: A Skin Conductance Response Study." *Psychophysiology* 22 (1985): 385–94.

Strickland, F. M. and B. C. Richardson. "Epigenetics in Human Autoimmunity. Epigenetics in Autoimmunity—DNA Methylation in Systemic Lupus Erythematosus and Beyond." *Autoimmunity* 41, no. 4 (2008): 278–86.

Travis, F. "Core and Matrix Thalamic Nuclei: Parallel Circuits Involved in Content of Experience and General Wakefulness." *NeuroQuantology* 12, no. 2 (2012): 1–6.

Travis, F., H. S. Harung, and Y. Lagrosen. "Moral Development, Peak Experiences and Brain Patterns in Professional and Amateur Classical Musicians: Support for a Unified Theory of Performance." *Consciousness and Cognition* 20 (2011): 1256–64.

Travis, F., D. A. Haaga, J. Hagelin, M. Tanner, A. Arenander, S. Nidich, C. Gaylord-King, S. Grosswald, M. Rainforth, and R. H. Schneider. "A Self-Referential Default Brain State: Patterns of Coherence, Power, and eLORETA Sources During Eyes-Closed Rest and Transcendental Meditation Practice." *Cognitive Processing* 11, no. 1 (2010): 21–30.

Travis, F., D. A. Haaga, J. Hagelin, M. Tanner, S. Nidich, C. Gaylord-King, S. Grosswald, M. Rainforth, and R. H. Schneider. "Effects of Transcendental Meditation Practice on Brain Functioning and Stress Reactivity in College Students." *International Journal of Psychophysiology* 71, no. 2 (2009): 170–76.

Travis, F. and C. Pearson. "Pure Consciousness: Distinct Phenomenological and Physiological Correlates of 'Consciousness Itself.'" *International Journal of Neuroscience* 100, nos. 1–4 (2000): 77–89.

Travis, F. and J. Shear. "Focused Attention, Open Monitoring and Automatic Self-Transcending: Categories to Organize Meditations from Vedic, Buddhist and Chinese Traditions." *Consciousness and Cognition* 19, no. 4 (2010): 1110–18.

Travis, F. and R. K. Wallace. "Autonomic and EEG Patterns During Eyes-Closed Rest and Transcendental Meditation (TM) Practice: The Basis for a Neural Model of TM Practice." *Consciousness and Cognition* 8, no. 3 (1999): 302–18.

Travis, F. and R. K. Wallace. "Autonomic Patterns During Respiratory Suspensions: Possible Markers of Transcendental Consciousness." *Psychophysiology* 34(1) (1997): 39–46.

Travis, F. T. "Transcendental Experiences During Meditation Practice." *Annals of the New York Academy of Sciences: Advances in Meditation Research: Neuroscience and Clinical Applications* 1307 (2014): 23–30.

Travis, F. T. *Your Brain Is a River, Not a Rock.* Fairfield, IA: Total Brain Publications, 2012.

Travis, F. T. and Y. Lagrosen. "Creativity and Brain-Functioning in Product Development Engineers: A Canonical Correlation Analysis." *Creativity Research Journal* 1040 (2014): 419–24.

Travis, F. T., J. Tecce, A. Arenander, and R. K. Wallace. "Patterns of EEG Coherence, Power, and Contingent Negative Variation Characterize the Integration of Transcendental and Waking States." *Biological Psychology* 61 (2002): 293–319.

Tsai, J. F., S. H. Jou, W. Cho, and C. M. Lin. "Electroencephalography When Meditation Advances: A Case-Based Time-Series Analysis." *Cognitive Processing* 14, no 4 (2013): 371–76.

Williamson, L. J. 2011. "Willoughby Britton at the Buddhist Geeks Conference, on the Problem with Meditation." *LA Weekly*, 2011. www.laweekly. com/public spectacle/2011/09/08/willoughby-britton-at-the-buddhist-geeks-conference-on-the-problem-with-meditation.

Zeidan, F., K. T. Martucci, R. A. Kraft, J. G. McHaffie, and R. C. Coghill. "Neural Correlates of Mindfulness Meditation-Related Anxiety Relief." *Social Cognitive and Affective Neuroscience* 23 (2013): 1–9.

THREE

Stress, Illness, and Transcendental Meditation: A Triad Worth Re-exploring

Deborah L. Bevvino, Ph.D., NP

In the United States, stress has become so ubiquitous that the phrase "I am so stressed out" is now recognized as a state of distress. We seem to take for granted that there is no way to escape the travails of chronic stress, as stated succinctly in a quote found in a British journal from fifty years ago: "Stress in addition to being itself, was also the cause of itself and the result of itself."[1]

For the most part, the majority of individuals who have experienced crisis and stress weather the experience with adequate physiological and psychological adaptation. In fact for some, stress is seen as a healthy response that enhances abilities, increases resources, and improves well-being. Positive change in the aftermath of a crisis can actually improve overall functioning and is referred to as "post-traumatic growth."[2] One needs only recognize the power of the human spirit after natural and human disasters. However, there are unique individual differences in vulnerabilities to the potential pathogenic effects of crisis and acute and or chronic stress.

Stress is now considered a public health crisis. For many, the adaptation to stress today is generally associated with frantic lives, poor coping, subsequent healthcare risks, and psychological and physical disorders. The healthcare risks of stress impose a significant toll on medical expenditures. Chronic stress is one of the most costly factors, with tobacco use, obesity, and inactivity exacting significant expenditures as well. The focus of the current healthcare system is on managing illnesses and not on prevention. Less than 6.5 percent of the U.S. healthcare budget is devoted to prevention.[3] The current healthcare system, more suited to be called an "illness medical system," is financially supported and medically focused on disease and tertiary care.

The survey "Stress in America—Missing the Healthcare Connection," conducted in 2012,[4] reported that "people are not receiving what they need from the healthcare providers to manage stress and address lifestyle and behavior changes to improve health." One of the least surprising findings of the survey was that 33 percent of Americans reported never discussing with their healthcare provider ways to manage stress. The United States spends more than any other country on healthcare and is a leader in both the quality and quantity of health research. Notably and unfortunately, these trends do not add up to better health outcomes.[5] When was the last time your physician inquired about your stress and discussed stress management? This chapter will present the epidemiology of stress, the impact of stress on the body, and the effect of TM on the stress response.

EPIDEMIOLOGY OF STRESS IN THE UNITED STATES

Since 2007, the American Psychological Association has commissioned an annual nationwide survey as part of its Mind/Body Health campaign to examine the state of stress across the country and understand its impact. A Stress in America Survey was conducted online in the United States on behalf of the American Psychological Association between August 3 and 31, 2013. Survey participants included 1,950 adults aged 18 or older and 1,018 teens aged 13 to 17. The Stress in America Survey measured attitudes and perceptions of stress among the general public and identified leading sources of stress, common behaviors used to manage stress, and the impact of stress on our lives. The results of the survey draw attention to the serious physical and emotional implications of stress and the inextricable link between the mind and body.[6]

Yet despite Americans' knowledge of the link between chronic stress and illness, the survey found that America is a culture of unhealthy stress. According to the Stress in America Survey, 78 percent of American adults reported a constant or increase in stress level over the past five years. Although American adults continue to report higher stress levels than what they believe to be healthy (5.1 versus 3.6 on a 10-point scale where 1 is "less or no stress" and 10 is "a great deal of stress"), most feel inadequate at managing it. When participants were asked about the level of stress they experienced over the previous month, 37 percent of adult participants reported that stress left them feeling overwhelmed. In addition, 30 percent felt that their stress level had a very strong impact on their physical health. And 30 percent reported that their level of stress had an impact on their mental health.[7]

According to the survey, while American adult stress levels may not be a surprise, the stress outlook for U.S. teens is daunting. American teens reported levels of stress that parallel those of adults. Teens reported stress levels far higher than they believe are healthy. Eighty-three percent of teens in this survey reported that stress levels during the school year far exceeded what they believed to be healthy (5.8 versus 3.9 on a 10-point scale) and exceeded the adults' average reported stress level of 5.1. Teens reported experiencing high stress levels during the summer months as well. Unfortunately, teens often have fewer coping mechanisms than adults for reducing stress, placing them at greater risk for subsequent illness. The impact of stress on teen physical health is clear. High stress levels can weaken immune systems and exhaust the body.[8] Healthy teens who experience consistently high levels of stress have higher levels of C-reactive protein, a marker of inflammation that has been associated with the development of cardiovascular disease.[9]

According to the Stress in America Survey, Millennials (18–34 years old) and Gen Xers (35–48 years old) reported higher average stress levels than other adults. Both groups reported that their stress levels had increased in the past year. Of interest is that Millennials were more likely than other generations to say they thought their stress would increase in the next year. In addition, the survey reported that across the country, adults, young adults, and teens reported doing a poor job managing their own stress. Only a small percentage of adults and teens who had tried to manage their stress were successful. The Stress in America Survey results portray a picture of high stress levels across Americans' lifespan, with minimal efficacy and effectiveness in stress reduction. Poorly managed stress seems to be the norm.

STRESS AND THE BRAIN

Why do some people get sick and others do not? The answer to this question is quite complex. Both the scientific literature as well as clinical practice suggest that "resiliency" and "vulnerability" to psychological and physical illnesses are a series of interactions between biology, temperament, personal characteristics, past and early childhood trauma, and experiences. The brain is both structurally and chemically shaped by biology, experiences, and the interaction of both. Brain regions such as the hippocampus, prefrontal cortex, and the amygdala respond to both acute and chronic stress. The same remarkable neuroendocrine, autonomic, immune, and cardiovascular adaptive and survival response to stress, once dysregulated by chronic stress, can be a precursor to poor health. According to the diathesis stress model,[10] stress is recognized as an important variable for consideration in susceptibility to illness. This model proposes that a person is more likely to suffer an illness if he or she has a particular *diathesis* (i.e., vulnerability or susceptibility) and is under a high level of stress.[11]

Unlike everyday stressors, which are managed with adequate coping behaviors, untreated chronic stress can result in serious health conditions, including anxiety, insomnia, muscle pain, high blood pressure, and a weakened immune system.[12] Research demonstrates that stress contributes to the development of major illnesses, such as heart disease, depression, and obesity.[4] It is now recognized that chronic stress contributes to overeating "comfort" foods, which contributes to the growing obesity epidemic.[13]

Research in the area of psychoneuroimmunology has long emphasized the importance of the mind-brain body relationship and its subsequent impact on physical and psychological well-being. Biological balance (homeostasis) is established through a cascade of hormones and interactions between the mind (psychology), the nervous system (neurology), and the immune system (immunology), hence the study of psychoneuroimmunology. The balance between these systems is paramount to good health and biological resiliency. It is thought that chronic stress may dysregulate one or all of these systems through a cascade of many complex reactions, setting up the body for ineffective or compromised functioning. The ongoing attempt to manage psychological and physiological chronic stress by personal behaviors such as smoking, drinking, inadequate sleep, and overeating is known as *allostatic load*. Allostasis is the physiological consequence of adapting to repeated or chronic stress in an effort to maintain homeostasis. Over time, the wear and tear (allostatic load) of this constant adaptation predisposes one to disease.[14]

There has been a renewed interest in the study of stress since the days of Hans Selye. The role of stress-induced neurocircuity remodeling is a new area of exploration. The brain is the central organ of stress. The genesis of stress starts in the brain and affects every organ. Neuroscience and the rapid progress of neuroimaging have promoted a greater interest in stress and mind-brain-body interactions. Structural and functional magnetic resonance imaging (fMRI) and positron emission tomography (PET scans) have advanced our understanding of how the brain responds to stimuli from the body, how the brain responds to stress, and how the brain responds to the expectation of pain.[15] There is a growing body of science attempting to understand how the stress of early adverse childhood experiences translates to altered brain development and subsequent cognitive, emotional, and physical disorders throughout life.[16] We now know that social environments impact brain systems. It is now possible to directly study neurobiological processes, including interactions between early traumatic experiences and genetic factors that play a role in manifestation of physical and emotional symptoms.

According to Emeran,[17] the brain is the key mediator in mind-brain-body interactions. For example, the brain-gut axis has long been an area of interest. Early investigations examined the effect of gut inflammation on the signaling system in the brain, as well as how gut inflammation changes brain responses to emotional stimuli. The severity and exacerbation of irritable bowel syndrome (IBS) may be strongly affected by the mind-brain-gut interactions. Early findings suggest that IBS may respond to both targeted pharmacological selective serotonin reuptake inhibitors (SSRIs) as well as non-pharmacological interventions such as yoga, meditation, and cognitive behavioral therapy.

The brain is sensitive to the exposure of chronic stress hormones during critical periods throughout the lifespan.[18] According to Lupien, the brain structures involved with cognition and mental health are affected. The specific effects on brain behavior and cognition are a function of both the timing and duration of the exposure to stress, the interaction between gene effects, and previous exposure to environmental adversity. For example, glucocorticoids are important for normal brain maturation. They initiate terminal maturation, remodel both axons and dendrites, and affect cell survival. However, elevated glucocorticoid levels, a result of chronic stress, impairs brain development. This has been demonstrated in the neurological and cognitive disturbance in the children of mothers who have experienced chronic psychological stress or adverse events, or who have received exogenous glucocorticoid during pregnancy.[19] Related research has demonstrated the negative impact of adverse childhood experiences (stress) on brain development and subsequent poor health behaviors and adult medical and psychological disorders. It has been suggested that chronic stress and trauma early in life compromise limbic-prefrontal cortex communication.[20] This compromised communication pathway impacts affective regulation and decision making. The Adverse Childhood Experience Study (ACE)[21] reports that early life stressors predispose one to brain changes, subsequent unhealthy lifestyle behaviors (poor decision making), and increased morbidity and mortality.[22] In addition, many adult diseases such as cardiovascular disease, chronic obstructive pulmonary disease, depression, and addiction have their origins in adverse early life experiences such as neglect and physical or sexual abuse.[23]

Chronic stress, gene expression, and environment all play a role in the expression of illness. However, the exact mechanism of how chronic stress causes illness, although widely held as common sense, is still under scientific scrutiny and remains elusive. Proposed frameworks include the hypothalamic-pituitary-adrenal axis and subsequent hormonal dysregulation, high levels and low levels of cortisol and subsequent inflammation, increased catecholamine production, higher oxidation stress, increased vagal tone, lower telomere activity, and shorter telomere length. Some known personality factors and protective factors of chronic stress include traits of hardiness[24] and optimism.[25] Cellular growth and activity such as telomere activity and length may impact health.[26]

The identification of protective behavioral strategies for decreasing stress has been challenging. The complexity and methodological issues of behavioral stress-management research have failed to provide consistent significant findings. The brain is the major organ of the stress response and is a mediator between the mind and the body; thus understanding the effect of stress on the brain could have implications for future mind-body treatments.

One of several behavioral strategies, Transcendental Meditation (TM®) now has a body of research that demonstrates its positive impact on the biological and physiological markers of stress reduction. Chapter 2 of this book presents a cogent explanation of the brain changes of TM.

PSYCHOSOCIAL STRESS, ILLNESS, AND TM

Of all the influences on our health and well-being, chronic stress is among the most ubiquitous. Stress can be defined as a mind-brain-body reaction to stimuli arising from the environment or from internal cues that are interpreted as disruptive of homeostasis.[27] Once the mind interprets a threat, real or perceived, the sympathetic nervous system—the activating part of the autonomic nervous—is turned on. Sympathetic projections originating in the brain exit the spine and branch out into the blood and nearly every organ. Nerve endings that project into the adrenal glands secrete adrenaline. Noradrenaline is secreted from other sympathetic projections to other organs and generates the fight or flight response, also known as the sympathetic adrenal medullary (SAM) response. In addition, once a stressor is sensed, the hypothalamus secretes corticotrophin releasing hormone (CRP) and other hormones into circulation via the anterior pituitary, causing the release of adrenocorticotropic hormone (ACTH). ACTH then triggers the release of glucocorticoids by the adrenal gland. This system is known as the hypothalamic-pituitary-adrenal (HPA) axis.[28]

Cortisol, the most important human glucocorticoid, is commonly known as the stress hormone and is elevated during acute stress. Cortisol regulates or supports a variety of important cardiovascular, metabolic, immunologic, and homeostasis functions.[29] The HPA axis functions to control adverse effects of acute stress via an exquisite negative feedback system that returns the body to a state of homeostasis. However, with persistent stress, chronic HPA dysregulation develops with prolonged cortisol elevation and imposes a cascade effect on related hormones that alter other neuroendocrine regulatory systems. This process leads to poor coping and negative health outcomes.

It is now known that the effects of psychological stress are associated with the body's ability to regulate the inflammatory response. Inflammation is, in part, regulated by the stress hormone, cortisol. Stress alters the effectiveness of cortisol to regulate the inflammatory response by decreasing tissue sensitivity to the hormone. In essence, immune cells become insensitive to the regulatory effects of cortisol. Chronic inflammation caused by lifestyle factors such as poor diet and stress, in part, keep cortisol levels high, which negatively impacts the immune system. An immune system responding to high levels of inflammation can lead to significant health problems. Inflammation is associated with a variety of chronic physical disorders such as cardiac disease, diabetes, IBS, and fibromyalgia.[30] Given the impact of chronic stress on homeostasis disruption and subsequent pathophysiological changes, alternative and behavioral interventions that alter the effects of chronic stress, are of import. The clinical effectiveness of behavioral approaches in reducing or preventing the cascade of neuroendocrine dysregulation would be beneficial for both physical and psychological health.

TM is described as a means of enhancing the growth of human awareness through higher states of human consciousness. It is the inner intelligence of the body that maintains optimal mental and physical functioning in life. These higher states of awareness (the transcending process) seem to confer greater abilities for successful interaction with both the internal (physiological) and external (social) environments.[31] In addition, TM allows the mind to appreciate subtle layers of the thinking process and subsequent appreciation for both external and external experiences. Positive external-environment effects may include improved interpersonal relationships and meeting the demands of life with less stress arousal. In effect, one begins to process information differently and creates different experiences. These new experiences can impact brain modeling and structure. Beneficial internal effects of TM include improved adaptive responses to the autonomic nervous system (ANS), neuroendocrine axis, and cardiovascular systems, thus decreasing allostatic load. High allostatic load caused by repeated or prolonged experience of stress predicts both cognitive and physical functioning decline and increased cardiovascular disease (CVD) events and risks.[32,33,34]

As previously noted, basic science and epidemiological studies have developed an impressive case that atherogenesis is essentially an inflam-

matory response to a variety of risk factors. Chronic stress has been identified as causing an increase in cortisol levels, making immune cells less
sensitive to the anti-inflammatory effect of cortisol, which in turn causes
vulnerability to a variety of diseases. The treatment of inflammation for
cardiac diseases has been primarily with pharmacological use of statins
that seem to reduce C-reactive protein. Theoretically, neutralizing the
stress response by decreasing an inflammation response could play a role
in prevention or in slowing the course of disease.

Research studies have demonstrated that TM produces the exact opposite physiological response of the stress response. Infante et al.[35] evaluated
the sympathetic adrenal medullary (SAM) functioning in 19 TM practitioners and a control sample of 16 healthy subjects who had not used any
previous relaxation techniques. TM practitioners who had been practicing
TM for over a year and groups were matched for state and trait anxiety
levels. Norepinephrine (NE), epinephrine (E), and dopamine (DA) were
measured at two different times of the day. Results indicated that morning
and evening NE levels ($p = 0.001$ and $p = 0.009$, respectively) and morning E levels were significantly lower in the TM group than in the control
group. No significant difference was found for catecholamine levels measured at different times of the day in the TM group, whereas a circadian
rhythm was found in the NE and DA plasma levels of the control group.
These findings held up when gender was analyzed separately. These
findings suggest that the regular practice of TM has a significant effect
on the SAM, specifically a low hormonal response to daily stress caused
by sympathetic tone regulation.[36] One should generalize cautiously from
these results because of the small sample size, however, these findings
support early findings in which low urinary levels of catecholamine metabolites and lower levels of cortisol and aldosterone were found in TM
practitioners.[37] Other findings suggest that TM reduces cortisol excretion
and several other biochemical indicators of stress.[38,39,40] Decreased blood
levels and cortisol excretion were reported in a random-assignment, longitudinal study of TM practitioners.[41]

Walton et al.[42] reported increased secretion of 5-hydroxyindoleacetic
acid (5-HIAA), a major metabolite of serotonin in individuals practicing TM. This increase in 5-HIAA has been shown to correlate with a
reduction in negative emotions such as anger and aggression. This biochemical change is cardio protective. In a cross-sectional comparison of
TM practitioners and non-meditating controls, the ratio of 5-HIAA to
cortisol showed a greater difference between the two groups than was
found for 5-HIAA or cortisol excretion alone. In addition, it has been
reported that the TM technique reduces baseline cortisol as well as average cortisol across stress sessions.[43] According to Walton et al.,[44] there

are over six hundred studies to date that have reported the beneficial, stress-reducing effects of TM.

Chronic stress has been linked to poor indices of cardiovascular health. Cardiovascular disease is the world's leading cause of death and disability, with daunting healthcare disparities.[45] Today, prevention of cardiovascular disease is a healthcare priority. It has been well documented[46] that acute emotional stress can trigger cardiovascular events. Community-wide events such earthquakes, riots, and stock-market volatility have increased cardiovascular events across the United States. In addition, certain sporting events, such as soccer matches in Europe, have been found to increase cardiac events and death rates. Tako-Tsubo, a stress-induced cardiomyopathy, though treatable, has been associated with significant cardiac EKGs and anatomical changes.

The impact of chronic stress is an equal cardiovascular risk factor. An article by Schneider et al.,[47] "Stress Reduction in the Prevention and Treatment of Cardiovascular Disease and African Americans: A Review of Controlled Research," presents a theoretical bio-behavioral model to illustrate a proposed causal relationship between psychosocial stress and cardiovascular disease clinical outcomes. This model illustrates the negative impact of psychological stressors such as low socioeconomic status, life events (divorce, job loss, bereavement), job stress, and perceived racism on subsequent anger, hostility, anxiety, and depression. These negative emotions trigger specific physiological changes, which include an increase in sympathetic tone, oxidation stress, thrombogenic factors, and neuroendocrine factors, and decreased parasympathetic tone. According to this model, these physiological changes cause specific cardiovascular risk factors, which include smoking, hypertension, hyperlipidemia, endothelial dysfunction, and atherosclerosis.[48]

According to Schneider et al., extensive random controlled trial reviews demonstrate that the TM technique can be clinically useful in decreasing systolic and diastolic pressures, lowering cholesterol and oxidized lipids, and helping smoking cessation. In addition, TM research has demonstrated a reduction in pathophysiological and neuroendocrine mechanisms such as reduced sympathetic arousal and cardiovascular reactivity that may reduce the risk of hypertension and subsequent cardiovascular disease. Lastly, as one might expect given the above findings, TM was effective in decreasing cardiac end points, including advanced progression of cardiovascular disease and subsequent mortality rates.[49] Walton et al.[50] also found in their review of random controlled trials, meta-analysis, and other controlled studies that TM reduces risk factors and can slow the progression of pathological changes such as reduction in blood pressure, medium carotid artery intima-medial thickness, myocardial ischemia, and left ventricular hypertrophy immortality. The magnitude of these effects compared positively with those of conventional interventions for secondary prevention.

Stress reduction is typically thought of as a viable, positive lifestyle change that may be beneficial in reducing high blood pressure in hypertensive patients. The physiological mechanism of different stress-reduction techniques may be similar. For example, it has been postulated that stress management and relaxation training may have common mechanisms such as reduction of sympathetic activity and slow, deep breathing. Slow, deep breathing, often associated with TM and mantra recitation, has been shown to induce a reduction in chemoreflex sensitivity and an increase in arterial baroreflex sensitivity coupled with increased parasympathetic and decreased sympathetic cardiovascular-like modulation. It is thought that the slow, deep breathing associated with TM and other modalities and not the unique features of TM is a catalyst for the events that may prove useful as a non-pharmacological approach to blood pressure reduction of hypertensive patients.[51]

The American Heart Association (AHA) has identified TM as the only meditating practice that lowers blood pressure. Due to mixed results and a paucity of available trials, other meditation techniques are not recommended in clinical practice to lower blood pressure, albeit other meditation techniques have been found to have a substantial positive impact on well-being. The AHA's scientific statement reports that lowering blood pressure by TM is associated with substantially reduced rates of heart attack and stroke. The AHA's scientific statement concludes that TM should be included in alternative treatments that are recommended for consideration in treatment plans for all individuals with blood pressure greater than or equal to 120/80 mmHg.[52]

Chapter 4 of this book presents a detailed and eloquent review of the impact of psychosocial stress on the cardiovascular system as well as the positive role TM has on cardiovascular health. The impact of chronic psychosocial stress, real or perceived, on the cellular biology has implications for cell senescence and longevity and health. Earlier interventions to neutralize the stress response and thus enhance cellular health could impact later onset of age-related diseases. In one study,[53] 58 healthy, premenopausal mothers who were biological mothers of either a healthy child (n = 19; the "control mothers") or a chronically ill child (n = 39; the "caregiver mothers") between the ages of 20 and 50 and free of chronic illness were studied. Mean telomere length and activity were measured. As expected, the average perceived stress level was significantly higher in the caregivers than in the control mothers. After controlling for age, findings suggested that the more years of caregiving, the shorter the mother's telomere, the lower the telomerase activity, and the greater the oxidation activity. These effects are known determinants of cell senescence and longevity.[54] Despite a small sample size, the findings warrant further research on the effects of chronic stress and cellular growth and activity. Longer telomeres are associated with fewer illnesses and a longer life.

Behavioral intervention programs that enhance resiliency or reverse the effects of stress can produce a variety of benefits to physical and mental health. An interesting attempt to identify the most efficacious of stress-management techniques to enhance resiliency was conducted by the military. A Medline review searched and screened 11,500 articles for relevance regarding soldiers' resiliency. Resiliency was defined as "the ability to meet challenges and bounce back after difficult experiences."[55] Criteria for inclusion in this study to identify the best stress-management program included efficacy, acceptability, quality control, and cost. In this review, a focus on discriminating among three types of meditation practices—TM, mindfulness meditation, and progressive relaxation—were examined. Results demonstrated that meditation as a whole had positive effects on stress management and subsequent soldiers' resiliency. Notably, TM had the most supporting data as a suitable option for stress reduction and increasing soldiers' resiliency, followed by mindfulness meditation and progressive relaxation.[56]

STRESS, TRANSCENDENTAL MEDITATION, AND CHILDREN

Anxiety and stress in school-age children in the wake of a rash of recent school violence and an atmosphere of high-performance expectations are ongoing problems. Adolescents experience high levels of stress, which take a toll on their physical and emotional well-being. Obesity and depression among adolescents is alarming. Stress in school settings, especially in the racial and ethnic minority population, is often compounded by violence, poverty, drug use, and association with gangs, which predispose students to high levels of stress and academic difficulty. African American adolescents often experience psychological stress by exposure to violence that increases the risk for depression, anger, post-traumatic stress, and subsequent academic and behavioral problems.[57,58,59]

There is a paucity of psychosocial intervention studies that have examined racial and minority school-related stress. A quasi-experimental study[60] of the effectiveness of TM on several measures of psychological distress and negative affect was conducted using the Strengths and Difficulties Questionnaire (SDQ), an emotional symptoms scale, the Spielberger State-Trait Inventory for Children, which measures student stress levels and anxiety, and the Mental Health Inventory (MHI), which is used to assess overall mental health and depressive symptoms.

A sample of 106 volunteers (68 meditating and 68 non-meditating) of secondary-school students who completed pre- and post-testing was included in the study. Students were sampled from four public secondary schools; however, no significant difference between group characteristics was observed. Eighty-seven of the students were from minority groups. An 8 × 4 MANOVA research design was conducted with two treatment groups, experimental and control, among four ethnicity groups: Hispanic, African American, American Indian, and other. A significant improvement (p = 0.037) was found on all study outcomes for the TM group compared to the control group over a four-month period. Decreasing the stress and distress of our children can have significant implications for the health of future generations.

CONCLUSION

High levels of stress dominate our culture and span our whole lives. Chronic stress is linked to the dysregulation of biological systems and poor coping strategies resulting in illness. High levels of stress impact the brain structure and function at critical periods of neurogenesis from neonate to the elderly.

The increase in neuroscience research is challenging the dualistic Cartesian medical model. Today there is a plethora of knowledge grounded in neuroscience that addresses the positive brain and behavioral changes with non pharmacological interventions such as meditation, cognitive behavioral therapy, dancing, and exercise.

The studies presented here suggest that TM is effective in reducing the toxic impact of stress after one to four months of practice. TM should be added to the repertoire of behavioral interventions, because it holds promise for combating the early neuroendocrine effects of prolonged stress, facilitates cardio protection, increases resiliency across the lifespan and with marginalized groups.

As with most research, particularly in social science, researcher and expectancy biases, robustness of interventions, and methodological problems exist. Collaboration and continued random controlled trials (RCT) with cross over research designs would continue to provide the importance of TM as a non-pharmacological treatment modality for optimal physical and emotional well being.

NOTES

1. American Institute of Stress, www.stress.org/what-is-stress/.

2. R. Tedeschi, C. Park, and L. Calhoun, *Posttraumatic Growth* (Mahwah, NJ: Lawrence Erlbaum Associates, 1980), 4.

3. D. R. Anderson, R. W. Whitmer, R. Z Goetz, R. J. Ozminkowski, J. Wasserman, S. Serxner, and the Health Enhancement Research Organization (HERO) Research Committee, "The Relationship between Modifiable Health Risks and Group Level Healthcare Expenditures," *Journal of Health Promotion* (2000): 49.

4. American Psychological Association, "The Stress in America—Missing the Healthcare Connection," *American Psychological* Association, www.apa.org/news/press/releases/stress/2012/full-report.

5. U.S Department of Health and Human Services, Health Resource and Services Administration, *U.S. Teens in Our World* (Rockville, MD: USC Department of Health and Human Services, 2003).

6. American Psychological Association, "The Stress in America."

7. Ibid.

8. C. McNeely and J. Blanchard, "Fifteen Years Explained: A Guide to Healthy Adolescent Development," paper presented at the Baltimore Center for Adolescent Health at Johns Hopkins Bloomberg School of Public Health, 2009.

9. A. J. Fuligini, E. H. Telzer, J. Bower, S. W. Cole, L. Kiang, M. R. Irwin, M. R., Kiang, "A Preliminary Study of Daily Interpersonal Stress and CV-reactive Protein Levels among Adolescents from Latin America and European Backgrounds," *Psychosomatic Medicine* (2009): 331.

10. "Diathesis-Stress Model," *International Encyclopedia of the Social Sciences.* www.encyclopedia.com/doc/1G23045300590.html.

11. Ibid.

12. A. Baum and D. Polsusnzy, "Health Psychology: Mapping Biobehavioral contributions to Health and Illness," *Annals Review of Psychology* 50 (1999): 137.

13. M. F. Dallman, N. C. Pecoraro, and S.E. la Fleur, "Chronic Stress and Comfort Foods: Self-medication and Abdominal Obesity," *Brain, Behavior, and Immunity* 19 (2005): 277.

14. *Medical Dictionary,* http://medical-dictionary.thefreedictionary.com/Allostatic+load.

15. *Research Media.* www.research-europe.com/index.php/international-innovation/.

16. J. P. Shonkoff, W. T. Boyce, and B. S. McEwan, "Neuroscience, Molecular Biology, and Childhood Roots of Health Disparity," *Journal of the American Medical Association* 301, no. 21 (2009): 2252.

17. *Research Media,* www.research-europe.com/index.php/international-innovation/.

18. S. Lupien, B. McEwan, M. Gunner, and C. Heim, "Effects of Stress throughout the Life Span on the Brain, Behavior, and Cognition," *Nature Reviews/Neuroscience* (2009): 434.

19. Ibid., 432.

20. K. H. Jung and V. Bhavya et al., "Decreased Expression of Synapses-related Gene and Synapses in Major Depressive Disorder," *Natural Medicine* (2012): 1416.

21. U.S. Department of Health and Human Services, Health Resource and Services Administration, *U.S. Teens in Our World* (Rockville, MD: USC Department of Health and Human Services, 2003).

22. V. J. Felitti, R. F. Anda, D. Nordenberg, D. F. Williamson, A. M. Spitz, V. Edwards, M. P. Koss, and S. James, "The Relationship of Childhood Abuse and Household Dysfunction to the Many Leading Causes of Deaths in Adults: The Adverse Childhood Experiences (ACE)," *American Journal of Preventive Medicine* 14, no. 4 (1998): 245.

23. R. F. Anda, A. Butchart, V. J. Felitti, and D. W. Brown, "Building a Framework for Global Surveillance of the Public Health: Implications of Adverse Childhood Adverse Childhood Experiences," *Preventive Medicine* 39, no. 1 (2010): 94.

24. S. Kobasa, "Stressful Life Events, Personality, and Health—Inquiry into Hardiness," *Personality and Social Psychology* 37, no. 1 (1979): 1.

25. C. S. Carver and M. F. Scheier, "Dispositional Optimism," *Trends in Cognitive Science* 18, no. 6 (2014): 3.

26. E. S. Epel, E. H. Blackburn, J. Lin, F. S. Dhabhar, N. E. Adler, and J. D. Morrow, "Accelerated Tolomere Shortening in Response to Life Stress," *Proceedings of the National Academy of Sciences USA* 101, no. 49 (2004): 17313.

27. *Research Media.* www.research-europe.com/index.php/international-inno vation/.

28. R. M. Sapolsky, *Why Zebras Don't Get Ulcers*, 3rd ed. (New York: Henry Holt and Company, 2004), 15.

29. S. Cohen, D. Janicki-Deverts, and D. Miller, "Psychological Stress and Disease," *Journal of the American Medical Association* 98, no. 14 (2007): 1685–87.

30. Ibid.

31. K. G. Walton, K. L Cavanaugh, and N. D. C. Pugh, "Effects of Group Practice of the Transcendental Meditation Program on Biochemical Indicators of Stress in Non-meditators: A Prospective Time Series Study," *Journal of Social Behavior and Personality* (2005): 342.

32. M. C. Dillbeck and D. W. Orme-Johnson, "Physiological differences betweeen Transcendental Meditation and Rest," *American Psychologist* (1987): 880.

33. R. R. Michaels, M. J. Huber, and D. S. McCann, "Evaluation of Transcendental Meditation as a Method of Reducing Stress." *Science* 195, no. 4245 (1976): 1242–44.

34. P. Mills, R. H. Schneider, D. Hill, K. G. Walton, and R. Keith Wallace, "Beta-adrenergic Receptor Sensitivity in Subjects Practicing Transcendental Meditation," *Journal of Psychosomatic Research* 34, no. 1 (1990): 29–33.

35. J. R. Infante, M. Torres-Avisbal, P. Pinel, J. A. Vallejo, F. Peran, F. Gonzalex, P. Conteras, C. Pacheco, A. Roldan, and J. M. Latre, "Catecholamine Levels in Practitioners of the Transcendental Meditation Technique," *Physiology & Behavior* 72 (2001): 144.

36. Ibid., 141.

37. K. G. Walton, N. D. C. Pugh, P. Gelderloos, and P. Macrae, "Stress Reduction and Preventing Hypertension: Preliminary Report for a Psychneurendocrine Mechanism." *Journal of Alternative and Complementary Medicine* 1, no. 3 (1995): 406.

38. R. Jevning, A. F. Wilson, and W. R. Smith, "Adrenocortical Activityl Activity During Meditation." *Hormones and Behavior* 99, no. 3 (1978): 58.

39. C. R. K. Maclean, K. G.Walton, S. R. Wenneberg. D. Levitsky, J. P. Manderino, R. Waziri, S. L. Hillis, and R. H. Schneider, "Effects of the Transcendental Meditation Program on Adaptive Mechanisms: Changes in Hormone Levels and Responses to Stress after 4 Months of Practice," *Psychoneuroendocrinology* 22, no. 4 (1997): 277–95.

40. K. G. Walton and N. D. C. Pugh, "Stress, Steroids, and 'Ojas': Neuroendocrine Mechanisms and Current Promise of Ancient Approaches to Disease Prevention," *Indian Jouranl Physiological Pharmacology* (1995): 3–36.

41. K. G. Walton, N. D. C. Pugh, P. Gelderloos, and P. Macrae, "Stress Reduction and Preventing Hypertension: Preliminary Report for a Psychneurendocrine Mechanism," *Journal of Alternative and Complementary Medicine* 39, no. 1 (1995): 263–83.

42. Ibid.

43. Ibid.

44. K. G. Walton, K. L. Cavanaugh, and N. D. C. Pugh, "Effects of Group Practice of the Transcendental Meditation Program on Biochemical Indicators of Stress in Non-meditators: A Prospective Time Series Study," *Journal of Social Behavior and Personality* (2005): 339–73.

45. R. H. Schneider, C. N. Alexander, J. Salerno, M. Rainforth, and S. Nidich, "Stress Reduction in the Prevention and Treatment of Cardiovascular Disease in African Americans: A Review of Controlled Research on that Transcendental Meditation Program," *Journal of Social Behavior and Personality* 18, no. 1 (2005): 160.

46. B. G. Schwartz, W. J. French, G. S. Mayeda, S. Burnstein, C. Economides, A. K. Bhandari, D. S. Cannon, and R. A. Kloner, "Emotional Stressors Trigger Cardiovascular Events." *International Journal of Clinical Practice* 66 (2012): 632–33.

47. R. H. Schneider, C. N. Alexander, J. Slaerno, M. Rainforth, and S. Nich, "Stress Reduction in the Prevention and Treatment of Cardiovascular Disease in African Americans: A Review of Controlled Research on the Transcendental Meditation Program." *Journal of Social Behavior and Personality* 18, no. 1 (2005): 163.

48. Ibid., 161.

49. Ibid., 163.

50. K. G. Walton, R. H. Schneider, J. Salerno, and S. Nidich, "Psychosocial Stress and Cardiovascular Disease, Part 3: Clinical and Policy Implications of Research on the Transcendental Meditation Program," *Behavioral Medicine* 30, no. 4 (2005): 173–83.

51. P. Gianfranco and A. Steptoe, "Stress Reduction and Blood Pressure Control in Hypertension: A Role for Transcendental Meditation?" *Journal of Hypertension* 22 (2004): 2059.

52. R. D. Brook et al., "Beyond Medications and Diet: Alternative Approaches to Lowering Blood Pressure, A Scientific Statement from the American Heart Association," *Hypertension* 61 (2013): 1360.

53. E. S. Epel, E. H. Blackburn, J. Lin, F. S. Dhabhar, N. E. Adler, J. D. Morrow, and R. M. Cawthon, "Accelerated Telomere Shortening in Response to Light Stress," *Proceedings of the National Academy of Sciences* (2004): 17312.

54. Ibid., 17313.

55. B. Rees, "Overview of Outcome Data of Potential Meditation Training for Soldier Resilience," *Military Medicine* 176, no. 11 (2011): 1232.

56. Ibid., 1242.

57. M. Hall, E. F. Cassidy, and H. C. Stevenson, "Acting 'Tough' in a 'Tough' World: An Examination of Fear among Urban African American Adolescents," *Journal of Black Psychology* (2008): 381–98.

58. M. I. Singer, T. M. Anglin, L. Y. Song, and L. Lunghofer, "Adolescents Exposure to Violence and Associated Symptoms of Psychological Trauma," *Journal of the American Medical Association* 273, no. 6 (1995): 477.

59. T. T. Massat, "Experiences of Violence, Post-traumatic Stress, Academic Achievement, and Behavioral Problems of Urban African American Children," *Child and Adolescent Social Work Journal* (2005): 367.

60. C. Elder, S. Nidich, R. Colbert, J. Heglin, J. Greshiled, L. Oviedo-Lim, D. R. Nidich, M. Rainforth, C. Jones, and D. Gerace, *Journal of Instructional Psychology* 38, no. 2 (2011): 109.

BIBLIOGRAPHY

American Institute of Stress. "What Is Stress?" www.stress.org/what-is-stress/.

American Psychological Association. *The Stress in America—Missing the Healthcare Connection.* www.apa.org/news/press/releases/stress/2012/full-report.pdf.

American Psychological Association. *Stress in America: Are Teens Adopting Adults' Stress Habits?* www.apa.org/news/press/releases/stress/2013/stress-report .pdf.

Anda, R. F., A. Fellitti, V.J . Butchart, and D. W. Brown. "Building a Framework for Global Surveillance of the Public Health: Implications of Adverse Effects of Childhood Experience." *American Journal of Preventive Medicine* 39, no. 1 (2010): 93–98.

Anderson, D. R., Whitmer, R. W., Goetzel, R. Z., Ozminkowski, R. J., Wasserman, J., and Serxner, S. "The Relationship between Modifiable Health Risks and Group Level Healthcare Expenditures." *Journal of Health Promotion* 15, no. 4 (2001): 45–52.

Baum, A. and D. Polsusnzy. "Health Psychology: Mapping Biobehavioral Contributions to Health and Illness." *Annals Review of Psychology* 15 (1999): 137–63.

Cantor, P. H. and P. Ernest. "Insufficient Evidence to Conclude Whether or Not Transcendental Meditation Lowers Blood Pressure: Results of a Systematic Review of Randomized Cinical Trials." *Journal of Hypertension* 22 (2004): 2049–54.

Cohen S., D. Janicki-Deverts, and D. Miller. "Psychological Stress and Disease." *Journal of the American Medical Association* 98, no. 14 (2007): 1685–687.

Cohen, S. *Carnegie Mellon News.* www.cmu.edu/news/stories/archives/2012/ april/april2_stressdisease.html.

Cole, S. W. "Elevating the Perspective on Human Stress on Genomes." *Psychoneuroendocrinology* 35 (2010): 955–62.

Cole, S. W. "Social Regulation of Human Gene Expression: Mechanisms and Implications for Public Health." *American Journal of Public Health* (2013): 84–92.

Dallman, M. F. "Chronic Stress in Obesity: A New View of Comfort Food." *Proceedings of the National Academy of Sciences USA* 100, no. 20 (2003): 11696–701.

Dillbeck M. C. and D. W.Orme-Johnson. "Physiological Differnces betweeen Transcendental Meditation and Rest." *American Psychologist* (1987): 879–81.

Emeran, M. *Interantional Innovation.* www.research-europe.com/index.php/international-innovation/.

Epel, E. S., E. H. Blackburn, J. Lin, F. S. Dhabhar, N. E. Adler, J. D. Morrow, and R. M. Cawthon. "Accelerated Telomere Shortening in Response to Light Stress." *Proceedings of the National Academy of Sciences USA* (2004): 17312–15.

Feletti, V. J., R. F. Anda, D. Nordenberg, D. F. Williamson, A. M. Spitz, V. Edwards, M. P. Ross, and J. S. Marks. "The Relationship of Childhood Abuse and Household Dysfunction to Many of the Leading the Causes of Deaths in Adults: The Adverse Childhood Experience Study." *Journal of Preventive Medicine* 14, no. 4 (1998): 245–58.

Fuligni, A. J, E. H. Telzer, J. Bower, S. W. Cole, L. Irwin, and M. R. Kiang. "A Preliminary Study of Daily Interpersonal Stress and CV-reactive Protein Levels among Adolescents from Latin America in European Background." *Psychosomatic Medicine* 71, no. 31 (2009).

Hall M. H., E. F. Cassidy, and H. C. Stevenson."Acting 'Tough' in a 'Tough' World: An Examination of Fear among Urban African American Adolescents." *Journal of Black Psychology* (2008): 381–98.

Heeringen, K. van. *The Neurobiological Basis of Suicide.* National Center for Biotechnology Information Bookshelf. www.ncbi.nlm.nih.gov/books/NBK107203/.

Infante, J. R., M. Torres-Avisbal, P. Pinel, J. A. Vallejo, F. Peran, F. Gonzalez, P. Contreras, C. Pacheco, A. Roldan, and J. M. Latre. "Catecholamine Levels in Practitioners of the Transcendental Meditation Technique." *Physiology and Behavior* 72 (2001): 141–46.

Jevning R, A. F.Wilson, and W. R. Smith. "Adrenocortical Activity During Meditation." *Hormones, Infants, and Behavior* 99, no. 3 (1978): 54–60.

Kang, H. J., H. Bhavya, T. R. Grazyna, and C. A. Licznerski et al. "Decreased Expression of Synapse-Related Genes and Loss of Synapses in Major Depressive Disorders." *Natural Medicine* 18, no. 9 (2012): 1413–17.

Kobasa, S. "Stessful Life Events, Personality, and Health: Inquiry into Hardiness." *Journal of Personality and Social Psychology* 37, no. 1 (1979): 1–11.

Levitsky, D. K. "Affects of Transcendental Meditation Program on Neuroendocrine Indicators of Chronic Stress." (1998).

Lupien, S. J, B. S. McEwen, M. R. Gunnar, and C. Hein. "Affects of Stress throughout the Lifespan on the Brain, Behavior and Cognition." *Nature Review Neuroscience* (2009): 434–45.

Maclean C., K. G. Walton, S. R. Wenneberg, D. K. Levitsky, J. P. Mandarino, R. Waziri, S. L. Hillis, and R. H. Schneider. "Effects of the Transcendental Meditation Program on Adaptive Mechanisms: Changes in Hormone Levels and Responses to Stress after 4 Months of Practice." *Psychoneuroendocrinology* 22, no. 4 (1997): 277–95.

McEwen, B. S. and M. Milluken. "Stress- and Allostasis-Induced Brain Pasticity." *Annual Review of Medicine* (2011): 431–45.

McNeely, C. and J. Blanchard. *15 Years Explained: A Guide to Healthy Adolescent Development.* Paper presented at the Center for Adolescent Health at Johns Hopkins Bloomberg School of Public Health, Baltimore, Maryland, 2009.

Michaels, R. R., M. J. Hube, and D. S. McCann. "Evaluation of Transcendental Meditation as a Method of Reducing Stress." *Science* 195, no. 4245 (1976): 1242–44.

Mills, T. J., R. H. Schneider, D. Hill, K. G. Walton, and R. K. Wallace. "Beta-adrenergic Receptor Sensitivity in Subjects Practicing Transcendental Meditation." *Journal of Psychosomatic Research* 34, no. 1 (1990): 29–33.

Orme-Johnson, D. W. and K. G. Walton. "All Approaches to Preventing and Reversing the Effects of Stress Are Not the Same." *American Journal of Health Promotion* 12, no. 5 (1998): 297–99.

Parati, G. and A. Steptoe. "Stress Reduction and Blood Pressure Control in Hypertension: A Role for Transcendental Meditation?" *Journal of Hypertension* 22, no. 4 (2004): 2057–60.

Rees, M. C. "Overview of Outcome Data of Potential Meditation Training for Soldier Resilience." *Military Medicine* 176, no. 11 (2011): 1232–42.

Sapolsky, R. *Why Zebras Don't Get Ulcers.* New York: St. Martin's Press, 2004.

Scheier, M. F. and C. S. Carver. "Optimism, Coping, Health Assessment, and Implications of Generalized Outcome Expectancy." *Health Psychology* 4, no. 3 (1985): 219–47.

Schneider, R. H., C. N. Alexander, C. N. Salerno, M. Rainforth, and S. Nidich. "Stress Reduction in the Prevention and Treatment of Cardiovascular Disease in African Americans: A Review of Controlled Research on the Transcendental Meditation Program." *Journal of Social Behavior and Personality* 18, no. 1 (2005): 159–80.

Shonkoff, J. P., W. T. Boyce, and B. S. McEwen. "Neuroscience, Molecular Biology and Childhood Roots of Health Disparity." *Journal of the American Medical Association* 301, no. 21 (2009): 2252–59.

Singer M. I, T. M. Anglin, L. Y. Song, and L. Lunghofer. "Adolescents Exposure to Violence and Associated Symptoms of Psychological Trauma." *Journal of the American Medical Association* 273, no. 6 (1995): 477–82.

Substance Abuse and Mental Health Adminstration. "Adverse Childhood Experiences." http://captus.samhsa.gov/prevention-practice/targeted-prevention/adverse-childhood-experiences/1.

Thompson, T. and C. Massat. "Experiences of Violence, Post-traumatic Stress, Academic Achievement, and Behavioral Problems of Urban African American Children." *Child and Adolescent Social Work Journal* (2005): 367–93.

U.S. Department of Health and Human Services, Health Resource and Services Administration. *U.S. Teens in Our World.* Rockville, MD: USC Department of Health and Human Services, 2003.

Walton, K. G., R. H. Schneider, S. I. Nidich, J. W. Salerno, C. K. Nordstrom, and C. N. Bairey Mertz. "Psychosocial Stress and Cardiovascular Disease Part 2: Ef-

fectiveness of the Transcendental Meditation Program in Treatment and Prevention." *Behavioral Medicine* 28, no. 3 (2002): 106–23.

Walton, K. G., R. H. Schneider, J. W. Salerno, and S. I. Nidich. "Psychosocial Stress
and Cardiovascular Disease Part 3: Clinical and Policy Implications of Research
on the Transcendntal Meditation Program." *Behavioral Medicine* 30, no. 4 (2005):
173–83.

Walton, K. G., K. L. Cavanaugh, and N. D. C. Pugh. "Effects of Group Practice of
the Transcendental Meditation Program on Biochemical Indicators of Stress in
Non-meditators: A Prospective Time Series Study." *Journal of Social Behavior and
Personality* (2005): 339–73.

Walton, K. G. and N. D. C. Pugh. "Stress, Steroids, and 'Ojas': Neuroendocrine
Mechanisms and Current Promise of Ancient Approaches to Disease Prevention." *Indian Journal Physiological Pharmacology* 39, no. 1 (1995): 3–36.

Walton, K. G., N. D. C. Pugh, P. Gelderloos, and P. Macrae. "Stress Reduction and
Preventing Hypertension: Preliminary Report for a Psychneurendocrine Mechanism." *Journal of Alternative and Complementary Medicine* 1, no. 3 (1995): 263–83.

SECTION II

RESEARCH

Medical Disorders

FOUR

Transcendental Meditation and Cardiovascular Health

Vernon A. Barnes, Ph.D.

INTRODUCTION

The pathogenesis and progression of cardiovascular disease is thought to be exacerbated by stress.[1] Research indicates that Transcendental Meditation (TM®) reduces acute and longitudinal sympathetic tone and stress reactivity. TM has been shown to decrease blood pressure, use of anti-hypertensive medication, angina pectoris, carotid atherosclerosis, and cardiovascular morbidity and mortality. In adolescents at risk for hypertension, TM reduces resting and ambulatory blood pressure, left ventricular mass, and cardiovascular reactivity to laboratory stressors. These findings have important implications for inclusion of TM in efforts to prevent and treat cardiovascular diseases and their clinical consequences.

The burden of cardiovascular disease (CVD) remains high, with one in three having CVD and one in three deaths from CVD in 2008, making it the leading cause of death in the United States.[2] The CVD cost burden is estimated at $298 billion, costs that are expected to triple by 2030.[3] Like most other diseases, CVD is multi-factorial in nature. Well-established, preventable CVD risk factors include dyslipidemia,[4] high blood pressure (BP),[5] smoking,[6] psychological distress and angry temperament,[7] metabolic syndrome,[8] obesity,[9] stress,[10] and physical inactivity.[11] Exposure to CVD risk factors during childhood and adolescence has been associated with the development of atherosclerosis later in life.[12] Modifying these risk factors by changes in lifestyle is expected to have beneficial effects in lowering CVD risk.[13]

Environmental and psychosocial stress plays a significant role in the development of essential hypertension (EH) by acting through both acute and long-term BP control mechanisms.[14] Stress is defined as a process in which environmental demands tax or exceed the adaptive capacity of an organism, resulting in physiological changes that, over time, may place an individual at risk for disease development.[15] The biobehavioral model of stress-induced hypertension incorporates both the acute phase of the stress response, which results in a rapid BP increase, and the chronic phase of the stress response, which acts to maintain elevated BP levels as long as physiologically needed to maintain homeostasis. Stress has been hypothesized to contribute to the development of CVD via a pathway of exaggerated cardiovascular reactivity[16] as well as by chronic sympathetic nervous system (SNS) activation.[17] The acute phase of the stress response involves complex neuroendocrine changes characterized by increased sympathetic activation.[18] Animal and human studies have demonstrated that exposure to chronic and acute stress augments SNS and hypothalamic-pituitary-adrenal activity, resulting in increased levels of catecholamines—including norepinephrine—and cortisol.[19] This results in a rapid rise in BP, predominantly due to increased vasoconstriction,[20] which increases total peripheral resistance.[21]

STRESS AND CVD

Exposure to stress results in SNS-mediated increases in BP to cope with the immediate need for an increased blood supply to the brain and body. It is well established that SNS activation in turn activates the renin-angiotensin-aldosterone system, which includes release of the potent vasoconstrictive hormone angiotensin II, which contributes to the acute rise in BP.[22] The recurrent and/or sustained exaggerated increases in BP responses to stress are associated with concomitant increases in cardiac and vascular wall tension.[23] It is hypothesized that over time this leads to secondary cardiovascular (CV) structural adaptation; that is, vascular and ventricular remodeling to help normalize wall tension.[18] An early sign of ventricular remodeling is increased left ventricular mass (LVM), which may lead to left ventricular hypertrophy, the strongest predictor of CV morbidity and mortality other than advancing age.[24] Research has shown that BP reactivity in youth predicts left ventricular hypertrophy, [25] and although not entirely consistent, several prospective studies observed that BP reactivity also predicts EH.[26]

Exaggerated CV reactivity to stress has been hypothesized[14] to play a particularly significant role in the development of EH due to exposure to both chronic and acute psychosocial and environmental stress.[27] Pediatric studies reported that exaggerated BP reactivity to laboratory behavioral stressors is an independent predictor of increases in measures of pre-clinical CVD.[28]

Chronic environmental stress is not easily altered, but the effects of stress can be ameliorated via behavioral stress reduction, i.e., changing how the individual responds to stressors to reduce negative impact on health. An individual's acute CV responses to stress can be moderated by psychological and lifestyle factors. For example, anger and hostility have been shown to be related to CV reactivity and a wide range of physical health problems including EH and CVD.[29] Similarly, coping styles (e.g., anger suppression), perceived environmental stress (e.g., unfair treatment), environmental noise,[30] and coping resources (e.g., social support) have been associated with resting BP and/or CV reactivity in adolescents and/or young adults.[31,32]

Evidence for the efficacy of certain non-pharmacological approaches to preventing and controlling EH has shown behavioral interventions to have great promise in reducing BP levels, improving stress-related coping skills, and alleviating psychosocial distress.[33] The benefits of psychosocial-behavioral interventions with respect to hypertension and coronary heart disease (CHD) have been demonstrated in a number of trials in adults.[34] Stress-reduction programs include those involving various methods of meditation, cognitive behavioral skills training, yoga, and muscle relaxation. This chapter is limited to examining applications of TM in prevention and treatment of EH and CVD.

One of the significant and unique aspects of the findings contained in this chapter is the wide range of subject populations involved, including minorities and youth. The wide implementation of a non-pharmacological BP-reducing intervention could potentially have an enormous impact on public health. Even a small downward shift in the distribution of BP of a few mmHg could potentially reduce the incidence of EH and related CVD.[35] The results of this chapter will provide insight into what has now become a very timely and important issue.

Psychological and Physiological Mechanisms Related to CVD

The hypothalamic-pituitary-adrenocortical axis provides mechanisms by which emotions and stress produce hormones that facilitate the stress response. For example, elevated baseline levels of plasma cortisol are associated with a greater prevalence of ischemic heart disease.[36] Prospective and randomized studies of TM indicate that it has acute as well as longitudinal effects on reducing baseline cortisol as well as average cortisol across stress sessions.[37] Aldosterone, a hormone that increases the absorption of sodium and water in the kidneys, decreases with TM, suggesting another mechanism by which TM may reduce blood volume and normalize BP.[38]

TM also increases levels of dehydroepiandrosterone sulfate,[37] an androgen hormone produced in the adrenal glands which at low levels is a significant predictor of CVD and ischemic heart disease.[39] The impact of TM on the sympathetic-adrenal-medulla system was studied by examining morning and evening norepinephrine levels, with a finding that morning epinephrine levels were significantly lower in the TM group compared with control subjects.[40] The implications are that patients will be benefited by reduced levels of stress hormones via TM.

A review of eight meta-analyses of a total of 587 studies on a wide variety of variables concluded that TM is more effective compared with clinically derived methods in reducing CVD risk factors.[41] TM has been shown to be more effective than treatment-as-usual and most alternative treatments, with greatest effects observed in individuals with high anxiety.[42] Evidence reviewed below indicates that TM benefits many of the risk factors that contribute to CVD in both adults (part 1) and adolescents (part 2).

PART 1: TM AND CARDIOVASCULAR RISK FACTORS IN ADULTS

The prevalence of EH in the United States is estimated at 27 percent with only 57 percent of these being treated and 29 percent unaware of their EH.[2] TM's effects in reducing BP in both hypertensive and pre-hypertensive individuals,[43-46] coupled with its additional benefits for health-related behaviors and well-being,[47-49] could be extremely valuable as part of a population strategy for CVD prevention.

Impact of TM on Hypertension

Anti-hypertensive drug therapy has been associated with intolerability of adverse side effects,[50] impaired quality of life concerns,[51] and lack of cost effectiveness.[52] BP control in treating hypertensives is thought to be unsatisfactory due to poor patient compliance (forgetfulness and/or ignorance), insufficient use of combination drug treatment, and other difficulties in achieving well-controlled BP.[53] Given the potential role of psychosocial stress in the development of EH, stress reduction with its lack of adverse side effects is a compelling option in the reduction of BP.

Research on TM and hypertension in adults originated in the early 1970s. Collectively, uncontrolled studies[54-56] reported a systolic blood pressure/diastolic blood pressure (SBP/DBP) mean decrease of 12.6/8.8 mmHg after a mean of six months of TM practice. Long-term practitioners of TM were found to have significantly lower BP compared with age-group-based population norms.[57] Recently, larger and better-controlled randomized clinical trials (RCTs) have corroborated these early observations.[43–47,58,59]

Alexander et al. conducted an RCT on TM by examining BP and other factors of 73 Boston-area subjects (mean age 81 years) assigned to TM, mindfulness training (which involved both a structured word-production task and an unstructured creative mental activity task), a TM analog (a mental relaxation technique), or an untreated control group. SBP in the TM and mindfulness training groups was significantly reduced compared the other groups.[47]

In a subsequent RCT, 127 older African Americans (mean age 67 years) were randomly assigned to TM, progressive muscle relaxation (PMR), or health education (HE) groups. Multiple baseline measurements were taken, and after three months of intervention, the 10.7 mmHg SBP decrease was significant for the TM group, compared to the PMR and HE groups.[44] In this study, TM was found to be more efficacious for those who were not on medication. Subgroup analyses suggested the effectiveness of TM for treating hypertension for both sexes and those in high and low EH risk categories of obesity, alcohol use, psychosocial stress, dietary sodium-to-potassium ratio, physical inactivity, and a multiple risk category.[59] TM decreased BP significantly more than HE for all six risk factors.

Wenneberg et al. assigned 66 normotensive 18-to-34-year-old men to either TM or an active control group modeled after the standard TM course to control for expectancy, instructor attention, and daily time commitment. After four months of treatment, ambulatory DBP decreased only in the high-compliance TM subgroup, suggesting a dose-response effect, such that greater benefit is accrued with regular practice.[58]

Schneider et al. randomly assigned 150 hypertensive African Americans (mean age 49 years) to TM, PMR, or HE groups. The trial examined an important clinical question, i.e., whether lifestyle modification programs would remain effective in reducing BP over one year in adult African Americans. The study decreased DBP significantly more in the TM group than in the PMR and HE groups, and there was a trend for a greater reduction in SBP. Importantly, there was a significant reduction in antihypertensive medication use in the TM group compared to the controls.[60]

Nidich et al. examined 298 university students, including 159 subjects at-risk for hypertension, and found a significant SBP/DBP decrease at three months for the high-risk TM group of 5.0/2.8 mmHg compared with an increase of 1.3/1.2 mmHg for the high-risk wait-list control subjects. The TM group also showed significant reductions compared with control subjects in total psychological distress, anxiety, depression, anger/hostility, and coping. Moreover, reductions in psychological distress and coping were significantly correlated with reductions in SBP and DBP.[61]

Anderson et al. examined nine RCTs and found that TM lowered BP an average of 4.7/3.2 mmHg compared with control groups.[62] Subjects ranged in age from adolescent (mean age 16 years) to senior (mean age 81 years) and included normotensive, prehypertensive, and hypertensive individuals. Subgroup analyses of four hypertensive groups and three high-quality studies showed similar BP reductions in all TM groups.

Rainforth et al. examined a variety of stress-reduction programs in hypertensive patients, evaluating studies that used active controls, adequate baseline measurement, and blinded BP assessment. BP decreases associated with biofeedback, relaxation-assisted biofeedback, PMR, and stress-management training were not statistically significant; however, TM significantly lowered SBP/DBP by 5.0/2.8 mmHg.[63] BP reductions of this magnitude are suggested to result in significant decreases in CVD risk.[64] As a result of reviewing eleven RCTs and two meta-analyses, the American Heart Association has recommended TM as an alternative method for lowering BP on a level equivalent to exercise and pharmacological treatment.[65]

Effects of TM on Tobacco and Alcohol Usage

The restorative rest produced by TM has been suggested to normalize neurochemical imbalances that motivate and are caused by substance abuse.[66] As a result, the physiological basis for craving is thought to decline, often accompanied by a decline in substance use.[67] A meta-analysis of 198 studies on behavioral techniques for reducing tobacco, alcohol, and drug consumption suggested that TM has substantially larger effect sizes in reducing harmful substance consumption compared to other techniques.[68] The findings also showed that patterns of abstinence were maintained for a longer time. A study with 295 university students showed a significant reduction in drinking rates in males.[69] A prospective study of 324 cigarette smokers found that 51 percent of those who reported full compliance with TM practice quit smoking after two years, compared to 21 percent for both partial TM adherents and non-TM controls. The TM program dispenses no advice to quit smoking.[70] Rather, reduction in smoking behavior subsequent to TM is thought to be motivated by reduced need for stimulation and increased sensitivity to the harmful effects of tobacco on the body.[71]

Acute Effects of TM on CV Function

The acute effect of TM upon CV function was examined in a preliminary study of thirty-two healthy middle-age adults without any history of vascular dysfunction.[72] Long-term TM practitioners (mean of twice-daily

TM for twenty-three years) were compared to a matched normotensive control group on CV function at rest and during twenty minutes of self-relaxation (eyes-closed rest for the control group versus TM for the TM group). The TM group exhibited significantly greater decreases in SBP and total peripheral resistance compared to self-relaxation in the control group. Vasoconstriction is a result of elevated SNS activity,[73] and a wide range of evidence shows TM produces acute and enduring reductions in SNS tone.[74] This suggests that decreases in SNS activity and hence vaso-constrictive tone during TM may be a hemodynamic mechanism responsible for reduction of high BP over time.

Reduction of Angina Pectoris, Carotid Atherosclerosis, and Functional Capacity in Heart Patients with TM

A single-blind prospective pilot study of angina pectoris reported that TM improved exercise tolerance, increased maximum workload, and delayed appearance of electrocardiographic abnormalities during exercise (delayed onset of ST segment depression) in 12 heart patients after 1 year of TM compared to 9 wait-listed controls.[75] An RCT of 60 hypertensive African American subjects examined the impact of TM on carotid intima-media thickness, a validated surrogate measure for coronary and cerebral atherosclerosis. The findings showed a decrease in carotid artery thickness in the TM group compared with an increase in the control group, suggesting that TM may reduce carotid atherosclerosis.[76] Changes of this magnitude predict an 11 percent reduction in myocardial infarction[77] and an 8–15 percent reduction in stroke.[78] A preliminary six-month RCT of African American patients (N = 23) hospitalized for chronic heart failure found significant improvement in functional capacity on a six-minute walk test in the TM group compared to HE controls. The study also found reduced depression, improvement in health-related quality of life, and a trend toward fewer re-hospitalizations in the TM group.[79]

Reduction in Cardiovascular Clinical Events with TM

Data from previous RCTs were combined in a retrospective study[80] that showed a 23 percent reduction in all-cause mortality compared to combined controls, a 30 percent reduction in the rate of CV mortality, and a 49 percent reduction in the rate of cancer mortality in the TM group. These findings provided support for an RCT supported by the National Institutes of Health (NIH) that was conducted with 201 African American CHD patients (M age = 59 years). Subjects were assigned to TM or control groups. At the five-year follow-up, there was a 47 percent reduction in the primary composite endpoints of all-cause mortality, non-fatal myocardial infarction, and non-fatal stroke and a 5 mmHg average reduction in SBP associated with a decrease in clinical events and significant reductions in psychological stress in the high-stress subgroup. Of the 51 primary end-point events during the study (30 deaths, 5 nonfatal myocardial infarctions, and 6 strokes), 20 were in the TM group and 31 in the HE group. The findings provide the strongest evidence to date that TM is useful in prevention of CHD mortality, myocardial infarction, and stroke.[81]

PART 2: BLOOD PRESSURE REDUCTION
IN PREHYPERTENSIVE ADOLESCENTS

Current treatments to control elevated BP and cholesterol are not typically effective in reducing morbidity and mortality.[82] Therefore, primary prevention of all major CVD risk factors starting early in life is critical. Hypertension is no longer considered an adult disease.[35] BP levels track relative to peers from late childhood onward,[83] and these levels may predict EH in young adulthood.[83,84] Children in the highest BP quintile are at greater risk to develop EH in early adulthood.[83,85] The incidence of EH has risen dramatically in recent years among youth,[35] increasing as much as sevenfold among minority populations, including African Americans, for whom rates are now estimated at 5–12 percent.[86] These rates in adolescents are expected to increase together with increases in obesity.[87] The number 2 cause of death in children under the age of fifteen is CVD.[88] In 1997 the NIH announced an initiative for pediatric intervention studies for primary prevention of CVD, which may benefit overall health and well-being and reduce healthcare costs.[89]

Impact of TM on Resting BP and BP Reactivity in Adolescents

A preliminary eight-week RCT examined the effects of TM on resting BP and BP reactivity in adolescents with high normal BP.[45] Thirty-five adolescents (ages 15–18 years) with resting SBP in the 85th to 95th percentiles were assigned to either TM (n = 17) or HE control (CTL; n = 18) groups. After two-months, the TM group exhibited a statistically significant 4.8 mmHg decrease in resting SBP from pre- to two-month post-intervention compared to an increase of 2.6 mmHg in the HE group. The TM group also exhibited greater decreases in SBP, heart rate, and cardiac output reactivity to the car-driving stressor, along with SBP reactivity to the social stressor interview, compared to the HE group. These findings should be viewed with caution due to the small sample size but suggest that lowering BP and reducing exaggerated CV reactivity to chronic stress may beneficially impact CV structure and function, thereby reducing CVD risk.[90]

Impact of TM on Ambulatory BP in Youth

A sixteen-week study was conducted with 156 pre-hypertensive African Americans (mean age = 16 yrs) with high normal SBP (85th to 95th percentile for their age group, i.e., 129/75 mmHg).[46] Subjects were identified via SBP screening conducted in schools and were assigned to TM or CTL groups following pre-testing. On school days, the TM group meditated for fifteen minutes each day at school under the daily supervision of a certified TM instructor. On weekends and after school, subjects practiced at home. Average self-reported compliance with TM at home was 75.9 percent. The CTL group participated in daily, fifteen-minute, CV HE sessions on school days. Reproducibility of ambulatory results have been validated in youth.[91,92] The study found decreased daytime ambulatory SBP and DBP in the TM group compared to controls by approximately 4 mmHg over the four-month intervention period, with a similar SBP decrease maintained at the follow-up four months later. These reductions in BP demonstrate a beneficial impact of TM during daytime when the at-risk youth would most likely be encountering stressful events.

Impact of TM on Left Ventricular Mass in Adolescents

Heart structure was examined in a sub-sample of the above-mentioned ambulatory BP study. The impact of TM on LVM was studied in 62 (30 TM; 32 health education CTL) pre-hypertensive African American youth. The echocardiographic-derived measure of LVM was measured before and after the four-month TM intervention and at the four-month follow-up via 2D guided M-mode echocardiography. Blinding of the sonographers to subjects' group classifications decreased likelihood of systematic bias in the measurements. The TM group exhibited a significantly greater decrease in LVM indexed by height at the four-month follow-up compared to the CTL group. The findings suggest that TM resulted in decreases in LVM index compared to CTL.[93] Interestingly, the findings also indicated that the TM group showed greater control of body weight, with a significant difference between the two groups at follow-up.[93]

The Safety of TM

The practice of TM is considered safe, and it can be performed without adopting any system of spirituality or belief. No serious adverse events were reported from reviews of twenty RCTs,[94] and no safety concerns were raised in a report with 813 studies of meditation practices for health, including TM.[95] Importantly, NIH-sponsored clinical trials conducted with TM have not observed any adverse effects from TM.

CONCLUSION

In summary, TM reduces resting and ambulatory BP and CV reactivity and lowers LVM in adolescents at-risk for hypertension. In adults with mild or moderate EH, TM decreases alcohol and tobacco use, BP, angina pectoris, carotid atherosclerosis, and CVD clinical events, and it improves CV function. The mechanism of the effects of TM appears to be through acute and longitudinal reductions in reactivity to stress and sympathetic tone.

Considerable compelling evidence for the efficacy of TM as an approach to preventing and controlling EH and CVD risk has also been documented in extensive reviews.[96–98] Evidence presented offers a basis for public health policies and clinical approaches that can greatly affect the incidence and consequences of EH and CVD in the population at large.[99] The effective implementation of such an approach depends to a large extent on the training and motivation of the healthcare administration. Intervention through stress reduction in youth and adults is suggested as a future direction for preventive cardiology.[100] Large-scale clinical trials are needed to see if this approach can reduce the incidence of CVD when applied on a widespread basis. The medical, financial, and humanitarian significance of such research can hardly be overestimated. The support and involvement of health professionals, educators, community organizations, industry, and government is necessary to support the adoption of healthy lifestyles for our society for succeeding generations.[101] If such improvements are replicated among other at-risk groups and in cohorts of CVD patients, this will have important implications for inclusion of this technique in efforts to prevent and treat CVD and its clinical consequences.

NOTES

1. This manuscript is an extended and updated version of a previously published manuscript: V. A. Barnes and D. W. Orme-Johnson, "Prevention and Treatment of Cardiovascular Disease in Adolescents and Adults through the Transcendental Meditation Program: A Research Review Update," *Current Hypertension Reviews* 8, no. 3 (2012): 227–42.

2. American Heart Association, "Heart Disease and Stroke Statistics—2012 Update: A Report from the American Heart Association," (2012).

3. P. A. Heidenreich, J. G. Trogdon, and O. A. Khavjou et al. "Forecasting the Future of Cardiovascular Disease in the United States: A Policy Statement from the American Heart Association," *Circulation* 123, no. 8 (2011): 933–44.

4. B. G. Talayero and F. M. Sacks, "The Role of Triglycerides in Atherosclerosis," *Current Cardiology Reports* 13, no. 6 (2011): 544–52.

5. J. Stamler, R. Stamler, and J. D. Neaton, "Blood Pressure, Systolic and Diastolic, and Cardiovascular Risks: U.S. Population Data," *Archives of Internal Medicine* 153, no. 5 (1993): 598–615.

6. J. E. Keil, S. E. Sutherland, and C. G. Hames et al., "Coronary Disease Mortality and Risk Factors in Black and White Men. Results from the Combined Charleston, South Carolina, and Evans County, Georgia, Heart Studies," *Archives of Internal Medicine* 155, no. 14 (1995): 1521–7.

7. J. E. Williams, F. J. Nieto, and C. P. Sanford et al., "Effects of an Angry Temperament on Coronary Heart Disease Risk: The Atherosclerosis Risk in Communities Study," *American Journal of Epidemiology* 154, no. 3 (2001): 230–5.

8. M. J. Sorrentino, "Implications of the Metabolic Syndrome: The New Epidemic," *American Journal of Cardiology* 96, no. 4A (2005): 3E–7E.

9. G. Reaven, F. Abbasi, and T. McLaughlin, "Obesity, Insulin Resistance, and Cardiovascular Disease," *Recent Progress in Hormone Research* 59 (2004): 207–23.

10. S. Lewis, "Broken Heart Syndrome: Perspectives from East and West." *Advances in Mind-Body Medicine* 21, no. 2 (2005): 3–5.

11. J. C. Eisenmann, "Physical Activity and Cardiovascular Disease Risk Factors in Children and Adolescents: An Overview," *Canadian Journal Cardiology* 20, no. 3 (2004): 295–301.

12. O. T. Raitakari, M. Juonala, and M. Kahonen et al., "Cardiovascular Risk Factors in Childhood and Carotid Artery Intima-Media Thickness in Adulthood: The Cardiovascular Risk in Young Finns Study," *Journal of the American Medical Association* 290, no. 17 (2003): 2277–83.

13. S. M. Grundy, J. I. Cleeman, and C. N. Merz et al., "Implications of Recent Clinical Trials for the National Cholesterol Education Program Adult Treatment Panel III Guidelines," *Journal of the American College of Cardiology* 44, no. 3 (2004): 720–32.

14. F. A. Treiber, H. Davis, and J. R. Turner, "Cardiovascular Responsivity to Stress and Preclinical Manifestations of Cardiovascular Disease in Youth," In *Health and Behavior in Childhood and Adolescence: Cross-Disciplinary Perspectives*, edited by L. Hayman, M. McMahon, and J. R. Turner (New York: Lawrence Erlbaum Associates, 2001).

15. S. Cohen, R. C. Kessler, and G. L. Underwood, "Strategies for Measuring Stress in Studies of Psychiatric and Physical Disorders," In *Measuring Stress*, edited by S. Cohen, R. C. Kessler, and L. Underwood Gordon, 3–26 (New York: Oxford University Press, 1995).

16. H. Snieder, G. Harshfield, and P. Barbeau et al., "Dissecting the Genetic Architecture of the Cardiovascular and Renal Stress Response," *Biological Psychology* 61, nos. 1–2 (2002): 73–95.

17. M. Esler, "The Sympathetic System and Hypertension," *American Journal of Hypertension* 13, no. 6 (2000): 99S–105S.

18. S. Julius and S. Nesbitt, "Sympathetic Overactivity in Hypertension: A Moving Target," *American Journal of Hypertension* 9, no. 11 (1996): 113S–20S.

19. W. R. Lovallo, *Stress and Health: Biological and Psychological Interactions* (Thousand Oaks, CA: Sage Publications, 2005).

20. F. C. Luft, C. E. Grim, and N. Fineberg et al., "Effects of Volume Expansion and Contraction in Normotensive Whites, Blacks, and Subjects of Different Ages," *Circulation* 59, no. 4 (1979): 643–50.

21. N. B. Anderson, "Ethnic Differences in Resting and Stress-Induced Cardiovascular and Humoral Activity," In *Handbook of Research Methods in Cardiovascular Behavioral Medicine*, edited by N. Schneiderman, S. M. Weiss, and P. G. Kaufman (New York: Plenum Press, 1989).

22. A. C. Guyton and J. E. Hall, *Textbook of Medical Physiology*, 11th ed. (Philadelphia: W. B. Saunders Company, 2005).

23. B. Folkow, "'Structural Factor' in Primary and Secondary Hypertension," *Hypertension* 16, no. 1 (1990): 89–101.

24. M. J. Koren, R. B. Devereux, and P. N. Casale et al., "Relation of Left Ventricular Mass and Geometry to Morbidity and Mortality in Uncomplicated Essential Hypertension," *Annals of Internal Medicine* 114, no. 5 (1991): 345–52.

25. K. A. Murdison, F. A. Treiber, and G. Mensah et al., "Prediction of Left Ventricular Mass in Youth with Family Histories of Essential Hypertension," *American Journal of Medical Science* 315, no. 2 (1998): 118–23.

26. K. A. Matthews, K. L. Woodall, and M. T. Allen, "Cardiovascular Reactivity to Stress Predicts Future Blood Pressure Status," *Hypertension* 22 (1993): 479–85.

27. R. Clark, N. B. Anderson, and V. Clark et al., "Racism as a Stressor for African Americans: A Biopsychosocial Model," *American Psychologist* 54, no. 10 (1999): 805–16.

28. F. A. Treiber, T. Kamarck, and N. Schneiderman et al., "Cardiovascular Reactivity and Development of Preclinical and Clinical Disease States," *Psychosomatic Medicine* 65, no. 1 (2003): 46–62.

29. T. Rutledge and B. E. Hogan, "A Quantitative Review of Prospective Evidence Linking Psychological Factors with Hypertension Development," *Psychosomatic Medicine* 64, no. 5 (2002): 758–66.

30. S. Stansfeld and R. Crombie, "Cardiovascular Effects of Environmental Noise: Research in the United Kingdom," *Noise Health* 13, no. 52 (2011): 229–33.

31. L. Musante, J. R. Turner, and F. A. Treiber et al., "Moderators of Ethnic Differences in Vasoconstrictive Reactivity in Youth," *Ethnicity & Disease* 6 (1996): 224–34.

32. L. B. Wright, F. Treiber, and H. Davis et al., "The Role of Maternal Hostility and Family Environment Upon Cardiovascular Functioning among Youth Two Years Later: Socioeconomic and Ethnic Differences," *Ethnicity & Disease* 8, no. 3 (1998): 367–76.

33. D. Labarthe and C. Ayala, "Nondrug Interventions in Hypertension Prevention and Control," *Cardiology Clinics* 20, no. 2 (2002): 249–63.

34. W. Linden, C. Stossel, and J. Maurice, "Psychological Interventions for Patients with Coronary Artery Disease," *Archives of Internal Medicine* 156, no. 7 (1996): 745–52.

35. P. Muntner, J. He, and J. A. Cutler et al., "Trends in Blood Pressure among Children and Adolescents," *Journal of the American Medical Association* 291, no. 17 (2004): 2107–13.

36. R. K. Pitman and S. P. Orr, "Twenty-Four-Hour Urinary Cortisol and Catecholamine Excretion in Combat-Related Posttraumatic Stress Disorder," *Biological Psychiatry* 27 (1990): 245–47.

37. K. G. Walton, and R. H. Schneider, S. I. Nidich et al., "Psychosocial Stress and Cardiovascular Disease Part 2: Effectiveness of the Transcendental Meditation Program in Treatment and Prevention," *Behavioral Medicine* 28 (2002): 106–123.

38. K. G. Walton, N. D. C. Pugh, and P. Gelderloos et al., "Stress Reduction and Preventing Hypertension: Preliminary Support for a Psychoneuroendocrine Mechanism," *Journal of Alternative and Complementary Medicine* 1, no. 3 (1995): 263–83.

39. E. Barrett-Connor, K. T. Khaw, and S. S. Yen, "A Prospective Study of Dehydroepiandrosterone Sulfate, Mortality, and Cardiovascular Disease," *New England Journal of Medicine* 315, no. 24 (1986): 1519–24.

40. J. R. Infante, M. Torres-Avisbal, P. V. Pinel, and J. A. Vallejo et al., "Catecholamine Levels in Practitioners of the Transcendental Meditation Technique," *Physiology & Behavior* 72, nos. 1–2 (2001): 141–46.

41. D. W. Orme-Johnson and K. G. Walton, "All Approaches of Preventing or Reversing Effects of Stress Are Not the Same," *American Journal of Health Promotion* 12, no. 5 (1998): 297–99.

42. D. W. Orme-Johnson and V. A. Barnes, "Effects of the Transcendental Meditation Technique on Anxiety: A Meta-analysis of Randomized Clinical Trials," *Journal of Complementary and Alternative Medicine* 20, no. 5 (2014): 330–41.

43. R. H. Schneider, C. N. Alexander, and J. Salerno et al., "Stress Reduction in the Prevention and Treatment of Cardiovascular Disease in African Americans: A Review of Controlled Research on the Transcendental Meditation (TM) Program," *Journal of Social Behavior and Personality* 17 (2005): 159–80.

44. R. H. Schneider, F. Staggers, and C. N. Alexander et al., "A Randomized Controlled Trial of Stress Reduction in the Treatment of Hypertension in African Americans over One Year," *American Journal of Hypertension* 18, no. 1 (2005): 88–98.

45. V. A. Barnes, F. A. Treiber, and H. Davis, "Impact of Transcendental Meditation on Cardiovascular Function at Rest and During Acute Stress in Adolescents with High Normal Blood Pressure," *Journal of Psychosomatic Research* 51, no. 4 (2001): 597–605.

46. V. A. Barnes, F. A. Treiber, and H. Davis, "Impact of Transcendental Meditation on Ambulatory Blood Pressure in African American Adolescents." *American Journal of Hypertension* 17, no. 4 (2004): 366–69.

47. C. N. Alexander, E. J. Langer, and R. I. Newman et al., "Transcendental Meditation, Mindfulness, and Longevity: An Experimental Study with the Elderly," *Journal of Personality and Social Psychology* 57, no. 6 (1989): 950–64.

48. C. N. Alexander, P. Robinson, and D. W. Orme-Johnson et al., "Effects of Transcendental Meditation Compared to Other Methods of Relaxation and Meditation in Reducing Risk Factors, Morbidity and Mortality," *Homeostasis* 35 (1994): 243–264.

49. K. Eppley, A. I. Abrams, and J. Shear, "Differential Effects of Relaxation Techniques on Trait Anxiety: A Meta-analysis," *Journal of Clinical Psychology* 45, no. 6 (1989): 957–74.

50. C. Bucca, "Take the Side-Effects of Drugs into Account," *Lancet* 364, no. 9441 (2004): 1285.

51. A. Bremner, "Antihypertensive Medication and Quality of Life—Silent Treatment of a Silent Killer?" *Cardiovascular Drugs and Therapy* 16, no. 4 (2002): 353–64.

52. E. Ambrosioni, "Pharmacoeconomics of Hypertension Management: The Place of Combination Therapy," *Pharmacoeconomics* 19, no. 4 (2001): 337–47.

53. G. Grassi, G. Seravalle, and G. Mancia, "Blood Pressure Control and Antihypertensive Treatment," *Current Vascular Pharmacology* 10, no. 4 (2012): 506–1.

54. H. Benson and R. K. Wallace, "Decreased Blood Pressure in Hypertensive Subjects Who Practiced Meditation," *Circulation* 45 and 46, suppl. 2 (1972): 516.

55. B. Blackwell, I. B. Hanenson, and S. S. Bloomfield et al., "Effects of Transcendental Meditation on Blood Pressure: A Controlled Pilot Experiment," *Psychosomatic Medicine* 37, no. 1 (1975): 86.

56. B. L. Agarwal and A. Kharbanda, "Effect of Transcendental Meditation on Mild and Moderate Hypertension," *Journal of the Association of Physicians of India* 29 (1981): 591–96.

57. R. K. Wallace, J. Silver, and P. J. Mills et al., "Systolic Blood Pressure and Long-Term Practice of the Transcendental Meditation and TM-Sidhi Programs: Effects of TM on Systolic Blood Pressure," *Psychosomatic Medicine* 45, no. 1 (1983): 41–46.

58. S. R. Wenneberg, R. H. Schneider, and K. G. Walton et al., "A Controlled Study on the Effects of Transcendental Meditation on Cardiovascular Reactivity and Ambulatory Blood Pressure," *International Journal of Neuroscience* 89 (1997): 15–28.

59. C. N. Alexander, R. H. Schneider, and F. Staggers et al., "Trial of Stress Reduction for Hypertension in Older African Americans Part II: Sex and Risk Subgroup Analysis," *Hypertension* 28 (1996): 228–37.

60. R. H. Schneider, C. N. Alexander, and F. Staggers et al., "A Randomized Controlled Trial of Stress Reduction for Hypertension in Older African Americans," *Hypertension* 26, no. 5 (1995): 820–27.

61. S. I. Nidich, M. V. Rainforth, and D. A. Haaga et al., "A Randomized Controlled Trial on Effects of the Transcendental Meditation Program on Blood Pressure, Psychological Distress, and Coping in Young Adults," *American Journal of Hypertension* 22, no. 12 (2009): 1326–31.

62. J. W. Anderson, C. Liu, and R. J. Kryscio, "Blood Pressure Response to Transcendental Meditation: A Meta-analysis," *American Journal of Hypertension* 21, no. 3 (2008): 310–16.

63. M. V. Rainforth, R. H. Schneider, and S. I. Nidich et al., "Stress Reduction Programs in Patients with Elevated Blood Pressure: A Systematic Review and Meta-analysis," *Current Hypertension Reports* 9 (2007): 520–28.

64. J. A. Staessen, L. Thijisq, and R. Fagard et al., "Effects of Immediate versus Delayed Antihypertensive Therapy on Outcome in the Systolic Hypertension in Europe Trial," *Journal of Hypertension* 22, no. 4 (2004): 847–45.

65. R. D. Brook, L. J. Appel, and M. Rubenfire et al., "Beyond Medications and Diet: Alternative Approaches to Lowering Blood Pressure, A Scientific Statement from the American Heart Association," *Hypertension* 61 (2013): 1360–83.

66. K. G. Walton and D. Levitsky, "A Neuroendocrine Mechanism for the Reduction of Drug Use and Addictions by Transcendental Meditation," In *Self Recovery — Treating Addictions Using Transcendental Meditation and Maharishi Ayur-Veda,* edited by D. F. O'Connell and C. N. Alexander, 89–118 (Binghamton, NY: Harrington Park Press, 1994).

67. M. A. Hawkins, "Effectiveness of the Transcendental Meditation Program in Criminal Rehabilitation and Substance Abuse Recovery: A Review of the Research," *Journal of Offender Rehabilitation* 36 (2002): 47–65.

68. C. N. Alexander, P. Robinson, and M. Rainforth, "Treating and Preventing Alcohol, Nicotine and Drug Abuse through Transcendental Meditation Technique: A Review and Statistical Analysis." In *Self Recovery — Treating Addictions Using Transcendental Meditation and Maharishi Ayur-Veda*, edited by D. F. O'Connell and C. N. Alexander, 13–88 (Binghamton, NY: Harrington Park Press, 1994).

69. D. A. Haaga, S. Grosswald, and C. Gaylord-King et al., "Effects of the Transcendental Meditation Program on Substance Use among University Students," *Cardiology Research and Practice* 537101 (2011): 1–8.

70. R. Roth, *Maharishi Mahesh Yogi's Transcendental Meditation* (Washington, DC: Primus, 1994).

71. A. Royer, "The Role of the Transcendental Meditation Technique in Promoting Smoking Cessation: A Longitudinal Study." In *Self Recovery — Treating Addictions Using Transcendental Meditation and Maharishi Ayur-Veda*, edited by D. F. O'Connell and C. N. Alexander, 221–42 (Binghamton, NY: Harrington Park Press, 1994).

72. V. A. Barnes, F. A. Treiber, and J. R. Turner et al., "Acute Effects of Transcendental Meditation on Hemodynamic Functioning in Middle-Aged Adults," *Psychosomatic Medicine* 61, no. 4 (1999): 525–31.

73. P. L. Ludmer, A. P. Selwyn, and T. L. Shook et al., "Paradoxical Vasoconstriction Induced by Acetylcholine in Atherosclerotic Coronary Arteries," *New England Journal of Medicine* 315, no. 17 (1986): 1046–51.

74. M. C. Dillbeck and D. W. Orme-Johnson, "Physiological Differences between Transcendental Meditation and Rest," *American Psychologist* 42 (1987): 879–81.

75. J. W. Zamarra, R. H. Schneider, and I. Besseghini et al., "Usefulness of the Transcendental Meditation Program in the Treatment of Patients with Coronary Artery Disease," *American Journal of Cardiology* 77, no. 10 (1996): 867–70.

76. A. Castillo-Richmond, R. Schneider, and C. Alexander et al., "Effects of Stress Reduction on Carotid Atherosclerosis in Hypertensive African Americans," *Stroke* 31, no. 3 (2000): 568–73.

77. J. T. Salonen and R. Salonen "Ultrasound B-Mode Imaging in Observational Studies of Atherosclerotic Progression," *Circulation* 87, suppl. 3 (1993): II56–II65.

78. D. H. O'Leary, J. F. Polak, and R. A. Kronmal et al., "Carotid-Artery Intima and Media Thickness as a Risk Factor for Myocardial Infarction and Stroke in Older Adults: Cardiovascular Health Study Collaborative Research Group," *New England Journal of Medicine* 340 (1999): 14–22.

79. R. Jayadevappa, J. C. Johnson, and B. S. Bloom et al., "Effectiveness of Transcendental Meditation on Functional Capacity and Quality of Life of African Americans with Congestive Heart Failure: A Randomized Control Study," *Ethnicity & Disease* 17, no. 1 (2007): 72–77.

80. R. H. Schneider, and C. N. Alexander, and F. Staggers et al., "Long-Term Effects of Stress Reduction on Mortality in Persons ≥55 Years of Age with Systemic Hypertension," *American Journal of Cardiology* 95, no. 9 (2005): 1060–64.

81. R. H. Schneider, C. E. Grim, and M. A. Rainforth et al., "Stress Reduction in the Secondary Prevention of Cardiovascular Disease: Randomized Controlled

Trial of Transcendental Meditation and Health Education in Blacks," *Circulation: Cardiovascular Quality and Outcomes* 5, no. 6 (2012): 750–58.

82. M. L. Daviglus, D. M. Lloyd-Jones, A. Pirzada, "Preventing Cardiovascular Disease in the 21st Century: Therapeutic and Preventive Implications of Current Evidence," *American Journal of Cardiovascular Drugs* 6, no. 2 (2006): 87–101.

83. W. Bao, S. A. Threefoot, and S. R. Srinivasan et al., "Essential Hypertension Predicted by Tracking of Elevated Blood Pressure from Childhood to Adulthood: The Bogalusa Heart Study," *American Journal of Hypertension* 8, no. 7 (1995): 657–65.

84. B. S. Alpert, J. K. Murphy, and F. A. Treiber, "Essential Hypertension: Approaches to Prevention in Children," *Medicine and Exercise in Nutrition and Health* 3 (1994): 296–307.

85. J. Lambrechtsen, and F. Rasmussen et al., "'Tracking Quartile' in Blood Pressure from Childhood to Adulthood: Odense Schoolchild Study," *Journal of Human Hypertension* 13, no. 6 (1999): 385–91.

86. International Pediatric Hypertension Association, "Blood Pressure Facts," www.pediatrichypertension.org.

87. M. Guillaume and P. Björntorp, "Obesity in Children," *Hormone and Metabolic Research* 28 (1996): 573–81.

88. American Heart Association, *Heart Disease and Stroke Statistics—2011 Update* (Dallas, TX: American Heart Association).

89. NIH Special Emphasis Panel on Intervention Studies in Children and Adolescents to Prevent Cardiovascular Disease, "Minutes of Meeting September 8–9, 1997" (Department of Health and Human Services, National Institutes of Health, National Heart, Lung, and Blood Institute, 1998).

90. T. G. Pickering, "Mental Stress as a Causal Factor in the Development of Hypertension and Cardiovascular Disease," *Current Hypertension Reports* 3, no. 3 (2001): 249–54.

91. V. A. Barnes, M. H. Johnson, and J. C. Dekkers et al., "Reproducibility of Ambulatory Blood Pressure Measures in African American Adolescents," *Ethnicity & Disease* 12, no. 4 (2002): 240–45.

92. V. A. Barnes, M. H. Johnson, and F. A. Treiber, "Temporal Stability of Twenty-Four-Hour Ambulatory Hemodynamic Bioimpedance Measures in African American Adolescents," *Blood Pressure Monitoring* 9, no. 4 (2004): 173–77.

93. V. A. Barnes, G. Kapuku, and F. A. Treiber, "Impact of Transcendental Meditation on Left Ventricular Mass in African American Adolescents," *Evidence-Based Complementary and Alternative Medicine*, article ID 923153 (2012): 1–6.

94. A. J. Arias, K. Steinberg, and A. Banga et al., "Systematic Review of the Efficacy of Meditation Techniques as Treatments for Medical Illness," *Journal of Alternative and Complementary Medicine* 12, no. 8 (2006): 817–32.

95. M. B. Ospina, T. K. Bond, and M. Karkhaneh et al., "Meditation Practices for Health: State of the Research," *Evidence Report/Technology Assessment* 155 (2007): 1–263.

96. D. W. Orme-Johnson, V. A. Barnes, and R. H. Schneider, "Transcendental Meditation for Primary and Secondary Prevention of Coronary Heart Disease." In *Heart & Mind: The Practice of Cardiac Psychology*, edited by R. Allan and J. Fisher, 365–79 (Washington, DC: American Psychological Association, 2011).

97. R. H. Schneider, C. N. Alexander, and R. K. Wallace, "In Search of an Optimal Behavioral Treatment for Hypertension: A Review and Focus on Transcendental Meditation," In *Personality, Elevated Blood, and Essential Hypertension,* edited by E. H. Johnson, W. D. Gentry, and S. Julius, 291–318 (Washington, DC: Hemisphere Publishing Corporation, 1992).

98. K. G. Walton, R. H. Schneider, and J. W. Salerno et al., "Psychosocial Stress and Cardiovascular Disease Part 3: Clinical and Policy Implications of Research on the Transcendental Meditation Program," *Behavioral Medicine* 30, no. 4 (2005): 173–83.

99. M. Lawrence, M. Arbeit, and C. C. Johnson et al., "Prevention of Adult Heart Disease Beginning in Childhood: Intervention Programs," *Cardiovascular Clinics* 21, no. 3 (1991): 249–62.

100. M. Lawrence, M. Arbeit, and C. C. Johnson et al., "Prevention of Adult Heart Disease Beginning in Childhood: Intervention Programs," *Cardiovascular Clinics* 21, no. 3 (1991): 249–62.

101. M. Lawrence, M. Arbeit, and C. C. Johnson et al., "Prevention of Adult Heart Disease Beginning in Childhood: Intervention Programs," *Cardiovascular Clinics* 21, no. 3 (1991): 249–62.

FIVE

Transcendental Meditation and the Prevention of Diabetes Mellitus and Other Disorders

David Lovell-Smith, Ph.D., M.B., CH.B., FRNZCGP

A pandemic of type-2 diabetes threatens to bankrupt Western industrialized nations. In 2012 in the United States alone, more than 22.3 million people (about 7 percent of the U.S. population) suffered from the disease at an estimated cost of $245 billion.[1]

Prevention has so far focused on dietary manipulation and exercise. On completing this chapter, the reader will have gained practical knowledge of the significant contribution that Transcendental Meditation (TM®) and its associated techniques from Maharishi Ayurveda can make in extending these measures to a more global prevention strategy.

TYPE-2 DIABETES—OVERVIEW

Glucose is an energy-rich substance, and its presence in the blood is a little like keeping propane inside the house. Injudicious handling can lead to calamitous complications. Raised blood glucose damages blood vessels so that every tissue in the body can be afflicted in diabetes. Heart attacks, strokes, amputations, kidney disease, and blindness are common complications.

In normal health, blood glucose concentration is kept within narrow limits by a feedback loop between blood glucose and insulin. As blood glucose rises, the pancreas responds by secreting insulin, which brings blood glucose back to within the safe range. Glucose enters the blood from ingested food, from the breakdown of liver glycogen stores, and from gluconeogenesis (the chemical conversion of non-carbohydrate carbon substrates such as pyruvate, lactate, and certain amino acids into glucose). Insulin lowers blood glucose by promoting muscle-cell uptake of glucose and by inhibiting liver glucose production. Food taken to excess can overpower the ability of the pancreas to clear glucose from the blood, leading to high peak and fasting blood-glucose concentrations. High blood-glucose, in turn, damages the insulin-producing beta cells of the pancreas, so the blood-glucose lowering ability of the pancreas is impaired. A vicious cycle ensues, insidious at first, then accelerating over time, leading to dangerously high blood-glucose concentrations. Compounding this process is the phenomenon of cellular insulin resistance. Glucose in excess is toxic to cells. In effect, cells say, "Stop sending us glucose! We have too much already." Pathways within the cell wall are activated to make the cell less sensitive to the effect of insulin. When cells are reluctant to accept glucose and a failing pancreas is increasingly powerless to force it upon them (and also increasingly powerless to stop the liver from secreting glucose), spiraling blood glucose concentrations inevitably ensue.

Transcendental Meditation Improves Insulin Resistance

TM acts to reverse this spiral through a number of mechanisms that will be detailed in this chapter. A direct effect of TM on insulin resistance has been shown in a randomized single-blind controlled trial[2] in which 103 subjects with stable coronary heart disease were assigned to either sixteen weeks of TM (N = 52; mean age 67.1 years) or health education matched for frequency and time (N = 51; mean age 67.1 years). Eighty-four subjects (82 percent) completed the study. Insulin resistance was determined by the homeostasis model assessment (HOMA). HOMA is a mathematical model of glucose/insulin interaction that allows determination of insulin resistance and beta-cell deficiency from measurement of fasting plasma insulin and glucose concentrations. In simple terms, it indicates how far down the slippery slope of insulin resistance and pancreatic insufficiency a patient has fallen.

Patients in the TM group showed improved fasting blood-glucose and insulin, and thus reduced insulin resistance. Of the eighty-four subjects who completed the study, eight had diabetes. The beneficial effect on insulin resistance remained both after removing diabetic patients from the analysis and on analyzing the diabetic patients alone. The authors pointed out that these physiological effects were accomplished without changes in body weight, medication, or psychosocial variables, and despite a marginally statistically significant increase in physical activity in the health education group.

TM also helps address the underlying issues that promote insulin resistance, namely our Western habits of diet and behavior. These include eating too much of the wrong foods, becoming stressed, and not getting enough exercise. Even in established diabetes, consideration of these precipitating factors remains important in managing the illness. Drugs should not be relied upon alone for they do not address the underlying causes of the disease.

Figure 5.1 outlines some of the habits and external pressures that shape our eating behaviors, and the subsequent misfortunes that befall us. These habits are deeply embedded in who we are and in the way we live; thus prevention and early treatment of this disease may seem daunting. As detailed below, pressure, stress, loneliness, and alienation can all be shown to lead to excessive food intake. The nuclear family and a culture in which individual freedoms are prized may be implicated in the sense of alienation that characterizes much of the Western way of life. Data from tribes un-acculturated to the Western lifestyle indicate a greater ability to keep glucose within normal limits,[3] an ability that decreases disastrously as more indigenous peoples accept Western habits. TM and dietary skills derived from Maharishi Ayurveda lend themselves well to assisting in a much-needed global approach that encompasses these deep psychological and sociological issues.

Underlying Causes of Type-2 Diabetes

STRESS, DEPRESSION, ANXIETY, AND LONELINESS

The word *stress* is commonly used to imply both stressful life events (*stressors*) and the body's physiological reaction to stressful events (in engineering terms, this would be called *strain*). Anxiety and depression are psychological affective states that often occur in reaction to stressful events.[4] They are generally agreed to be distinct from each other. The conditions overlap significantly, however, and frequently occur together.[5] Depressive symptoms include feelings of sadness, emptiness, hopelessness, helplessness, despair, anger, and low energy. Anxiety can be regarded as a marked apprehension concerning the future, resulting from perceived inability to predict, control, or obtain desired results in forthcoming situations.[6] Loneliness has been defined as "a distressing feeling that accompanies the perception that one's social needs are not being met by the quantity or especially the quality of one's social relationships."[7]

STRESS, ANXIETY, DEPRESSION, AND LONELINESS RAISE BLOOD GLUCOSE

The stress hormones cortisol, adrenalin, and noradrenalin enhance the release of glucose from stored liver and muscle glycogen, presumably to prepare the body for imminent energy expenditure. Cortisol antago-

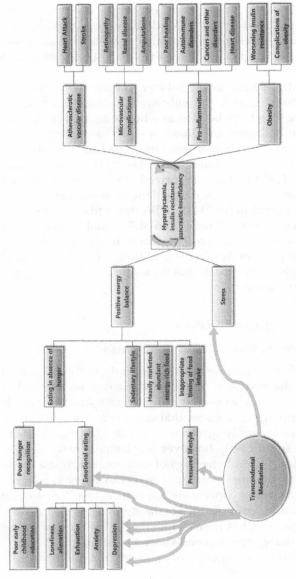

Figure 5.1. Causes and complications of hyperglycemia and insulin resistance.

Note: The current "epidemic of diabetes" is usually attributed to an increasingly sedentary yet stressful lifestyle coupled with an abundance of palatable and highly marketed energy-rich food. The primary care therapist/physician needs to be part endocrinologist, gastroenterologist, immunologist, psychologist, life-coach, dietician, sports doctor, sociologist, confidant and friend. Fortunately Transcendental Meditation and Maharishi Ayurveda have benefits across many disciplines to assist in this. © David Lovell-Smith 2014.

nizes the effect of insulin; stress has been shown to be associated with poor glycaemic control in diabetes[8]; depression has been found to be associated with impaired glucose utilization[9]; and loneliness has been associated with raised cardiovascular-system risk factors, including glycated hemoglobin in young adults.[10] Taken together, stress, depression, anxiety, and loneliness increase the probability of the pre-diabetic state and type-2 diabetes.

The stress response was first characterized by Selye,[11] who recounts how as a young medical student he noticed that the many and varied patients presented by his professors all seemed to have one thing in common: *They all looked ill.* It was this observation of a nonspecific response to illness that led Selye in his quest for the biochemistry of stress, which he defined as the "non-specific response of the body to any demand placed upon it."

When explaining the stress response to patients, it can be helpful to compare it to the use of a credit card. Both are handy, but prolonged misuse exacts a heavy toll. Selye extended Cannon's work and identified a general adaptation syndrome (GAD), which includes three phases of the stress response. During the first phase, alarm, the body prepares itself for fight or flight by secreting catecholamines (the card is pulled out of the wallet). In the second phase, adaptation, the body resists the demands placed upon it by producing cortisol (the bills are paid). Then comes the reckoning. The third phase is exhaustion, a kind of aging process due to wear and tear imposed by the stress hormones themselves and associated with raised blood glucose (the exorbitant interest charge on a misused credit card). In a society in which stressful situations occur frequently, the stress response is prevalent. It is a potent risk factor not only for impaired glucose tolerance but also for other components of the metabolic syndrome (including impaired lipid metabolism, obesity, and hypertension), which in turn predict not only type-2 diabetes but also cardiovascular disease and all-cause mortality.[12]

Evidence That TM Lowers Cortisol

In a study of fifteen long-term regular practitioners of TM compared to fifteen non-meditating controls, a rapid and significant decline (27 percent) in cortisol was found during the practice of TM.[13] The authors commented that a 27 percent decline of plasma cortisol concentration over a thirty-minute period is consistent with complete inhibition of pituitary-adrenal activity. In other words, in at least some of the long-term practitioners, during TM the adrenal gland was completely switched off. This is akin to cutting up the credit card and throwing it away, at least for the period of the meditation.

The effect of TM on stress hormones is sustained. In a prospective, randomized blind study,[14] twenty-nine healthy 18-to-32-year-old men were subjected to various stressful laboratory tests before instruction and four months after instruction in either TM or a stress education class. The TM group decreased significantly from pre-test to post-test in baseline cortisol and in overall mean cortisol.[15]

Emotional Eating Increases Energy Intake

In addition to the direct physiological effect of the stress hormones in raising blood glucose, psychological reactions to stress contribute by promoting increased energy intake, leading to raised blood glucose. Negative emotions that can initiate over-eating cover virtually the entire spectrum, including sadness, anxiety, frustration, loneliness, anger, disgust, fear, and grief. Overeating for emotional reward or as a strategy to cope with such emotions in susceptible individuals is well documented.[16,17] Such overeating is regulated by the hedonic system, which frequently overrides homeostatic hunger/satiety food intake regulation,[18] thus obscuring the experience or recognition of internal visceral states, including physical hunger.[19] Food cravings are often associated with intake of highly palatable, energy-dense "comfort" foods such as chocolate and carry-out foods.[20] It has been postulated that the ingestion of carbohydrate-rich meals in some depressed individuals increases brain serotonin via an effect of insulin on the serotonin precursor tryptophan.[21] Such "carbohydrate cravers" experience a temporary lift in mood; however, both energy-dense and high-carbohydrate foods come at the expense of energy balance and at the risk of increasing insulin resistance.

Transcendental Meditation Alleviates Anxiety and Negative Emotions

Chapter 6 of this volume deals in detail with the effect of TM on anxiety. A salient study in this area is a meta-analysis of 143 randomized controlled trials on trait anxiety by Eppley et al.,[22] which showed that TM was superior to other techniques studied in reducing trait anxiety. Commenting on a later meta-analysis conducted by Sedlmeier et al., Orme-Johnson and Dillbeck found a significant improvement in a composite index of trait anxiety, negative emotion, neuroticisim, self-concept, and self-realization in all meditations, with the greatest effect size deriving from TM.[23] Brooks et al. found significant reductions in depression, anxiety, and emotional numbness among Vietnam War veterans practicing TM.[24] In a recent randomized controlled trial, Elder et al. surveyed employees of a residential therapeutic school for students with behavioral problems. Employees were randomly assigned to either instruction in TM or a wait-list control group. After four months, the employees instructed in TM reported reduced stress, depression, and burnout as indicated by standard self-report measures.[25] Putting the results of these studies together, it can be concluded that practitioners of TM do not need to produce high levels of cortisol to cope with stress. The credit card can be used wisely.

MAHARISHI AYURVEDA: BRIEF OVERVIEW

Dietary Skills of Maharishi Ayurveda Help Prevent Diabetes

TM combined with diet advice based on Maharishi Ayurveda is a powerful combination in the prevention and treatment of early type-2 diabetes. Maharishi Ayurveda, a reinterpretation of the classical system of health from India, recognizes three elements in food intake: the food, the eater, and the relationship between them. These will be detailed in turn.

THE FOOD—SHOULD BE UNPROCESSED, SHOULD BE LIGHT

Undoubtedly the nature of the food ingested plays a major role in the genesis of diabetes. In Western dietetics, the optimum composition and quantity of food consumed by diabetic patients has been exhaustively researched. In Maharishi Ayurveda, food is prescribed by body type according to the theory of the three doshas: Vata, Pitta, and Kapha. It is beyond the scope of this chapter to expand on Tri-dosha theory and the dietary recommendations that follow from it.[26] However, it is interesting that type-2 diabetes is in most cases considered a Kapha disorder. The Kapha-reducing diet consists of light, non-energy-dense, non-sweet, low-glycaemic foods such as green vegetables, beans, and pulses. This is consistent with the recommendations of most Western dieticians.

Recently attention has focused once again on the dangers of widespread excessive consumption of sucrose and refined carbohydrates with a relative absence of dietary fiber ("fast food").[27] Calls for regulations to restrict the rampant sale of sugar-added foods reflect a widespread concern about processed foods in general. Many people have limited access to unprocessed foods because of their high cost, even if such foods are available. At the same time, these people are under advertising pressure from skilled food-industry marketers to favor processed foods. Add to that the possibility that, at least for some people, sugar can become an addictive substance,[28] and whole populations may be in no position to choose food that is not diabetogenic.[29] Individuals have no choice but to eat what is available, and according to one view, our only recourse is to embark on the hugely challenging task of convincing governments to curb the activities of a food industry reluctant to change its ways. In mitigation of this rather bleak outlook, TM offers to assist in addiction and dependency (see chapter 8, this volume), allowing individuals greater scope to make better food choices. In addition, Maharishi Ayurveda offers strategies to make best use of what food is available. This latter is a powerful approach and will be outlined next.

THE EATER—SHOULD BE PREPARED FOR DIGESTION

Maharishi Ayurveda holds that "it is not what one eats but what one digests." The eater must be in a fit state to ingest food. In particular, the physiological state of hunger must be present. Thus an important principle of Maharishi Ayurveda is that we eat at meal times but only if physically hungry.

HUNGER RECOGNITION

"Junk food when eaten while hungry could do you more good than the best whole food eaten when you are not." When I tell patients this, the idea is not to encourage them to eat junk food but to highlight the vital importance of eating only when one is prepared to digest (of course it is ideal to eat whole foods when hungry). One is prepared to digest only when one is physically hungry. Physical hunger here means the experience of an actual physical sensation. I have termed this the "empty hollow sensation" (EHS). The EHS is unrecognized by many people. Other interoceptive perceptions are commonly taken to represent physical hunger. These may be anxiety, thirst, other vague, nonspecific sensations, or simply the desire to eat in complete absence of any physical sensation.

Health researchers from a number of disciplines have converged upon this idea that hunger is poorly recognized. One of the first was the psychiatrist Hilda Bruch, who in 1969 wrote, "Hunger awareness is not innate biological knowledge . . . learning is necessary [for it] to become organized into recognizable patterns."[30]

Non-recognition of hunger, according to Bruch and later workers, owes to faulty childhood education. Infants' perception of hunger is forestalled, owing to regimented feeding regimes early in life.[31,32,33] Other researchers argue that the recognition of hunger is "intuitive" but forgotten in the course of development.[34,35] Much work has been done identifying extrinsic factors that override, forestall, or replace hunger.[36] Such factors include eating with other people,[37] social norms,[38] abundance of palatable food,[39] and sophisticated food marketing of convenience food.[40] Whether hunger must be learned, or whether it is innate but later overshadowed, all agree that "eating in the absence of hunger"[41] is detrimental to health.

Training people to recognize hunger has been developed by Mario Ciampolini and the author.[42] The author's approach[43] involves helping people to accurately identify hunger, using a clear terminology to tease out the manifold experiences that have been associated with hunger. Ciampolini's method[44] employs the measurement of blood glucose as an objective hunger marker.

Ciampolini et al. has demonstrated that physical hunger is associated with low blood-glucose concentrations.[45] Many people habitually eat when not experiencing hunger and therefore at high blood-glucose concentrations.[46] Initiating a meal when the EHS is present is therefore desirable, since by starting low, blood glucose during and after the meal is less likely to peak to unsafe levels.

Much of the focus of diabetes control has been in avoiding post-prandial blood-glucose highs. The usual strategy has been to measure one- or two-hour post-prandial blood glucose and then to try to adjust dietary content and portion size in such a way as to minimize a post-prandial peak. This policy of "going slow," involving low-glycemic-index food and small meal portions, has been well publicized and understood. Only recently has the importance of "starting low" received attention.

HUNGER RECOGNITION IMPROVES INSULIN SENSITIVITY

Training in perception of physical hunger has resulted in improved insulin sensitivity in non-diabetic subjects as demonstrated by Ciampolini et al.[47] In a randomized controlled trial, 120 subjects were assigned to hunger recognition training or were non-trained controls. Insulin sensitivity was calculated from blood glucose and insulin measurements before training and at five months after training. Significant decreases were found in insulin sensitivity, insulin and blood-glucose peaks, glycated hemoglobin, and pre-meal blood glucose when compared to control subjects. Significant decreases occurred in energy intake, body mass index (BMI), and body weight when compared to control subjects.

In a related study on weight[48] using a larger sample size, Ciampolini et al. identified a group of subjects who, although not obese by BMI criteria, nevertheless habitually ate at high blood-glucose concentrations and lost weight after training in hunger recognition. This is an at-risk group for diabetes hitherto unrecognized.

It is common for untrained patients to "think" they are hungry, and it can be revelatory for some to discover that they are, in fact, experiencing no physical abdominal sensations. TM can help here. Transcending is a process of refining the perception of a thought until the thought is left altogether. During this process, the mind becomes accustomed to subtle perceptions. I have observed that people who meditate regularly are able to differentiate more accurately between the experience of physical hunger and other nonspecific sensations.

The strategy that emerges from the above discussion is to eat only when your blood glucose is likely to be low. The Maharishi Ayurveda principles of eating only when physically hungry and never when anxious or upset (when stress hormones are high) are two ways to accomplish this. The time of day at which food is eaten and the timing of sleep are also important as will be discussed in the next section. It's not only what you eat but how and when.

RELATIONSHIP BETWEEN EATER AND FOOD:
RECOMMENDED DAILY ROUTINE

Daily routine, known as *Dinacharya*, is central to Maharishi Ayurveda. Several principles of Dinacharya are of direct relevance to the prevention and management of diabetes type-2.

1. Eat only when hungry.
2. Eat in a settled atmosphere; never eat when anxious or upset.
3. Lunch should be the main meal of the day.
4. The evening meal should be light.
5. Do not eat after 7 p.m.
6. Breakfast is optional depending upon hunger.
7. Be in bed by 10 p.m.

These principles are helpful in assisting the body maintain safe blood-glucose concentrations, yet they are so simple that they may be easily dismissed.

Growth hormone (GH), produced by the pituitary gland, stimulates growth and metabolism in muscle, bone, and cartilage cells. It promotes growth in children and regeneration of tissues in adults. It is maximally secreted between the hours of 10 p.m. and 2 a.m.[49] and may have an important role in the regenerative capacity of sleep. Sleep between 10 p.m. and 2 a.m. thus has an important function that "night owls" miss out on. Hence the instruction to be in bed, lights out, by 10 p.m.

Growth hormone significantly elevates blood-glucose concentration by decreasing insulin sensitivity in the liver and peripheral tissues such as muscle.[50] This, and the action of other hormones such as cortisol, contributes to what is known as the "dawn effect." The dawn effect explains why people with type-1 diabetes may be puzzled to find their blood glucose has gone high overnight without their having eaten anything. Eating a large, late meal, say at 9 or 10 p.m., will produce a glucose peak between 11 p.m. and midnight, just as growth hormone is peaking.

Thus it is logical to eat the largest meal at midday and have just soup or some other light dish in the early evening. The hormone cortisol peaks in the early morning hours, with a brisk increase shortly after waking in most people (the cortisol awakening response).[51] This is presumably in anticipation of the demands of the coming day. Cortisol remains high for an hour or so, thus elevated blood-glucose coincides with breakfast time. This helps explain why breakfast has been traditionally regarded in Maharishi Ayurveda as optional. Breakfast should be eaten only if hunger indicates that blood glucose is sufficiently low to warrant it. In the absence of hunger, breakfast best consists of a cup of tea or hot water. This advice flies in the face of conventional wisdom but is logical when one considers hunger as the body's request for food. If the body is not asking for food, then why eat?

Chronic, partial sleep-deprivation is now endemic. The prevalence of artificial lighting, longer work days and commuting, an increase in evening work, and frequent late-night computer and Internet sessions are thought to account for the dramatically lowered mean sleep duration seen in the United States over the past thirty-five years (8 to 8.9 hours in 1960 down to 7 hours in 1995).[52] Short sleep duration has been shown to be an independent risk factor for type-2 diabetes.[53] Sleep restriction, even in the short term, is thought to lead to increased sympathetic tone and elevated blood cortisol concentrations, in turn leading to decreased carbohydrate tolerance and increased insulin resistance. Curtailing sleep has been shown to promote excessive energy intake from meals and snacks.[54] Long-term sleep restriction could therefore be expected to lead to type-2 diabetes. Anxiety and poor sleep patterns frequently coexist. TM can help by decreasing anxiety and subsequently regulating sleep.

A recent case from my practice illustrates the value of following the above principles.

Mrs. J. A. was a 64-year-old nurse who kept good health until November 2013, when her hospital ward merged with another. She suddenly found herself in an unfamiliar and less-congenial work environment. For the first time since her early training, she was obliged to work night shifts, a transition she found challenging and stressful in the later stages of her career. In the pre-Christmas rush she grabbed food when she could and often ate late at night. On Christmas morning 2013, having worked through the night, and in a stressed and exhausted state, she nodded off for a second at the wheel of her car and crashed into an unoccupied car, extensively damaging both vehicles. She was admitted to the hospital where her injuries were found to be minor, but she was noted to have a blood-glucose concentration of 19 mmol/l (342 g/dL). A charge of careless use of a vehicle, an impending court appearance, and an indifferent response from her employer compounded her stress. Metformin was recommended; however, she decided to first try to correct her blood glucose by non-pharmacological means.

During a consultation at my practice, she could not remember ever feeling hungry and stated that she simply ate out of habit. She had learned TM in the past but had become irregular in the practice. I trained her in hunger recognition, encouraged her to become more regular in her TM, and wrote a note requesting her employer that she be excused from night work. She was encouraged to perform light exercise and to avoid food containing refined sugar. She was also asked to measure her fasting blood-glucose each morning with a sample of two-hour post-prandial readings.

Five days later she wrote the following e-mail (all readings in mmol/l).

> I have been following the regime [of hunger recognition] you suggested.
> My blood sugars appear to be coming down steadily. The following are on consecutive days:
> Morning fasting: 12.6, 9.6, 6.1, 7.0, 6.5
> Two-hours after meal: 9.6, 9.5, 9.2, 7.8, 8.5, 8.4, 7.7, 7.0
> I have started some exercise and am beginning to feel more energy.
> [My employer] has accepted your letter, and I have attended my court appearance. Life seems a bit more rosy!

When I saw her six weeks later, her readings were as follows: Morning fasting: 4.8, 7.3, 7.7, 6.3, 6.7, 6.9, 5.6; two-hour post-prandial: 8.0, 7.2, 8.1, 7.6, 9.8 (she had attended a friend's party), 8.0.

She had lost fifteen pounds in weight and had incidentally noticed that her troublesome symptoms of reflux had disappeared. She also noticed that her sleep had improved and she was no longer waking at 3 a.m. She commented that she had had to wait for a few days on a very light diet before experiencing physical hunger, and she stated, "Now I recognize that feeling, the food tastes so much better!"

Mrs. J. A. was severely glucose intolerant. She was stressed and her sleep patterns were disrupted. She was eating habitually, having forgotten what the sensation of hunger was like. With correction of her principal stressors, reinstatement of TM, regulation of her sleep, correction of diet, the addition of some light exercise, and attention to eating in accordance with hunger, she forestalled a dangerous slide into type-2 diabetes.

Resolution of her reflux esophagitis was a surprise for her. This had troubled her for several years. Improvements in reflux, heartburn, indigestion, and gastritis are routinely observed when food intake is timed with physical hunger. It is common for patients to express delight at how well they feel overall. Often an apparently trivial, nonspecific symptom, such as waking in the morning feeling groggy and dull, has simply been accepted as "life." It can be a revelation that the dull feeling is connected to eating too much food, too late at night, in the absence of hunger. Once the connection is made, it becomes much easier for the patient to comply with the principles.

Improved Control of Type-1 Diabetes

The control of blood glucose in type-1 diabetes has traditionally been difficult for patient and therapists alike. Even the most conscientious patients, those who follow their physician's guidelines to the letter, suffer discouraging peaks and troughs in blood-glucose concentration that seem to follow no logical pattern.

Traditional treatment of type-1 diabetes has been based on an assumption that has held sway for eighty years: *To keep blood glucose more or less constant, we should keep constant all known factors that affect blood glucose, including insulin dose, food intake, and exercise.*

Hunger recognition overthrows that assumption and leads to a new set of principles that are summarized in table 5.1.

The last two principles in table 5.1 are increasingly recognized in current treatment; however, they are not always fully appreciated by patients. Many patients still think of insulin as a medicine they must take in equal quantities each day and of exercise as a thing to be avoided lest it induce a frightening "hypo."

Using these principles, I have found type-1 diabetes to be much easier to control.[55] The vicious circle that otherwise can so easily develop is broken, a circle in which food taken mindlessly "according to the clock" seems to require a hefty dose of insulin to inject it into the cells. This leads to further food intake to mop up what later turns out to be an insulin excess, the whole process leading to spiraling food intake and insulin dosage.

Of course, blood-glucose monitoring is essential when making major adjustments to food intake and insulin dosage. Adoption of these new principles should always be done with the support of a medical pro-

Table 5.1. Old Principles and New Principles in the Management of Type-1 Diabetes

Old Principle	New Principle
Eat frequently—Many snacks.	Eat only when experiencing physical hunger.
Keep food intake per meal constant.	Adjust food intake according to hunger (and contentment at the end of the meal).
Keep insulin dose more-or-less constant.	Adjust insulin dose according to food intake.
Maintain a constant exercise regime.	Exercise when desired or convenient, but adjust insulin dose accordingly.

fessional. Existing guidelines for the management of fasting diabetic patients[56] can be usefully adapted by the professional even though strict fasting is not being advocated here. Professionals should be sure that a patient is motivated and ready to learn a new skill. In type-2 diabetes, oral hypoglycaemic medications can cause hypoglycemia, and dosage should be adjusted if food intake is decreased. In both types of diabetes, it is necessary to check that a patient recognizes an impending hypoglycemic episode and knows how to forestall it. Old principles are often deeply embedded so that a patient may easily slip into familiar habits. Thus vigilance is required in type-1 diabetes to ensure that patients fully understand that food and insulin are a "balancing act" and that if food intake is lowered without a corresponding lowering of insulin dose, then a "hypo" will follow. It should also be made clear to the patient that once the sensation of hunger is felt, there is no value in continued fasting. He or she should eat. Provided these precautions are taken, hunger recognition followed by insulin according to food intake typically results in much lower doses of daily insulin, avoidance of obesity, and patients who have a greater sense of control over their illness.

Maharishi Ayurveda Alleviates Diabetes Complications

ATHEROSCLEROTIC VASCULAR DISEASE

TM and associated Maharishi Ayurveda techniques have been shown to directly affect the outcomes of insulin resistance, often referred to as the *metabolic syndrome*. The benefits of TM in cardiovascular disease have been dealt with in chapter 4. A salient study here is that of Schneider et al.,[57] a randomized controlled trial in which TM was associated with 48 percent fewer deaths from all causes, heart attacks, and strokes among African Americans practicing TM over a five-year period.

OBESITY

In an unpublished study, Schneider found that over an eight-month period, pre-hypertensive African American adolescents practicing TM (n = 30) gained significantly less weight and BMI than a health education control group (n = 32). Using the dietary skills of Maharishi Ayurveda, I have helped numerous patients lose weight. The following recent case is illustrative.

Mr. D. O., a forty-year-old music teacher, became concerned about his weight in January 2013 when his doctor warned him of his susceptibility to diabetes. His weight was 251 pounds and his BMI was 33.3. He had already lost some weight using dietary restraint and was apprehensive that he would not only be unable to lose further weight but also that he would be unable to sustain the improvement he had already made. He adopted Maharishi Ayurveda dietary skills in March 2013. In July his weight was 229 pounds, and by October it had fallen to 220 pounds (BMI 29.2), a 31-pound loss over nine months. The patient commented,

> Prior to starting I was already reducing portion sizes, but it never occurred to me to actually wait until I was hungry before eating again. Now I have adjusted to [that] the whole process is pretty much effortless. I simply eat when I need to, and don't when I don't. I have a lot more energy (mental and physical) and my stress response has decreased—even before I started meditating. When I do eat, I eat slowly and I do love it—but I eat a lot less volume than I did before embarking on this process.

Hunger Recognition Reduces Subclinical Inflammation

Every clinician knows that uncontrolled diabetes is associated with poor healing. However, it is now understood that even mild insulin resistance is associated with alterations in intestinal microflora[58] and resultant subclinical inflammation.[59,60] This continuous inflammatory stimulation has been associated with functional deterioration of the immune system and has been implicated in illnesses associated with inflammation. These may include arthritis, inflammatory bowel disease and other autoimmune illnesses, allergy, cardiovascular diseases, musculoskeletal disorders, polycystic ovary syndrome, and some malignancies.[61]

Ciampolini et al. has shown that in children with irritable bowel syndrome and celiac disease, the bacterial count (mainly streptococci and staphylococci) per gram of mucosa for all subjects was 24 times higher after a 20-hour fast than after a 26-hour fast; for celiac sufferers, the bacterial count was 39 times higher.[62] In a further study, Ciampolini et al. showed that training in hunger recognition (a kind of "appropriate fast") successfully eradicated *Helicobacter Pylori* (as indicated by seroconversion) in 15 of 24 trained subjects compared to only 3 of 23 control subjects.[63]

How did hunger recognition clear the stomach of harmful bacteria? During the experience of physical hunger (EHS), powerful, wave-like contractions of the distal stomach and duodenum occur, known as "phase III contractions."[64] These contractions are thought to have a "housekeeping" function in that they sweep the bowel clear of pathogenic bacteria, debris, and indigestible food remnants. Their removal eliminates or greatly attenuates the cause of subclinical inflammation. In my clinical practice, training in hunger recognition (and ensuring that EHS is present for most meals) has resulted in encouraging improvements in some cases of immune-associated disorders, including rheumatoid arthritis,[65] Crohn's disease, and Graves's disease. The following two cases from my medical practice, in which the combination of regularly practiced TM and

Maharishi Ayurveda dietary skills have resulted in prolonged remission, are illustrative and provide a stimulus for further research in this area.

CROHN'S DISEASE

In August 2005, B. B., a fourteen-year-old boy, was brought to the clinic showing a 6–8 week history of blood per rectum, a 4.5-pound weight loss in the previous month, fatigue, and abdominal pain after eating. Investigations showed elevated inflammatory markers (ESR, 47 mm/hr; C-reactive protein [CRP], 53mg/L), and a biopsy confirmed he had Crohn's disease, with extensive involvement of the colon and small intestine. A specialist physician advised long-term prednisone "because of the extreme nature of his condition." I found out that B. B. frequently ate in the absence of any sensation that could be related to hunger. B. B. underwent training in hunger recognition and was also advised to restart his practice of TM, which he had allowed to lapse.

B. B. has had only one episode of (mild) abdominal pain since, no vomiting, and no rectal bleeding. The loose stools persisted for about two weeks and have recurred mildly only a few times since. His ESR has been within the normal range as well, and his CRP, which, like the ESR, fell precipitously (see figure 5.2), has been within acceptable range. Episodes of higher CRP coincide with a return of loose stool—on one occasion with

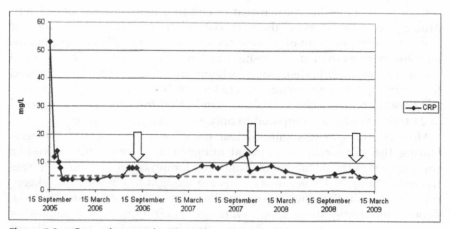

Figure 5.2.   C-reactive protein, Mr B.B.

Note: CRP fell precipitously soon after Mr B.B. resumed Transcendental Meditation and learned hunger recognition. CRP reached the normal range within 2 months (normal range is less than 5 mg/L as indicated by the dashed line). Since then it has been within an acceptable range. The improvements seen in September 2006, November 2007 and January 2009 (arrows) coincide with revision of his eating skills. © David Lovell-Smith 2010.

abdominal pain—and invariably with a lapse in his hunger recognition. Revision of his eating skills was followed by an improvement in CRP (see arrows, figure 5.2). B. B. has since put on weight; he was 113.5 pounds soon after presentation, and his present weight is 155 pounds. He has resumed his studies and he runs and plays rugby.

Is B. B. cured of Crohn's disease? From a Western point of view, the illness has been sufficiently improved to remove the overt signs and symptoms that would constitute a diagnosis of Crohn's disease and to release him from danger of further complications. His consulting physician understandably expressed concern that "in the long term his quite severe Crohn's disease is going to run a frequent relapsing course and have a high risk of developing complications such as strictures, etc." At the time of writing, B. B. is now eight years post-treatment without any significant relapse. In view of his episodic elevation of CRP, B. B. remains under follow-up. Six stages in pathogenesis are described in the Vedic system. Only in the last two stages do signs and symptoms recognizable as disease appear. From the viewpoint of Maharishi Ayurveda, B. B. has not yet been fully cured, but he has moved from the very dangerous stage 6 (disruption of function), to stages 1–4 in which signs and symptoms are nonspecific.

A great deal more research is needed before the encouraging results seen in this and other cases of inflammatory bowel disease in my practice can be generalized. What can be said with certainty is that had B. B. not taken the opportunity to employ TM and the Maharishi Ayurveda dietary skills, he would certainly have been exposed to high and frequent doses of powerful and damaging anti-inflammatory medication. He would also very likely have required surgery.

GRAVES'S DISEASE

Mrs. J. V., age fifty-five, entered the clinic in January 2003 complaining of loose stool and feeling hot, tense, and anxious. She also experienced a constant feeling of urgency, "as if late for a bus." She complained that she felt as if something were stuck in her throat at about the level of the thyroid cartilage. She was soon found to be thyrotoxic and was referred for a specialist's opinion. In the meantime, she was advised in dietary skills essentially identical to those given to B. B. She was also encouraged to restart her practice of TM. Within a month she noticed that she could sleep under a bed cover for the first time in many years and that her throat symptoms had disappeared.

Since May 2003 to the time of writing, Mrs. J. V. has been euthyroid. Carbimazole, a drug that reduces the production of the thyroid hormones, was prescribed for a month in March 2003 after she developed atrial fibrillation. However, she reverted to sinus rhythm before the drug had time to exert an effect and has had no further episodes. The drug was withdrawn when blood-free thyroxine (T4) came into normal range. Her thyroid stimulating hormone (TSH), previously suppressed by high T4, increased to normal concentrations eight months after dietary skills were instigated.

The progression of Mrs. J. V.'s T4 is shown in figure 5.3. This is an uncommonly quick remission for someone in her age group and cannot be accounted for by just one month of carbimazole. The thyroid specialist's letter stated, "At least 12 and probably 18 months of low dose carbimazole would be appropriate to see if she goes into long-term remission . . . radioiodine would be appropriate if she does not remit." About 10–20 percent of all patients with Graves's disease may have a spontaneous remission within the first year of diagnosis; however, the remission is frequently not permanent. A ten-year remission, while theoretically not impossible, is rare. After six weeks of treatment, the patient stated, "I feel so good now. I wake up in the morning feeling really good, really ready for the day. I did not realize you could feel that good."

The next section explores this global effect of TM and Maharishi Ayurveda.

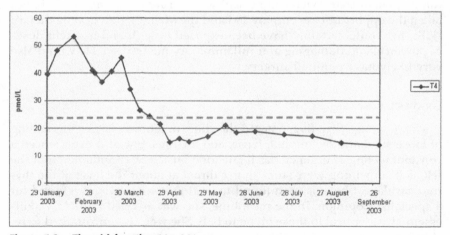

Figure 5.3. Thyroid function Mrs J.V.

Note: The current "epidemic of diabetes" is usually attributed to an increasingly sedentary yet stressful lifestyle coupled with an abundance of palatable and highly marketed energy-rich food. The primary care therapist/physician needs to be part endocrinologist, gastroenterologist, immunologist, psychologist, lifecoach, dietician, sports doctor, sociologist, confidant and friend. Fortunately Transcendental Meditation and Maharishi Ayurveda have benefits across many disciplines to assist in this. © David Lovell-Smith 2014.

Global Effect of TM and Maharishi Ayurveda

As Selye himself put it, "Research already conducted shows that the physiological effects of TM are exactly the opposite to those identified by medicine as being characteristic of the body's effort to meet the demands of stress."[66]

The clinician should therefore not be surprised to discover that meditating patients have a common tendency to feel and look well. One of the joys of prescribing this technique is that in contrast to the usual practice of identifying a disease and then treating that disease specifically, TM and associated Maharishi Ayurveda strategies enhance health in a global fashion. It is common for a patient to learn TM for high blood pressure, then to discover that headaches have disappeared. Patients sleep more soundly and get on better with family and coworkers. Although this book sets out mainly to present evidence for the efficacy of TM in specific disease conditions, the value of this nonspecific tendency toward wellness must not be undervalued. Improvements in a wide spectrum of illnesses have been indicated by a large-scale cohort study that compared five years of medical insurance utilization among 2,000 regular participants in TM against 600,000 members of the same insurance carrier.[67] Admissions per 1,000 were lower for the TM group for all of seventeen major medical treatment categories, including benign and malignant tumors (–55.4 percent), heart disease (–83.7 percent), infectious diseases (–30.4 percent), mental disorders (–30.6 percent), and diseases of the nervous system (–87.3 percent).

Individual case histories, while they cannot be generalized, do provide an impetus for further formal study and should not be discounted, particularly when the result does not follow the expected natural history of the illness in question.[68] I have, for example, noted sustained improvements in severe migraines over years in a series of patients. Three middle-age female patients—all of whom had suffered from severe, frequent, and debilitating migraine headaches since their teens—were instructed in TM. These patients experienced almost complete relief and were able to discontinue medication.[69] One patient commented,

> When there is a migraine coming on [and I meditate], there is a great feeling that everything is coming into harmony, a feeling of letting go, almost as if your brain is changing, calming down, evening out.

Another intractable migraine sufferer, who presented in his early thirties, has been followed for twenty-one years and has remained migraine-free apart from one episode associated with the near collapse of his marriage. He comments on the global effects,

I've always been the sort of guy who's into V8s and restoring American cars but now I'm noticing things I didn't notice before, like the beauty of the mountains. The clarity of vision is amazing. Losing the migraines was wonderful but it's all these other offshoots that are really so great."

Numerous phase-1 studies indicate promising areas for further research. In a recent six-month single-blind randomized controlled study,[70] twenty-two subjects suffering from AIDS were assigned to either TM or a healthy-eating education control group. According to an array of psychological testing instruments, significant improvements in vitality, mental health, social function, and general health were found in the group practicing TM. Other areas deserving further study include asthma,[71] insomnia,[72] periodontal health,[73] pain,[74] and amelioration of the aging process.[75,76]

Spiritual Considerations

LONELINESS, ALIENATION

Reference has been made to the sense of dislocation in Western society and its role in the genesis of type-2 diabetes. Numerous studies have suggested that TM improves interpersonal relationships, leading to an improved sense of social adequacy, increased ability to appreciate others, decreased social introversion, and an increased capacity for warm, interpersonal relationships. An interesting cross-sectional study is that of Gelderloos et al.,[77] in which practitioners of TM and the more advanced TM-Sidhi program showed greater facility than controls on five dimensions.

1. Unifying ability—the ability to integrate self with others, work ideals, or "deeper" levels of the self.
2. Autonomy—self-sufficiency, self-reliance, self-referral, self-determination, freedom and independence, and control or mastery of a situation.
3. Intrinsic spirituality—reported experience of a relationship to the "Absolute," transcendence, or God, and a strong orientation toward higher values in life.
4. Creativity—a high level of originality, spontaneity, liveliness, dynamism, or increasing growth or development.
5. Directedness—an articulated and differentiated purposefulness, a clear perception of where one is going and what one is doing.

The primary care physician may not be used to dealing with these aspects of a patient's life, preferring to leave them to psychologists, counselors, or priests. However, illness, its causes and complications, respects no boundaries of profession, and the complete treatment of diabetes should involve the integration of such mental and spiritual dimensions.

UNIVERSAL HARMONY

Of particular importance is the spiritual dimension. To fully prevent diabetes, we need to heal deeply, from within. Until four hundred years ago, health meant universal harmony, the individual attuned to the underlying unity of the cosmos and therefore attuned to all that lies within and without. It was considered self-evident that the spiritual, mental, and physical dimensions were linked and intrinsic to health. The philosophy of dualism (often attributed to Descartes) allowed a split between mind and body. This, along with a concession from the Church that sanctioned the dissection of the human body, eventually led to the body becoming the domain of science, while spiritual matters remained the sole preserve of the Church.[78] The rift between body and spirit has not been fully healed, even now. How often do questions about spirituality form part of a standard history in a primary care consultation? The reader may bridle at the suggestion, arguing that the spiritual side of life is a very personal thing and no business of the physician. This is a valid point of view, at least as far as present cultural expectations go. No physician wants to jar a patient's sensibilities or offend their expectations. Yet how far are those expectations a legacy of a historical accident, a compromise between scientists and the Church, made long ago? How much loneliness and agony of soul owes to coyness on the part of the profession to approach the spiritual basis of a patient's life? To what degree do such emotions play out in the human body? It is a fraught area and one which many practitioners prefer to avoid.

TM can address these issues. When prescribing TM, it is not necessary to discuss spirituality, although that can be done if the patient is open to it. It is certainly not necessary to change a patient's system of belief. TM is purely a technique and does not involve belief of any kind. Transcending does, however, broaden the practitioner's inner and outer capacity to experience. It allows the mind to appreciate more subtle layers of the thinking process, resulting in greater appreciation of all things subtle, inside and out, and an integration of those things with the Self. It is not uncommon for practitioners to report a greater appreciation of their spiritual path, whether that be Christianity,[79] Buddhism,[80] Hinduism, or any other spiritual system. An atheist practicing TM may not necessarily espouse a belief in God but is very likely to report greater appreciation of self, of others, and of nature—a kind of humanistic pantheism that embraces many of the moral virtues associated with the established religions. In its integrating tendency, not on the level of belief but on the level of *experience*, Transcendental Meditation offers to finally heal a four-hundred-year-old wound.

CONCLUSION

TM and Maharishi Ayurveda are invaluable tools in preventing diabetes and its complications. Maharishi Ayurveda cuts a path through the jungle of dietary injunctions to provide simple, logical advice that can be applied easily and goes to the heart of glycaemic control. TM has been shown not only to have a direct effect upon insulin resistance but also to reach deeply into the psychological and social causes that lie beneath it. The ramifications are broad. Together these techniques have the potential to alleviate some of the greatest scourges of Western industrialized nations: diabetes, heart disease, cancer, and strokes, as well as some of the most intractable of the inflammatory conditions. In doing all these things, nevertheless, the greatest contribution of these techniques is to uplift the spirit and heal the soul.

NOTES

1. American Diabetes Association, "Economic Costs of Diabetes in the U.S. in 2012," *Diabetes Care* 36, no. 4 (2013).

2. M. Paul-Labrador, D. Polk, J. H. Dwyer, I. Velasquez, S. Nidich, M. Rainforth, R. H. Schneider, and C. N. Bairey Merz, "Effects of a Randomized Controlled Trial of Transcendental Meditation on Components of the Metabolic Syndrome in Subjecs with Coronary Heart Disease," *Archives of Internal Medicine* 166 (2006): 1222.

3. R. S. Spielman, S. S. Fajans, J. V. Neel, S. Pek, J. C. Floyd, and W. J. Oliver, "Glucose Tolerance in Two Unacculturated Indian Tribes of Brazil," *Diabetologia* 23, no. 2 (1982): 92.

4. R. Finlay-Jones and G. W. Brown, "Types of Stressful Life Event and the Onset of Anxiety and Depressive Disorders," *Psychological Medicine* 11, no. 4 (1981): 812.

5. S. Toker, A. Shirom, I. Shapira, S. Berliner, and S. Melamed, "The Association between Burnout, Depression, Anxiety, and Inflammation Biomarkers: C-Reactive Protein and Fibrinogen in Men and Women," *Journal of Occupational Health Psychology* 10, no. 4 (2005): 347.

6. L. D. Kubzansky, I. Kawachi, S. T. Weiss, and D. Sparrow, "Anxiety and Coronary Heart Disease: A Synthesis of Epidemiological, Psychological, and Experimental Evidence," *Annals of Behavioral Medicine* 20, no. 2 (1998): 47.

7. L. C. Hawkley and J. T. Cacioppo, "Loneliness Matters: A Theoretical and Empirical Review of Consequences and Mechanisms," *Annals of Behavioral Medicine* 40, no. 2 (2010): 218.

8. S. Ranabir and K Reetu, "Stress and Hormones," *Indian Journal of Endocrinology and Metababolism* 15, no. 1 (2011).

9. A. Winokur, G. Maislin, J. L. Phillips, and J. D. Amsterdam, "Insulin Resistance after Oral Glucose Tolerance Testing in Patients with Major Depression," *American Journal of Psychiatry* 145, no. 3 (1988): 329.

10. A. Caspi, H. Harrington, T. E. Moffitt, B. J. Milne, and R. Poulton, "Socially Isolated Children 20 Years Later: Risk of Cardiovascular Disease," *Archives of Pediatrics and Adolescent Medicine* 160, no. 8 (2006): 809.

11. H. Selye, *The Stress of Life* (New York: McGraw-Hill, 1965).

12. K. Raikkonen, K. A. Matthews, and L. H. Kuller, "Depressive Symptoms and Stressful Life Events Predict Metabolic Syndrome among Middle-Aged Women: A Comparison of World Health Organization, Adult Treatment Panel III, and International Diabetes Foundation Definitions," *Diabetes Care* 30, no. 4 (2007): 872.

13. R. Jevning, A. F. Wilson, and W. R. Smith, "The Transcendental Meditation Technique, Adrenocortical Activity, and Implications for Stress," *Experientia* 34, no. 5 (1978): 619.

14. C. R. MacLean, K. G. Walton, S. R. Wenneberg, D. K. Levitsky, J. V. Mandarino, R. Waziri, and R. H. Schneider, "Altered Responses of Cortisol, GH, TSH and Testosterone to Acute Stress after Four Months' Practice of Transcendental Meditation (TM)," *Annals of the New York Academy of Sciences* 746 (1994): 384.

15. Because the sample sizes for these studies are relatively small, the significant p values imply a large effect size; however, these p values are somewhat fragile when it comes to generalizability, since the presence of "outliers" in a small sample might unduly influence the p value. In the first study on cortisol quoted above, the authors helpfully state that "cortisol concentration declined in four controls, increased in six and was unchanged in five" whereas in the TM practitioners, it "declined in 12 of the 15 subjects and remained constant or increased slightly in the remaining three." Although further studies are needed to confirm this, examination of the data at least in this study supports the idea that lowering of cortisol is likely to be experienced by most meditators.

16. J. Slochower, S. P. Kaplan, and L. Mann, "The Effects of Life Stress and Weight on Mood and Eating," *Appetite* 2, no. 2 (1981): 122.

17. M. Macht, "How Emotions Affect Eating: A Five-Way Model," *Appetite* 50, no. 1 (2008): 2.

18. H. Zheng and H.-R. Berthoud, "Eating for Pleasure or Calories," *Current Opinion in Pharmacology* 7, no. 6 (2007): 610.

19. T. van Strien and M. A. Ouwens, "Effects of Distress, Alexithymia and Impulsivity on Eating," *Eating Behaviors* 8, no. 2 (2007): 256.

20. A. J. Hill, "The Psychology of Food Craving," *Proceedings of the Nutrition Society* 66, no. 2 (2007): 279.

21. J. J. Wurtman, "Depression and Weight Gain: The Serotonin Connection," *Journal of Affective Disorders* 29, nos. 2–3 (1993): 186–87.

22. K. R. Eppley, A. I. Abrams, and J. Shear, "Differential Effects of Relaxation Techniques on Trait Anxiety: A Meta-analysis," *Journal of Clinical Psychology* 45, no. 6 (1989).

23. D. W. Orme-Johnson and M. C. Dillbeck, "Methodological Concerns for Meta-analyses of Meditation: Comment on Sedlmeier et al. (2012)," *Psychological Bulletin* 140, no. 2 (2014): 613.

24. J. S. Brooks and T. Scarano, "Transcendental Meditation in the Treatment of Post-Vietnam Adjustment," *Journal of Counseling and Development* 64, no. 3 (1985): 213.

25. C. Elder, S. I. Nidich, F. Moriarty, and R. J. Nidich, "Effect of Transcendental Meditation on Employee Stress, Depression, and Burnout: A Randomized Controlled Study," *Permanente Journal* 18, no. 1 (2014): 21.

26. H. Sharma and C. Clark, *Contemporary Ayurveda*, ed. Marc Micozzi (New York: Churchill Livingstone, 1998), 36.

27. E. Isganaitis and R. H. Lustig, "Fast Food, Central Nervous System Insulin Resistance, and Obesity," *Arteriosclerosis, Thrombosis and Vascular Biology* 25, no. 12 (2005): 2451–62.

28. N. M. Avena, P. Rada, and B. G. Hoebel, "Evidence for Sugar Addiction: Behavioral and Neurochemical Effects of Intermittent, Excessive Sugar Intake," *Neuroscience & Biobehavioral Reviews* 32, no. 1 (2008): 20–39.

29. R. H. Lustig, *Fat Chance* (London: HarperCollins, 2014), 48–63.

30. H. Bruch, "Hunger and Instinct," *Journal of Nervous and Mental Disease* 149, no. 2 (1969): 93.

31. L. L. Birch, J. O. Fisher, and K. Krahnstoever Davison, "Learning to Overeat: Maternal Use of Restrictive Feeding Practices Promotes Girls' Eating in the Absence of Hunger," *American Journal of Clinical Nutrition* 78, no. 2 (2003): 215–20.

32. J. L. Carper, J. O. Fisher, and L. L. Birch, "Young Girls' Emerging Dietary Restraint and Disinhibition Are Related to Parental Control in Child Feeding," *Appetite* 35 (2000): 121–29.

33. C. Harshaw, "Alimentary Epigenetics: A Developmental Psychobiological Systems View of the Perception of Hunger, Thirst and Satiety," *Developmental Review* 28, no. 4 (2008): 541–69.

34. L. C. Avalos and T. L. Tylka, "Exploring a Model of Intuitive Eating with College Women," *Journal of Counseling Psychology* 53, no. 4 (2006): 486.

35. M. Ciampolini, "Infants Do Request Food at the Hunger Blood Glucose Level, but Adults Don't Any More," *Appetite* 46 (2006): 345, abstract.

36. S. Schachter, "Obesity and Eating: Internal and External Cues Differentially Affect the Eating Behavior of Obese and Normal Subjects," *Science* 161, no. 843 (1968): 753.

37. V. I. Clendenen, C. P. Herman, and J. Polivy, "Social Facilitation of Eating among Friends and Strangers," *Appetite* 23, no. 1 (1994): 7.

38. C. P. Herman, N. E. Fitzgerald, and J. Polivy, "The Influence of Social Norms on Hunger Ratings and Eating," *Appetite* 41, no. 1 (2003): 18.

39. H. -R. Berthoud, "Interactions between the 'Cognitive' and 'Metabolic' Brain in the Control of Food Intake," *Physiology and Behavior* 91, no. 5 (2007): 495.

40. L. S. Lieberman, "Evolutionary and Anthropological Perspectives on Optimal Foraging in Obesogenic Environments," *Appetite* 47, no. 1 (2006): 4.

41. J. O. Fisher and L. L. Birch, "Eating in the Absence of Hunger and Overweight in Girls from 5 to 7 Years of Age," *American Journal of Clinical Nutrition* 76, no. 1 (2002): 226.

42. M. Ciampolini, H. D. Lovell-Smith, T. Kenealy, and R. Bianchi, "Hunger Can Be Taught: Hunger Recognition Regulates Eating and Improves Energy Balance," *International Journal of General Medicine* 2013, no. 6 (2013): 465–67.

43. H. D. Lovell-Smith, T. Kenealy, and S. Buetow, "Eating When Empty Is Good for Your Health," *Medical Hypotheses* 75 (2010): 172.

44. M. Ciampolini and R. Bianchi, "Training to Estimate Blood Glucose and to Form Associations with Initial Hunger," *Nutrition & Metabolism* 3, no. 42 (2006): 2–3.

45. Ibid., 6.

46. M. Ciampolini, Lovell-Smith, Kenealy, and Bianchi, "Hunger Can Be Taught," 469.

47. M. Ciampolini, H. D. Lovell-Smith, R. Bianchi, B. de Pont, M. Sifone, M. van Weeren, W. de Hahn, L. Borselli, and A. Pietrobelli, "Sustained Self-Regulation of Energy Intake: Initial Hunger Improves Insulin Sensitivity," *Journal of Nutrition and Metabolism*, www.ncbi.nlm.nih.gov.cmezproxy.chmeds.ac.nz/pmc/articles/P.M.C2915650/.

48. M. Ciampolini, H. D. Lovell-Smith, and M. Sifone, "Sustained Self-Regulation of Energy Intake, Loss of Weight in Overweight Subjects, Maintenance of Weight in Normal-Weight Subjects," *Nutrition & Metabolism* 7, no. 4 (2010), www.nutritionandmetabolism.com/content/7/1/4.

49. K. C. Yuen, L. E. Chong, and M. C. Riddle, "Influence of Glucocorticoids and Growth Hormone on Insulin Sensitivity in Humans," *Diabetic Medicine* 30, no. 6 (2013): 657.

50. G. Perriello, P. De Feo, E. Torlone, C. Fanelli, F. Santeusanio, P. Brunetti, and G. B. Bolli, "Nocturnal Spikes of Growth Hormone Secretion Cause the Dawn Phenomenon in Type 1 (Insulin-Dependent) Diabetes Mellitus by Decreasing Hepatic (and Extrahepatic) Sensitivity to Insulin in the Absence of Insulin Waning," *Diabetologia* 33, no. 1 (1990): 56.

51. E. Fries, L. Dettenborn, and C. Kirschbaum, "The Cortisol Awakening Response (CAR): Facts and Future Directions," *International Journal of Psychophysiology* 72, no. 1 (2009): 68.

52. J-P. Chaput, J-P. Despres, C. Bouchard, A. Astrup, and A. Tremblay, "Sleep Duration as a Risk Factor for the Development of Type 2 Diabetes or Impaired Glucose Tolerance: Analyses of the Quebec Family Study," *Sleep Medicine* 10, no. 8 (2009): 919.

53. Ibid., 923.

54. A. V. Nedeltcheva, J. M. Kilkus, J. Imperial, K. Kasza Kasza, D. A. Schoeller, and P. D. Penev, "Sleep Curtailment Is Accompanied by Increased Intake of Calories from Snacks," *American Journal of Clinical Nutrition* 89, no. 1:129.

55. H D. Lovell-Smith, "Diabetes: Let the Body Speak Its Mind," *New Zealand Family Physician* 3 (1996): 39.

56. E. Hui, V. Bravis, M. Hassanein, W. Hanif, R. Malik, T. A. Chowdhury, M. Suliman, and D. Devendra, "Management of People with Diabetes Wanting to Fast During Ramadan," *BMJ* 340 (2010): 1407.

57. R. H. Schneider, C. E. Grim, M. V. Rainforth, T. Kotchen, S. I. Nidich, C. Gaylord-King, J. W. Salerno, J. M. Kotchen, and C. N. Alexander, "Stress Reduction in the Secondary Prevention of Cardiovascular Disease: Randomized, Controlled Trial of Transcendental Meditation and Health Education in Blacks," *Circulation: Cardiovascular Quality and Outcomes* 5, no. 6 (2012): 750–58.

58. W. R. Russell, L. Hoyles, H. J. Flint, and M. E. Dumas, "Colonic Bacterial Metabolites and Human Health," *Current Opinion in Microbiology* 16, no. 3 (2013): 249.

59. C. G. Gustavsson and C. D. Agardh, "Markers of Inflammation in Patients with Coronary Artery Disease Are Also Associated with Glycosylated Haemoglobin A1c within the Normal Range," *European Heart Journal* 25, no. 23 (2004): 2120.

60. B. Vozarova, C. Weyer, R. S. Lindsay, R. E. Pratley, C. Bogardus, and P. A. Tataranni, "High White Blood Cell Count Is Associated with a Worsening of

Insulin Sensitivity and Predicts the Development of Type 2 Diabetes," *Diabetes* 51, no. 2 (2002): 455.

61. Z. T. Bloomgarden, "Insulin Resistance: Causes and Consequences," *International Review of Neurobiology* 65 (2005): 1–24.

62. M. Ciampolini, S. Bini, and A. Orsi, "Microflora Persistence on Duodeno-jejunal Flat or Normal Mucosa in Time after a Meal in Children," *Physiology and Behavior* 60, no. 6 (1996): 1553.

63. M. Ciampolini, L. Borselli, and V. Giannellini, "Attention to Metabolic Hunger and Its Effects on Helicobacter Pylori Infection," *Physiology and Behavior* 70, nos. 3–4 (2000): 293.

64. G. J Sanger, P. M. Hellstrom, and E. Naslund, "The Hungry Stomach: Physiology, Disease and Drug Development Opportunities," *Frontiers in Pharmacology* 1 (2011), www.ncbi.nlm.nih.gov/p.m.c/articles/P.M.C3174087/.

65. H. D. Lovell-Smith, "Rheumatoid Arthritis and Maharishi Ayur-Veda (Letter)," *New Zealand Medical Journal* 105 (1992): 42.

66. H. Selye, "An Interview with the 'Father of Stress' About TM," www.tm.org/blog/people/interview-with-father-of-stress/.

67. D. W. Orme-Johnson, "Medical Care Utilization and the Transcendental Meditation Program," *Psychosomatic Medicine* 49, no. 5 (1987): 493.

68. L. Lasagna, "Sounding Boards, Historical Controls: The Practitioner's Clinical Trials," *New England Journal of Medicine* 307, no. 21 (1982): 1339.

69. H. D. Lovell-Smith, "Transcendental Meditation and Three Cases of Migraine," *New Zealand Medical Journal* 98 (1985): 443–45.

70. S. Chhatre, D. S. Metzger, I. Frank, J. Boyer, E. Thompson, S. Nidich, L. J. Montaner, and R. Jayadevappa, "Effects of Behavioral Stress Reduction Transcendental Meditation Intervention in Persons with HIV," *AIDS Care—Psychological and Socio-Medical Aspects of AIDS/HIV* 25, no. 10 (2013): 1294.

71. A. F. Wilson, R. Honsberger, J. T. Chiu, and H. S. Novey, "Transcendental Meditation and Asthma," *Respiration* 32, no. 1 (1975): 74–80.

72. J. W Fuson, "The Effect of the Transcendental Meditation Program on Sleeping and Dreaming Patterns," in *Scientific Research on the Transcendental Meditation and TM-Sidhi Programme*, ed. Roger Chalmers (The Netherlands: MVU Press, 1976), 880–96.

73. G. Seiler and V. Seiler, "The Effects of Transcendental Meditation on Periodontal Tissue," *Journal of the American Society of Psychosomatic Dentistry and Medicine* 26, no. 1 (1979): 8–12.

74. D. W. Orme-Johnson, R. H. Schneider, Y. D. Son, S. I. Nidich, and Z. Hee Cho, "Neuroimaging of Meditation's Effect on Brain Reactivity to Pain," *NeuroReport* 17, no. 12 (2006): 1359–63.

75. C. N. Alexander, E. J. Langer, R. I. Newman, H. M. Chandler, and J. L. Davies, "Transcendental Meditation, Mindfulness, and Longevity: An Experimental Study with the Elderly," *Journal of Personality and Social Psychology* 57, no. 6 (1989): 950–64.

76. R. H. Schneider, C. N. Alexander, J. W. Salerno, D. K. Robinson Jr, J. Z. Fields, and S. I. Nidich, "Disease Prevention and Health Promotion in the Aging with a Traditional System of Natural Medicine: Maharishi Vedic Medicine," *Journal of Aging and Health* 14, no. 1 (2002): 57–58.

77. P. Gelderloos, H. J. Hermans, H. H. Ahlscrom, and R. Jacoby, "Transcendence and Psychological Health: Studies with Long-Term Participants of the Transcendental Meditation and TM-Sidhi Program," *Journal of Psychology* 124, no. 2 (1990): 177–97.

78. E. J. Cassel, "The Nature of Suffering and the Goals of Medicine," *New England Journal of Medicine* 306, no. 11 (1982): 640.

79. A. B. Smith, *A Key to the Kingdom of Heaven* (Cornwall, UK: Hartnolls, 1993), 35–39.

80. R. H. Roth, "Thousands of Buddhist Monks in Asia Learn Transcendental Meditation," Maharishi Foundation USA, www.tm.org/blog/meditation/buddhist-monks/.

BIBLIOGRAPHY

Alexander, C. N., E. J. Langer, R. I. Newman, H. M. Chandler, and J. L. Davies. "Transcendental Meditation, Mindfulness, and Longevity: An Experimental Study with the Elderly." *Journal of Personality and Social Psychology* 57, no. 6 (December 1989): 950–64.

Association, A. D. "Economic Costs of Diabetes in the U.S. in 2012." *Diabetes Care* 36, no. 4 (April 2013): 1033–46.

Avalos, L. C. and T. L. Tylka. "Exploring a Model of Intuitive Eating with College Women." *Journal of Counseling Psychology* 53, no. 4 (October 2006): 486–97.

Avena, N. M., P. Rada, and B. G. Hoebel. "Evidence for Sugar Addiction: Behavioral and Neurochemical Effects of Intermittent, Excessive Sugar Intake." *Neuroscience & Biobehavioral Reviews* 32, no. 1 (2008): 20–39.

Berthoud, H. -R. "Interactions between the 'Cognitive' and 'Metabolic' Brain in the Control of Food Intake." *Physiology & Behavior* 91, no. 5 (2007): 486–98.

Birch, L. L., J. O. Fisher, and K. K. Davison. "Learning to Overeat: Maternal Use of Restrictive Feeding Practices Promotes Girls' Eating in the Absence of Hunger." *American Journal of Clinical Nutrition* 78, no. 2 (August 2003): 215–20.

Bloomgarden, Z. T. "Insulin Resistance: Causes and Consequences." *International Review of Neurobiology* 65 (2005): 1–24.

Brooks, J. S. and T. Scarano. "Transcendental Meditation in the Treatment of Post-Vietnam Adjustment." *Journal of Counseling & Development* 64, no. 3 (November 1985): 212–15.

Bruch, H. "Hunger and Instinct." *Journal of Nervous and Mental Disease* 149, no. 2 (August 1969): 91–114.

Carper, J. L., J. O. Fisher, and L. L. Birch. "Young Girls' Emerging Dietary Restraint and Disinhibition Are Related to Parental Control in Child Feeding." *Appetite* 35 (2000): 121–29.

Caspi, A., H. Harrington, T. E. Moffitt, B. J. Milne, and R. Poulton. "Socially Isolated Children 20 Years Later: Risk of Cardiovascular Disease." *Archives of Pediatrics & Adolescent Medicine* 160, no. 8 (August 2006): 805–11.

Cassel, E. J. "The Nature of Suffering and the Goals of Medicine." *New England Journal of Medicine* 306, no. 11 (1982): 639–45.

Chaput, J-P., J-P. Despres, C. Bouchard, A. Astrup, and A. Tremblay. "Sleep Duration as a Risk Factor for the Development of Type 2 Diabetes or Impaired Glucose Tolerance: Analyses of the Quebec Family Study." *Sleep Medicine* 10, no. 8 (September 2009): 919–24.

Chhatre, S., D. S. Metzger, I. Frank, J. Boyer, E. Thompson, S. A. Nidich, L. J. Montaner, and R. Jayadevappa. "Effects of Behavioral Stress Reduction Transcendental Meditation Intervention in Persons with HIV." *AIDS Care—Psychological and Socio-Medical Aspects of AIDS/HIV* 25, no. 10 (October 2013): 1291–97.

Ciampolini, M. "Infants Do Request Food at the Hunger Blood Glucose Level, but Adults Don't Any More (Abstract)." *Appetite* 46 (2006): 345.

Ciampolini, M. and R. Bianchi. "Training to Estimate Blood Glucose and to Form Associations with Initial Hunger." *Nutrition & Metabolism* 3, no. 42 (2006).

Ciampolini, M., S. Bini, and A. Orsi. "Microflora Persistence on Duodenojejunal Flat or Normal Mucosa in Time after a Meal in Children." *Physiology & Behavior* 60, no. 6 (December 1996): 1551–56.

Ciampolini, M., L. Borselli, and V. Giannellini. "Attention to Metabolic Hunger and Its Effects on Helicobacter Pylori Infection." *Physiology & Behavior* 70, nos. 3–4 (August–September 2000): 287–96.

Ciampolini, M., H. D. Lovell-Smith, R. Bianchi, B. de Pont, M. Sifone, M. van Weeren, W. de Hahn, L. Borselli, and A. Pietrobelli. "Sustained Self-Regulation of Energy Intake: Initial Hunger Improves Insulin Sensitivity." *Journal of Nutrition and Metabolism* (2010), DOI: 10.1155/2010/286952, www.ncbi.nlm.nih.gov.cmezproxy.chmeds.ac.nz/pmc/articles/P.M.C2915650/.

Ciampolini, M., H. D. Lovell-Smith, T. Kenealy, and R. Bianchi. "Hunger Can Be Taught: Hunger Recognition Regulates Eating and Improves Energy Balance." *International Journal of General Medicine* 2013, no. 6 (2013): 465–78.

Ciampolini, M., H. D. Lovell-Smith, and M. Sifone. "Sustained Self-Regulation of Energy Intake. Loss of Weight in Overweight Subjects. Maintenance of Weight in Normal-Weight Subjects." *Nutrition & Metabolism* 7, no. 4 (2010). doi:10.1186/1743707574., www.nutritionandmetabolism.com/content/7/1/4.

Clendenen, V. I., C. P. Herman, and J. Polivy. "Social Facilitation of Eating among Friends and Strangers." *Appetite* 23, no. 1 (August 1994): 1–13.

Elder, C., S. I. Nidich, F. Moriarty, and R. J. Nidich. "Effect of Transcendental Meditation on Employee Stress, Depression, and Burnout: A Randomized Controlled Study." *Permanente Journal* 18, no. 1 (2014): 19–23.

Eppley, K. R., A. I. Abrams, and J. Shear. "Differential Effects of Relaxation Techniques on Trait Anxiety: A Meta-analysis." *Journal of Clinical Psychology* 45, no. 6 (1989): 957–74.

Finlay-Jones, R. and G. W. Brown. "Types of Stressful Life Event and the Onset of Anxiety and Depressive Disorders." *Psychological Medicine* 11, no. 4 (November 1981): 803–15.

Fisher, J. O. and L. L. Birch. "Eating in the Absence of Hunger and Overweight in Girls from 5 to 7 Years of Age." *American Journal of Clinical Nutrition* 76, no. 1 (July 2002): 226–31.

Fries, E., L. Dettenborn, and C. Kirschbaum. "The Cortisol Awakening Response (Car): Facts and Future Directions." *International Journal of Psychophysiology* 72, no. 1 (Apr 2009): 67–73.

Fuson, J. W. "The Effect of the Transcendental Meditation Program on Sleeping and Dreaming Patterns." In *Scientific Research on the Transcendental Meditation and TM-Sidhi Programme*, edited by Roger Chalmers, 880–96. The Netherlands: MVU Press, 1976.

Gelderloos, P., H. J. Hermans, H. H. Ahlscrom, and R. Jacoby. "Transcendence and Psychological Health: Studies with Long-Term Participants of the Transcendental Meditation and TM-Sidhi Program." *Journal of Psychology* 124, no. 2 (March 1990): 177–97.

Gustavsson, C. G. and C. -D. Agardh. "Markers of Inflammation in Patients with Coronary Artery Disease Are Also Associated with Glycosylated Haemoglobin A1c within the Normal Range." *European Heart Journal* 25, no. 23 (December 2004): 2120–24.

Harshaw, C. "Alimentary Epigenetics: A Developmental Psychobiological Systems View of the Perception of Hunger, Thirst and Satiety." *Developmental Review* 28, no. 4 (December 2008): 541–69.

Hawkley, L. C. and J. T. Cacioppo. "Loneliness Matters: A Theoretical and Empirical Review of Consequences and Mechanisms." *Annals of Behavioral Medicine* 40, no. 2 (October 2010): 218–27.

Herman, C. P., N. E. Fitzgerald, and J. Polivy. "The Influence of Social Norms on Hunger Ratings and Eating." *Appetite* 41, no. 1 (August 2003): 15–20.

Hill, A. J. "The Psychology of Food Craving." *Proceedings of the Nutrition Society* 66, no. 2 (May 2007): 277–85.

Hui, E., V. Bravis, M. Hassanein, W. Hanif, R. Malik, T. A. Chowdhury, M. Suliman, and D. Devendra. "Management of People with Diabetes Wanting to Fast During Ramadan." *BMJ* 340 (2010): 1407–11.

Isganaitis, E. and R. H. Lustig. "Fast Food, Central Nervous System Insulin Resistance, and Obesity." *Arteriosclerosis, Thrombosis & Vascular Biology* 25, no. 12 (December 2005): 2451–62.

Jevning, R., A. F. Wilson, and W. R. Smith. "The Transcendental Meditation Technique, Adrenocortical Activity, and Implications for Stress." *Experientia* 34, no. 5 (1978): 618–19.

Kubzansky, L. D., I. Kawachi, S. T. Weiss, and D. Sparrow. "Anxiety and Coronary Heart Disease: A Synthesis of Epidemiological, Psychological, and Experimental Evidence." *Annals of Behavioral Medicine* 20, no. 2 (1998): 47–58.

Lasagna, L. "Sounding Boards. Historical Controls: The Practitioner's Clinical Trials." *New England Journal of Medicine* 307, no. 21 (1982): 1339–40.

Lieberman, L. S. "Evolutionary and Anthropological Perspectives on Optimal Foraging in Obesogenic Environments." *Appetite* 47, no. 1 (2006): 3–9.

Lovell-Smith, H. D. "Diabetes: Let the Body Speak Its Mind." *New Zealand Family Physician* 3 (1996): 37–39.

———. "Rheumatoid Arthritis and Maharishi Ayur-Veda (Letter)." *New Zealand Medical Journal* 105 (1992): 42.

———. "Transcendental Meditation and Three Cases of Migraine." *New Zealand Medical Journal* 98 (1985): 443–45.

Lovell-Smith, H. D., T. Kenealy, and S. Buetow. "Eating When Empty Is Good for Your Health." *Medical Hypotheses* 75 (2010): 172–78.

Lustig, R. H. *Fat Chance*. London: HarperCollins, 2014.

Macht, M. "How Emotions Affect Eating: A Five-Way Model." *Appetite* 50, no. 1 (January 2008): 1–11.

MacLean, C. R., K. G. Walton, S. R. Wenneberg, D. K. Levitsky, J. V. Mandarino, R. Waziri, and R. H. Schneider. "Altered Responses of Cortisol, GH, TSH and Testosterone to Acute Stress after Four Months' Practice of Transcendental Meditation (TM)." *Annals of the New York Academy of Sciences* 746 (November 30 1994): 381–84.

Nedeltcheva, A. V., J. M. Kilkus, J. Imperial, K. K. Kasza, D. A. Schoeller, and P. D. Penev. "Sleep Curtailment Is Accompanied by Increased Intake of Calories from Snacks." *American Journal of Clinical Nutrition* 89, no. 1, 126–33.

Orme-Johnson, D. "Medical Care Utilization and the Transcendental Meditation Program." *Psychosomatic Medicine* 49, no. 5 (September–October 1987): 493–507.

Orme-Johnson, D. W. and M. C. Dillbeck. "Methodological Concerns for Meta-Analyses of Meditation: Comment on Sedlmeier et al. (2012)." *Psychological Bulletin* 140, no. 2 (March 2014): 610–16.

Orme-Johnson, D. W., R. H. Schneider, Y. D. Son, S. I. Nidich, and Z. -H. Cho. "Neuroimaging of Meditation's Effect on Brain Reactivity to Pain." *NeuroReport* 17, no. 12 (August 21 2006): 1359–63.

Paul-Labrador, M., D. Polk, J. H. Dwyer, I. Velasquez, S. I. Nidich, M. Rainforth, R. H. Schneider, and C. N. B. Merz. "Effects of a Randomized Controlled Trial of Transcendental Meditation on Components of the Metabolic Syndrome in Subjects with Coronary Heart Disease." *Archives of Internal Medicine* 166 (2006): 1218–24.

Perriello, G., P. De Feo, E. Torlone, C. Fanelli, F. Santeusanio, P. Brunetti, and G. B. Bolli. "Nocturnal Spikes of Growth Hormone Secretion Cause the Dawn Phenomenon in Type 1 (Insulin-Dependent) Diabetes Mellitus by Decreasing Hepatic (and Extrahepatic) Sensitivity to Insulin in the Absence of Insulin Waning." *Diabetologia* 33, no. 1 (January 1990): 52–59.

Raikkonen, K., K. A. Matthews, and L. H. Kuller. "Depressive Symptoms and Stressful Life Events Predict Metabolic Syndrome among Middle-Aged Women: A Comparison of World Health Organization, Adult Treatment Panel III, and International Diabetes Foundation Definitions." *Diabetes Care* 30, no. 4 (April 2007): 872–77.

Ranabir, S. and K. Reetu. "Stress and Hormones." *Indian Journal of Endocrinology and Metabolism* 15, no. 1 (2011): 18–22.

Roth, R. H. "Thousands of Buddhist Monks in Asia Learn Transcendental Meditation." Maharishi Foundation USA, www.tm.org/blog/meditation/buddhist-monks/.

Russell, W. R., L. Hoyles, H. J. Flint, and M. E. Dumas. "Colonic Bacterial Metabolites and Human Health." *Current Opinion in Microbiology* 16, no. 3 (June 2013): 246–54.

Sanger, G. J., P. M. Hellstrom, and E. Naslund. "The Hungry Stomach: Physiology, Disease and Drug Development Opportunities." *Frontiers in Pharmacology* 1 (2011): 145, DOI:10.3389/fphar.2010.00145, www.ncbi.nlm.nih.gov/pmc/articles/ P.M.C3174087/.

Schachter, S. "Obesity and Eating: Internal and External Cues Differentially Affect the Eating Behavior of Obese and Normal Subjects." *Science* 161, no. 843 (August 23 1968): 751–56.

Schneider, R. H., C. N. Alexander, J. W. Salerno, D. K. Robinson Jr., J. Z. Fields, and S. I. Nidich. "Disease Prevention and Health Promotion in the Aging with a Traditional System of Natural Medicine: Maharishi Vedic Medicine." *Journal of Aging and Health* 14, no. 1 (February 2002): 57–78.

Schneider, R. H., C. E. Grim, M. V. Rainforth, T. Kotchen, S. I. Nidich, C. Gaylord-King, J. W. Salerno, J. M. Kotchen, and C. N. Alexander. "Stress Reduction in the Secondary Prevention of Cardiovascular Disease: Randomized, Controlled Trial of Transcendental Meditation and Health Education in Blacks." *Circulation: Cardiovascular Quality and Outcomes* 5, no. 6 (November 2012): 750–58.

Seiler, G., and V. Seiler. "The Effects of Transcendental Meditation on Periodontal Tissue." *Journal of the American Society of Psychosomatic Dentistry and Medicine* 26, no. 1 (1979): 8–12.

Selye, H. "An Interview with the 'Father of Stress' about TM." www.tm.org/blog/people/interview-with-father-of-stress/.

———. *The Stress of Life*. New York: McGraw-Hill, 1965.

Sharma, H. and C. Clark. *Contemporary Ayurveda*. Edited by Marc Micozzi New York: Churchill Livingstone, 1998.

Slochower, J. "Emotional Labeling and Overeating in Obese and Normal Weight Individuals." *Psychosomatic Medicine* 38, no. 2 (March–April 1976): 131–39.

Slochower, J., S. P. Kaplan, and L. Mann. "The Effects of Life Stress and Weight on Mood and Eating." *Appetite* 2, no. 2 (June 1981): 115–25.

Smith, A. B. *A Key to the Kingdom of Heaven*. Cornwall, UK: Hartnolls, 1993.

Spielman, R. S., S. S. Fajans, J. V. Neel, S. Pek, J. C. Floyd, and W. J. Oliver. "Glucose Tolerance in Two Unacculturated Indian Tribes of Brazil." *Diabetologia* 23, no. 2 (August 1982): 90–93.

Toker, S., A. Shirom, I. Shapira, S. Berliner, and S. Melamed. "The Association between Burnout, Depression, Anxiety, and Inflammation Biomarkers: C-Reactive Protein and Fibrinogen in Men and Women." *Journal of Occupational Health Psychology* 10, no. 4 (October 2005): 344–62.

Van Strien, T. and M. A. Ouwens. "Effects of Distress, Alexithymia and Impulsivity on Eating." *Eating Behaviors* 8, no. 2 (April 2007): 251–57.

Vozarova, B., C. Weyer, R. S. Lindsay, R. E. Pratley, C. Bogardus, and P. A. Tataranni. "High White Blood Cell Count Is Associated with a Worsening of Insulin Sensitivity and Predicts the Development of Type 2 Diabetes." *Diabetes* 51, no. 2 (February 2002): 455–61.

Wilson, A. F., R. Honsberger, J. T. Chiu, and H. S. Novey. "Transcendental Meditation and Asthma." *Respiration* 32, no. 1 (1975): 74–80.

Winokur, A., G. Maislin, J. L. Phillips, and J. D. Amsterdam. "Insulin Resistance after Oral Glucose Tolerance Testing in Patients with Major Depression." *American Journal of Psychiatry* 145, no. 3 (March 1988): 325–30.

Wurtman, J. J. "Depression and Weight Gain: The Serotonin Connection." *Journal of Affective Disorders* 29, nos. 2–3 (October–November 1993): 183–92.

Yuen, K. C., L. E. Chong, and M. C. Riddle. "Influence of Glucocorticoids and Growth Hormone on Insulin Sensitivity in Humans." *Diabetic Medicine* 30, no. 6 (June 2013): 651–63.

Zheng, H., and H.-R. Berthoud. "Eating for Pleasure or Calories." *Current Opinion in Pharmacology* 7, no. 6 (2007): 607–12.

SECTION II

RESEARCH

Mental Health Disorders

Six

Transcendental Meditation Research on Anxiety and Anxiety Disorders

Sarina Grosswald, Ed.D., David F. O'Connell, Ph.D., M.S., CFC, DABPS, and James Krag, M.D.

Anxiety disorders continue to be the most common class of mental disorders in the general population. Lifetime prevalence estimates for all anxiety disorders combined are reported to be 16.6 percent, with specific phobias, social anxiety disorder, and post-traumatic stress disorder (PTSD) having the highest lifetime prevalence.[1,2] These disorders affect 40 million adult Americans, or 19 percent of the adult American population, with an estimated annual cost of over $42 billion in the United States.

Anxiety disorders are characterized by excessive, irrational fear, and dread. They can be extremely crippling and disabling and can significantly affect daily functioning. Generalized anxiety disorder anxiety (GAD), for example, shows only a 20 percent chance of full recovery, and 20–40 percent of patients with GAD report a suicide attempt. The causes of anxiety disorders are unknown but are thought to involve a complex interplay of familial, genetic, personality psychodevelopmental, and environmental triggers; a history of trauma and associated factors, such as age and gender; and certain medical conditions and medications. Researchers have implicated certain areas of the brain, such as the amygdala and the hippocampus, as well as dysregulation in brain neurotransmitters in the meditation of anxiety. However at this point, the exact causes of anxiety disorders remain unknown although risk factors such as those previously mentioned are viewed as playing a role in the etiology and expression of disorders of anxiety.

Symptoms of anxiety include muscle tension, worry, restlessness, irritability, difficulty concentrating, and sleep disturbance. Anxiety symptoms tend to rise and fall over time, and they can be intermittent or chronic. Many patients experience *subsyndromal* anxiety—anxiety just below the diagnostic threshold—alternating with periods of remission. Anxiety disorder symptoms often overlap, with depression being a common comorbidity. Co-occurring disorders lead to a wide variety of clinical syndromes and presentations.[3]

RESEARCH ON TRANSCENDENTAL MEDITATION AND ANXIETY

The results of four decades of research have shown definitively that the regular practice of Transcendental Meditation (TM®) can result in significant deceases in both trait and state anxiety and in other symptoms of psychopathology.

Most of the research on TM and anxiety focuses on *trait anxiety*. Trait anxiety is defined as a stable, enduring tendency to attend to, experience, and report negative emotions, including fear, worry, and tension across many situations and contexts. It is considered a feature or component of an individual's personality. *State anxiety*, in contrast, refers to a temporary response of fear, discomfort, and other negative symptoms, usually in response to a threatening stimulus, and it passes when the threat is removed. The distinction between trait and state anxiety is used rarely in the clinical treatment. Nearly all of the *DSM-V* anxiety disorders would likely be considered examples of trait anxiety since they are chronic and cause clinically significant problems and even disability.

Early studies with hospitalized psychiatric patients demonstrated that psychiatric patients who learned TM, including patients with serious psychotic disorders such as schizophrenia, when compared with matched controls who received standard hospital treatments, showed significant decreases in anxiety and improvements in other indicators of psychopathology, including Minnesota Multiphasic Personality Inventory (MMPI) scores, nursing note evaluations of psychopathology, general condition, and decreases in need for sleep and psychiatric medications.[4,5] The authors also concluded that TM had no adverse effects on the patients.

The majority of the TM treatment group, 40 percent of whom were psychotic, reported that the calming effects of meditation played a significant role in their recovery. TM was accepted more readily and with longer periods of compliance by patients than either EEG alpha rhythm enhancement or progressive muscle relaxation.

A study of 372 high school students practicing TM demonstrated that TM resulted in lower anxiety levels and improvement on cognitive tasks compared with napping.[6] Shapiro and Walsh reported that the practice of TM led to significantly reduced anxiety relative to controls.[7]

Other research showed that racial and ethnic minority groups are particularly subject to high levels of stress due to exposure to violence, pressures associated with acculturation, and the educational process. A 2012 study was the first to evaluate the effects of TM on psychological distress across diverse racial and ethnic minority student groups.[8] Results from 106 secondary-school students (68 meditating, 38 non-meditating) showed significant reductions in general psychological distress and trait anxiety.

TRANSCENDENTAL MEDITATION COMPARED TO OTHER TECHNIQUES

When the first research was conducted on TM in the early 1970s, there was a common hypothesis that all techniques of meditation and relaxation would produce similar reductions in sympathetic arousal, and therefore all techniques should be equally effective. For many researchers and clinicians, this proposal soon became accepted as proven. However, this hypothesis has not withstood the test of scientific scrutiny. In fact, it has been shown that some techniques actually increase stress.

Different types of meditation, relaxation, and mental techniques involve varying types of mental activity and instructions. Therefore it can be expected that different techniques will activate the brain and body uniquely, giving different ranges and types of effects and experiences. A systematic review of independent outcomes[9] found that TM was twice as effective in reducing anxiety than other approaches, including other forms of meditation, progressive muscle relaxation, and techniques used to induce the relaxation response. Only TM showed a positive correlation between duration of regular practice and anxiety reduction. These findings of the greater effectiveness of TM held up even when only the strongest and most rigorous studies were examined.

In 2013, an extensive meta-analysis (see figure 6.1) looked at eight psychological variables.[10] The authors reported very strong effects of TM on reducing trait anxiety compared with other meditation techniques, noting that this result was consistent with a previous meta-analysis showing that TM produced superior effects on reducing trait anxiety. It is interesting to note that TM showed substantially greater effects than other approaches across seven of the eight variables measured, including trait anxiety. However, in the single variable of state anxiety, the combined category "Other Meditation" showed greater effect.

As noted, state anxiety represents a temporary response to a perceived stressor that subsides when the stressor is gone, while trait anxiety reflects overall tendency toward anxiousness as a personality trait, and the anxiety is more intense. It may be surmised that almost any relaxing experience at a specific point in time, such as massage or listening to re-

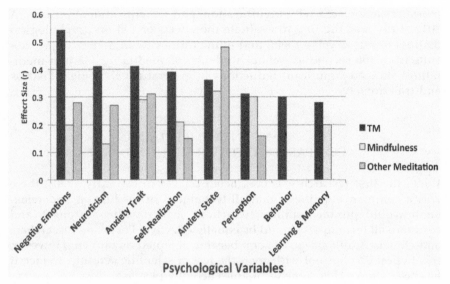

Figure 6.1.   Meta-Analysis of 163 Studies
Source: Sedimeier, D., Eberth, J., Schwartz, M., Zimmerman, D., Haarig, F., Jaeger, R. and Kunze, S. The psychological effects of meditation: a meta-analysis. Psychological Bulletin. 19 (2012).

laxing music, can reduce temporal anxiety. However, the ability to change underlying chronic anxiety is more difficult, and when accomplished, as with TM, it can have greater implications for mental health, well-being, and quality of life.

In a medical textbook on cardiovascular health, Dornelas,[11] citing a systematic review and meta-analysis,[12] concluded that the practice of TM has significant, beneficial effects on reducing anxiety and psychosocial stress. Chen et al. reported similar results for TM in another meta-analysis of the impact of various forms of meditation on anxiety.[13]

In a recent meta-analysis, Orme-Johnson and Barnes[14] examined research on TM and trait anxiety based solely on research reports using randomized controlled experimental designs that met rigorous criteria. They reviewed sixteen studies on TM and anxiety with 1,295 subjects. Results indicated that subjects with the highest levels of anxiety, the 90th percentile according to the measures used in the study, reduced their anxiety levels to the 57th percentile. The TM subjects did better relative to controls on most measures. Progressive muscle relaxation (PMR) did as well as TM in subjects with lower levels of anxiety. However, PMR does not show the other mental health and cognitive benefits found in the regular practice of TM.

Most of the research on TM and anxiety focuses on trait anxiety rather than on specific anxiety disorders, such as obsessive compulsive disorder, phobias, GAD, social anxiety disorder, and panic disorder. Several anecdotal reports and patient testimonials report the practice of TM results in reducing or relieving the symptoms of some of these disorders.

Objective measures show long-term, sustained effects from the practice of TM. The physiological effects seen with TM—reduced respiratory rate, skin conductance, plasma lactate, cortisol—are the opposite of those produced by anxiety. The effect of TM on stress-related risk conditions, for example high blood pressure and heart disease, of which anxiety is a key psychological component, further validates the technique's beneficial effects on stress reduction.

RESEARCH ON TM AND THE MANAGEMENT OF PTSD

PTSD is a particularly debilitating anxiety-related disorder. PTSD is complicated by the fact that it frequently occurs in conjunction with related disorders such as depression, substance abuse, problems of memory and cognition, and other physical and mental problems. The disorder is also associated with impairment of the person's ability to function in social or family life, causing occupational instability, marital problems, family discord, and divorces. The impairment caused by PTSD substantially affects work, social relationships, and family life.

An estimated 7.8 percent of Americans will experience PTSD at some point in their lives, with women (10.4 percent) twice as likely as men (5 percent) to have PTSD. About 3.6 percent of American adults ages 18 to 54 (5.2 million people) have PTSD during the course of a given year. The struggles of soldiers returning from deployments in Iraq and Afghanistan have raised awareness of the disorder and the extent of the debilitation it can cause. Though estimates of prevalence among Iraq and Afghanistan veterans vary from as low as 3 percent to as high as 30 percent, as many as twenty-two veterans take their own life every day, highlighting the effects of war on mental health.

PTSD can occur at any age, including during childhood. Each year in the United States, more than 5 million children are exposed to some form of extreme traumatic experience. These traumatic events include natural disasters, such as tornados, floods, and hurricanes; motor vehicle accidents; life-threatening illness and associated painful experiences, such as cancer or burns; and witnessing violence in the home or community. Over 30 percent of these traumatized children develop a clinical syndrome with emotional, behavioral, cognitive, social, and physical symptoms significant enough to be diagnosed as PTSD.

The neurobiology of PTSD differs from that of a normal response to fear or stress. The primary distinction is continued recurrence of the stress response well after the stressor or fear is no longer physically present.

As well as psychological symptoms, clinical PTSD is marked by clear neurobiological and physiological changes. The neurobiology is complex, involving dysregulation of neurotransmitters, such as serotonin and norepinephrine, as well as the sympathetic nervous system (fight or flight) and HPA axis. Dysfunction in these systems may lead to disturbances in the processes of perception, learning, and memory.

Alterations are seen in both the central and autonomic nervous systems, causing altered brainwave activity, decreased volume of the hippocampus, and abnormal activation of the amygdala. Both the hippocampus and the amygdala are involved in the processing and integration of memory. The amygdala has also been found to be involved in coordinating the body's fear response.

Psychophysiological alterations associated with PTSD include hyperarousal of the sympathetic nervous system, increased sensitivity of the startle reflex, and sleep abnormalities. The core symptoms are reliving the experience through nightmares or flashbacks, having difficulty sleeping, feeling detached and estranged from activity or other people, and experiencing impairment of daily life.

The first study of TM as an intervention for PTSD was conducted with Vietnam combat veterans.[15] This randomized controlled trial showed a 52 percent reduction in anxiety symptoms, a 46 percent reduction in depression, and a 40 percent reduction in PTSD symptoms after three months' practice of the technique. There were also dramatic reductions in insomnia and use of alcohol. The control group showed little to no improvement. A small pilot study of Iraq and Afghanistan veterans showed similar results: 48 percent reduction in PTSD symptoms, an 87 percent improvement in depression, and significant improvements in quality of life after two months' practice of TM.[16]

In a study reported by the University of Minnesota and the Minneapolis Veterans Affairs Medical Center, seventeen subjects received instruction in TM. At the eight-week follow-up, the eight subjects for whom the researchers had both pre- and post-test data averaged a 14-point decrease on the Post Traumatic Stress Disorder Checklist—Military (PCL-M; $p = 0.0011$).[17] A study of Congolese refugees further demonstrated the strong effects of TM for PTSD. In a matched single-blind pilot study of Congolese refugees in Uganda, a group of twenty-one who learned TM was matched with a control group on age, sex, and baseline scores on the Post Traumatic Stress Disorder Checklist—Civilian (PCL-C).[18] At post-test, the PCL-C scores in the control group trended upward. In contrast, the PCL-C scores in the TM group went from 65 on average at baseline, indicating severe post-traumatic stress symptoms, to below 30 on average after 30 days of TM, and the scores remained low at 135 days.

A reduction in symptoms was even more dramatic in a follow-up study.[19] Eleven subjects who were waitlist controls from the original study were taught TM. Measurements of PTSD symptoms were taken at baseline and at 10 days and 30 days post-instruction. Average PCL–C scores dropped 29.9 points, from 77.9 to 48.0 in 10 days, then dropped another 12.7 points to 35.3 at 30 days.

Pain often accompanies PTSD, and stress exacerbates pain. TM has been shown to have an effect on the brain's response to pain. A study of long-term TM meditators (thirty years of practice) found a 40–50 percent reduction in the brain's reactivity to pain, particularly in the frontal cortex and the anterior cingulate.[20] After practicing TM for five months, the control group also demonstrated 40–50 percent decreased pain reactivity. This is particularly interesting in light of the overlap of brain systems that mediate physical pain and social/psychological pain.[21]

While to date there are no published studies on the effect of TM on pain in the presence of PTSD, there are numerous anecdotal reports of reduction in pain. As one example, before learning TM, a soldier in an Army traumatic-brain-injury clinic reported baseline pain at a rating of 8 on a scale of 10. A few days after practicing TM, he reported his pain at 3.

APPLICATIONS OF TM FOR ANXIETY TREATMENT

TM is easily learned in a seven-step process. TM centers are found in most major American, Canadian, and European cities, as well as in several third-world countries. It can be "prescribed" by a healthcare clinician, which can result in a significant fee reduction of several hundred dollars. TM is very easy, and patients regularly report great satisfaction in learning and practicing this mental technique.

CASE STUDIES

The following brief case presentations from one of our clinical practices illustrate the improvement in patient functioning that can result from TM.

Case 1

A nineteen-year-old college student suffering from severe, chronic, disabling GAD and panic disorder showed poor response to cognitive-behavioral and client-centered psychotherapy as well as several minor tranquilizers and antidepressants. At the time, he was being maintained on diazepam, 10 mg, po, tid with modest results. He reported growing alcohol use to control anxiety. After one month of practicing TM, his panic attacks, which had occurred several times a day, subsided. He reported a dramatic drop in worrisome thoughts. Within three months of meditation practice, his anxiety levels dropped so low that his medication was withdrawn without ill effects. At a six-month follow-up, he was essentially free of all symptoms of both anxiety disorders. He was able to avoid inpatient treatment and ongoing pharmacotherapy, and he finished his third year of college with a 3.75 cumulative grade-point average.

Case 2

A twenty-two-year-old, male suffering from severe social anxiety disorder and obsessive compulsive disorder presented for outpatient treatment. He reported nearly continual obsessive thoughts about violence and fears of engaging in violent behaviors. He countered the thoughts while playing hard rock music on his iPhone. This was followed by repeated listening to more hard rock to cancel out, in his mind, disturbing violent lyrics in songs he was playing. He had a compulsion to avoid driving on certain stretches of road near his home. His obsessions and compulsion became continual, requiring him to drop out of college. He was maintained on Zoloft 200 mg, po, qd with only slight effects.

After three months of cognitive-behavioral therapy and response prevention and exposure techniques with inadequate response, he learned TM. Results were immediate. Though he reported thinking violent thoughts while meditating, he had little or no negative affective reaction to them. This began to generalize to activity outside of meditation. The compulsion to listen to hard rock music as a ritual to lower anxiety markedly diminished. His avoidant behavior while driving was entirely extinguished with continued regular meditation and therapeutic directions to confront feared driving routes by driving them repeatedly. After four months of meditation practice, his obsessions and compulsions and reports of anxiety were nearly nonexistent. He returned to college. The dosage of his Zoloft was reduced by 50 percent. He continued in psychotherapy with reports of growing effectiveness of this process.

Case 3

A twenty-four-year-old unemployed Army National Guard veteran entered treatment following two deployments to Afghanistan and Iraq. He saw significant combat and sustained serious injuries, consequently resulting in chronic pain. His diagnoses were PTSD and major depression. He reported continuous suicidal and self-destructive thoughts and urges, escalating alcohol abuse, insomnia, and flashbacks several times daily. He had one inpatient psychiatric stay and was given trials on several antidepressants and antianxiety agents with poor results.

After six weeks of psychotherapy, he learned TM through the David Lynch Foundation Operation Warrior Wellness program. Results came quickly. He reported growing "inner peace," less anger and agitation, and better sleep within one week of learning TM. He referred to his twice-daily meditation sessions as "my safe place." After four months of TM practice and psychotherapy, he reported an absence of suicidal thoughts, improved mood, markedly decreased flashbacks, as well as greater interest in social relationships and his daily activities. He got a job and began a distance-learning degree program majoring in psychology. At a ten-month follow up, he reported being symptom free and was compliant with regular TM.

HOW DOES TM WORK?

In the stress response, the brain floods with adrenaline. The lungs pump faster, and the heart starts to race. Blood pressure rises, stimulating the muscles and sharpening the mind on a single reference point: the stressor. The stomach gets "jumpy," and the release of endorphins numbs the body. Appetite, libido, and the immune system shut down. All the energy normally directed to these functions is redirected to the muscles. This is the fight or flight response. This response gives a person the strength to do extraordinary feats.

Once the stress or challenge is removed, the nervous system returns to baseline . . . or should. The ability to achieve stability through change is critical to survival. But the price of this constant accommodation to stress can be overload, causing wear and tear on the system. Over time, stress and the continuing physiological response to it can become debilitating. The system breaks down.

This kind of stress causes neurobiological, physiological, and psychological changes that easily trigger the fight or flight response, even when it is not needed. The brain chemistry is actually altered. Disruption in these systems can cause hypervigilance. It is the source of "re-experiencing." This also explains the startle reflex, such as jumping to reach for a weapon at the sound of a loud noise or the inability to control an anger response. Chronic stress, being in the fight or flight response mode for an extended period, can recalibrate the stress response, making it difficult to return to baseline, thus causing the body to lose physical and emotional resilience.

TM can help restore the resilience. TM creates a physiological response opposite to the stress response. During the practice of TM, the mind settles down, experiencing quieter states of awareness. Mental activity becomes less and less until one *transcends* active thought. The state of *pure consciousness* predominates (see chapter 1, this volume). This is considered the simplest form of awareness: a restful, wakeful, integrated, hypometabolic state.[22,23] In this state, the mind goes beyond the objects of awareness, such as thoughts, feelings, physical sensations and impulses, and the consciousness is left alone to experience its own nature; that is, consciousness *becomes conscious of itself*. This is an inherently peaceful, even blissful state of awareness.

As the mind settles down, the body becomes deeply relaxed. As the thinking process continues to refine through the technique, the mind transcends mental activity to experience deep silence. This produces a unique state of consciousness: transcendental consciousness (TC).

In TC, the mind is alert, while the body is deeply relaxed. The body settles into deep rest—the heart rate slows, the breathing slows and becomes shallower, blood pressure is reduced, and the flow of blood to the arms and legs is reduced, similar to how the body is during sleep—but the mind remains alert and aware. During these periods of transcendence, deep stresses are dissolved.

The brain chemistry is also changed. Cortisol is reduced, decreasing stress, anxiety, fear, and anger. Serotonin is increased, improving mood, anxiety, and depression. Adrenaline levels become balanced, improving overall thinking, attention, focus, planning, and organization. The intellect and logic are more functional; consequently, the person is able to recognize, for example, and mentally process a trashcan as a trashcan and not, for example, as an improvised explosive device (IED).

With regular practice of TM, stress is reduced, mood is naturally elevated, and the brain functions optimally. In other words, the individual can bounce back, being more resilient. Overtime, this resilience is sustained longer and longer after the meditation session. As a result of reduced stress, the person feels more relaxed throughout the day and usually has more energy. His or her anger begins to dissipate, and normal emotions return.

The experience of transcending is accompanied by a number of psychophysiological changes in the brain and body as documented by a wealth of research studies. Effects include

- reduced breath rate
- slower heart rate
- decreased serum cortisol
- increased serum serotonin
- decreased blood lactate
- reduced autonomic arousal

- reduced systolic and diastolic blood pressure
- normalization of the HPA axis
- increased EEG brain-wave coherence

These changes are to be expected to some degree in any technique that leads to lower autonomic and CNS arousal and a reduction in accompanying symptoms and signs of pathological anxiety. The additional psychophysiological changes and enhancement of cognitive, affective, and perceptual processes resulting from the practice of the technique are impressive.[24]

Perhaps the most widely documented and important effect of TM is the integration and balance of brain functioning, expressed as EEG coherence among all brain regions.[25-28] This global neurophysiological coherence, unique to TM, is correlated with greatly increased, organized, and enhanced cognitive abilities, including increased

- creativity
- academic performance
- neurological efficiency
- concept learning
- moral reasoning
- IQ
- affective stability
- problem-solving ability
- field independence

These changes, unique to TM, are coextensive with the reduction in anxiety reported in this chapter and may account, in part, for the added effectiveness of TM relative to other approaches.[29] As anxiety levels subside, creativity, intellectual problem-solving, cognitive and perceptual flexibility, and other executive functions are allowed to expand. As a result, the practice of TM is a useful tool to assist the meditating patient in developing better coping skills and raising his or her overall level of psychological functioning (see chapter 8, this volume).

CONCLUSION

Mental health disorders represent a significant problem today, with their prevalence continuing to increase. Anxiety is a major contributing factor to these rising numbers. The research findings on TM, as well as the anecdotal stories of sometimes life-transforming improvements, have significant implications for the management of anxiety disorders. Additionally, patients with anxiety and anxiety disorders rarely present for treatment with only one psychiatric disorder; most have two or more diagnosable disorders that can complicate the assessment and treatment of the patient. The presence of psychiatric comorbidity typically demands a more complex, varied treatment approach.

The research and clinical findings support TM as an effective treatment for many co-occurring psychiatric disorders. The inclusion of TM in the patient's treatment plan can be a particularly cost effective and significantly less time-intensive means for the greatest symptom reduction or for remission in the shortest period of time.

Given the research presented here, further study not only on the effects of TM on anxiety disorders, but also on the study of the combined effects on anxiety of TM with conventional treatments and with newer medications and various forms of psychotherapy is a worthwhile endeavor. In addition, exploring newly developed therapies derived from the ancient Vedic tradition from which TM originates[30] is an important, promising, and worthy effort.

NOTES

1. R. Kessler, "Lifetime Morbid Risk of Anxiety and Mood Disorders in the U.S.," *International Journal of Psychiatric Methods in Research* 21, no. 3 (2012): 164–86.

2. E. M. Goldner, P. H. Waraich, and J. M. Somers, "Prevalence and Incidence Studies of Anxiety Disorders," *Canada Journal of Psychology* 51, no. 2 (2006): 100–13.

3. S. M. Stahl, *Essential Psychopharmacology—Neuroscientific Basis and Practical Applications* (New York: Cambridge University Press, 2000).

4. B. C. Glueck and C. F. Stroebel, "Biofeedback and Meditation in the Treatment of Psychiatric Illness," *Comprehensive Psychiatry* 16, no. 4 (1975): 4.

5. B. C. Glueck and C. F. Stroebel, "Meditation in the Treatment of Psychiatric Illness," *Meditation: Classic and Contemporary Perspectives* (New York: Alden Publications, 1984).

6. E. M. Sibinga and K. J. Kemper, "Complementary, Holistic and Integrative Medicine: Meditation Practice for Pediatric Health," *Pediatrics in Review/American Academy of Pediatrics* 31, no. 12 (2012): e95–e96.

7. S. L. Shapiro and R. Walsh, "An Analysis of Recent Meditation Research and Suggestions for Future Directions," *Humanistic Psychologist* 31, nos. 2–3 (2003): 69–90.

8. C. Elder, S. Nidich, S. Colbert, J. Hagelin, L. Grayshield, D. Oviedo-Lim, M. Rainforth, C. Jones, and D. Gerace, "Reduced Psychological Distress in Racial and Ethnic Minority Students Practicing the Transcendental Meditation Program," *Journal of Instructional Psychology* 38, no. 2 (2011): 109–16.

9. K. Eppley, A. I. Abrams, and J. Shear, "Differential Effects of Relaxation on Trait Anxiety: A Meta-analysis," *Journal of Clinical Psychology* 45, no. 6 (1989): 957–74.

10. D. Sedlmeier, Eberth, Schwartz, Zimmerman, F. Haarig, S. Jaeger, and S. Kunze, "The Psychological Effects of Meditation: A Meta-analysis," *Psychological Bulletin* 138, no. 6 (2012): 1139.

11. E. M. Dornelas, "The Effects of Yoga and Meditation on Cardiovascular Aging," *Stress Proof the Heart: Behavioral Interventions for Cardiac Patients*, ed. E. M. Dornelas (New York: Springer Science+Business Media, 2012), 227.

12. M. V. Rainforth, R. H. Schneider, S. I. Nidich, G. King, J. W. Salerno, and J. W. Anderson, "Stress Reduction Programs in Patients with Elevated Blood Pressure: A Systematic Review and Meta-analysis," *Current Hypertension Reports* 9, no. 6 (2007).

13. K. W. Chen, C. C. Berger, D. P. Forde, J. F. Magidson, L. Dachman, and C. W. Leguez, "Meditative Therapies for Reducing Anxiety: A Systematic Review and Meta-analysis of Randomized, Controlled Trials," *Depression and Anxiety* 29, no. 7 (2012): 11–12.

14. D. W. Orme-Johnson and V. Barnes, "Effects of Transcendental Meditation Practice on Trait Anxiety: A Meta-analysis of Controlled Trials," *Journal of Alternative and Complementary Medicine* 19, no. 10 (2013).

15. J. S. Brooks and T. Scarano, "Transcendental Meditation in the Treatment of Post–Viet Nam Adjustment," *Journal of Counseling and Development* 64 (1985).

16. J. Rosenthal, S. Grosswald, R. Ross, and N. Rosenthal, "Effects of Transcendental Meditation (TM) in Veterans of Operation Enduring Freedom (OEF) and Operation Iraqi Freedom (OIF) with Posttraumatic Stress Disorder (PTSD): A Pilot Study," *Military Medicine* 176, no. 6 (2011).

17. K. O. Lim, G. Lamberty, M. Kukowski, P. Thuras, C. Erbes, and M. Polusny, "Transcendental Meditation for the Treatment of PTSD in Veterans," presentation at the 52nd Annual Meeting of the American College of Neuropharmacology, Hollywood, FL, December 8–12, 2013.

18. B. Rees, F. Travis, D. Shapiro, and R. Chant, "Reduction in Post-traumatic Stress Symptoms in Congolese Refugees Practicing Transcendental Meditation," *Journal of Traumatic Stress* 26 (2013).

19. B. Rees, F. Travis, D. Shapiro and R. Chant, "Significant Reduction in Post-traumatic Stress Symptoms in Congolese Refugees within 10 Days of Transcendental Meditation Practice," *Journal of Traumatic Stress Studies* 27 (2014).

20. D. W. Orme-Johnson, R. H. Schneider, Y. D. Son, S. Nidich, and Z. H. Cho, "Neuroimaging of Meditation's Effect on Brain Reactivity to Pain," *NeuroReport* 17, no. 12 (2006).

21. N. I. Eisenberger, M. D. Lieberman, and K. D. Williams, "Does Rejection Hurt? An FMRI Study of Social Exclusion," *Science* 302, no. 5643 (2003): 290–92.

22. R. K. Wallace, "Physiological Effects of Transcendental Meditation," *Science* 167 (1970).

23. R. K. Wallace, H. Benson, and A. F. Wilson, "Wakeful Hypometabolic Physiological State," *American Journal of Physiology* 221 (1971).

24. S. L. Shapiro, "Meditation and Positive Psychology," In *Oxford Handbook of Positive Psychology*, ed. S. Lopez et al. (New York: Oxford University Press, 2009).

25. D. W. Orme-Johnson and C. T. Haynes, "EEG Phase Coherence, Pure Consciousness, Creativity and TM/Sidhi Experiences," *International Journal of Neuroscience* 13 (1981).

26. M. C. Dillbeck and E. C. Bronson, "Short-term Longitudinal Effects of the Transcendental Meditation Technique on EEG Power and Coherence," *International Journal of Neuroscience* 14 (1981).

27. M. C. Dillbeck and S. Araas-Veseley, "Participation in the Transcendental Meditation Program and Frontal EEG Coherence During Concept Learning," *International Journal of Neuroscience* 29 (1986).

28. F. Travis and A. Arenander, "Cross-sectional and Longitudinal Study of the Effects of Transcendental Meditation Practice on Interhemispheric Frontal Asymmetry and Frontal Coherence," *International Journal of Neuroscience* 116 (2006).

29. K. Eppley, A. I. Abrams, and J. Shear, "Differential Effects of Relaxation on Trait Anxiety: A Meta-analysis," *Journal of Clinical Psychology* 45, no. 6 (1989): 957–74.

30. R. W. Boyer, *Vedic Principles of Therapy: A Holistic Consciousness-Based Approach* (Malibu, CA: Institute for Advanced Research, 2012).

BIBLIOGRAPHY

Boyer, R. W. *Vedic Principles of Therapy: A Holistic Consciousness-Based Approach.* Malibu, CA: Institute for Advanced Research, 2012.

Brooks, J. S. and Scarano, T. "Transcendental Meditation in the Treatment of Post-Viet Nam Adjustment." *Journal of Counseling and Development* 64 (1985): 212–14.

Chen, K. W., Christine, C., Berger, E. M., Forde, D., Magidson, J., Dachman, L., and Leguez, C. W. "Meditative Therapies for Reducing Anxiety: A Systematic Review and Meta-analysis of Randomized, Controlled Trials." *Depression and Anxiety* 29, no. 7 (2012): 1, 11–12.

Dillbeck, M. C. "The Effects of the Transcendental Meditation Technique on Anxiety Levels." *Journal of Clinical Psychology* (1977): 1076–78.

Dillbeck, M. C. and Araas-Veseley, S. "Participation in the Transcendental Meditation Program and Frontal EEG Coherence During Concept Learning." *International Journal of Neuroscience* 29 (1986): 45–55.

Dillbeck, M. C., and Bronson, E. C. "Short-term Longitudinal Effects of the Transcendental Meditation Technique on EEG Power and Coherence." *International Journal of Neuroscience* 14 (1981): 147–51.

Dornelas, E. M. "The Effects of Yoga and Meditation on Cardiovascular Aging." In *Stress Proof the Heart: Behavioral Interventions for Cardiac Patients*, edited by E. M. Dornelas. New York: Springer Science+Business Media, 2010.

Elder, C., Nidich, S., Colbert, R., Hagelin, J., Grayshield, L., Oviedo-Lim, D., Nidich, S., Rainforth, M., Jones, C., and Gerace, D. "Reduced Psychological Distress in Racial and Ethnic Minority Students Practicing the Transcendental Meditation Program." *Journal of Instructional Psychology* 38, no. 2 (2011): 109–16.

Eppley, K., Abrams, A. I., and Shear, J. "Differential Effects of Relaxation Techniques on Trait Anxiety: A Meta-analysis." *Journal of Clinical Psychology* 45, no. 6 (1989): 957–74.

Glueck, B. C., and Stroebel, C. F. "Biofeedback and Meditation in the Treatment of Psychiatric Illness." *Comprehensive Psychology* 16, no. 4 (1975).

Glueck, B. C., and Stroebel, C. F. "Meditation in the Treatment of Psychiatric Illness." *Meditation: Classic and Contemporary Perspectives* (New York: Alden Publications, 1984).

Goldner, E. M., Waraich, P. H., and Somers, J. M. "Prevalence and Incidence Studies of Anxiety Disorders: A Systematic Review of the Literature." *Canada Journal of Psychology* 51, no. 2 (2006): 100–13.

Haratani, T., and Hewmi, T. "Effects of Transcendental Meditation on Mental Health of Industrial Workers." *Japanese Journal of Industrial Health* 32 (1990): 656.

Lim, K. O., Lamberty, G., Kuskowski, M., Thuras, P., Erbes, C., and Polusny, M. "Transcendental Meditation for the Treatment of PTSD in Veterans." Presentation at the 52nd Annual Meeting of the American College of Neuropharmacology, Hollywood, FL, December 8–12, 2013.

Kessler, R. C., Sampson, N. A., Wittchen, H. U., Petukwa, M., and Zaslasky, A. M. "Lifetime Morbid Risk of Anxiety and Mood Disorders in the US." *International Journal of Methods in Psychiatric Research* 21, no. 3 (2012): 164–86.

Orme-Johnson, D. W., and Barnes, V. "Effects of Transcendental Meditation Practice on Trait Anxiety: A Meta-analysis of Controlled Trials." *Journal of Alternative and Complementary Medicine* 19, no. 10 (2013): 1–12.

Orme-Johnson, D. W., and Haynes, C. T. "EEG Phase Coherence, Pure Consciousness, Creativity and TM/Sidhi Experiences." *International Journal of Neuroscience* 13 (1981): 211–17.

Rainforth, M. V., Schneider, R. H., Nidich, S. I., Gaylord-King, C., Salerno, J. W., and Anderson, J. W. "Stress Reduction Programs in Patients with Elevated Blood Pressure: A Systematic Review and Meta-analysis." *Current Hypertension Reports* 9, no. 6 (2007): 520–28.

Rees, B., Travis, F., Shapiro, D., and Chant, R. 2013. "Reduction in Posttraumatic Stress Symptoms in Congolese Refugees Practicing Transcendental Meditation." *Journal of Traumatic Stress* 26 (2013): 295–98.

Rees, B., Travis, F., Shapiro, D., and Chant, R. "Significant Reduction in Posttraumatic Stress Symptoms in Congolese Refugees within 10 Days of Transcendental Meditation Practice." *Journal of Traumatic Stress* 27 (February 2014): 112–15.

Rosenthal, J., Grosswald, S., Ross, R., and Rosenthal, N. "Effects of Transcendental Meditation (TM) in Veterans of Operation Enduring Freedom (OEF) and Operation Iraqi Freedom (OIF) with Posttraumatic Stress Disorder (PTSD): A Pilot Study." *Military Medicine* 176, no. 6 (2011): 626–30.

Sedlmeier, D., Eberth, J., Schwartz, M., Zimmerman, D., Haarig, F., Jaeger, S., and Kunze, S. "The Psychological Effects of Meditation: A Meta-analysis." *Psychological Bulletin* 138, no. 6 (2012): 1139–17.

Shapiro, S. L., and Walsh, R. "An Analysis of Recent Meditation Research and Suggestions for Future Directions." *Humanistic Psychologist* 31 nos. 2–3 (2003): 86–114.

Shapiro, S. L. "Meditation and Positive Psychology." In *Oxford Handbook of Positive Psychology*, edited by S. Lopez and C. R. Synders, 601–10. New York: Oxford University Press, 2009.

Sibinga, E. M., and Kemper, K. J. "Complementary, Holistic and Integrative Medicine: Meditation Practice for Pediatric Health." *Pediatrics in Review/American Academy of Pediatrics* 31, no. 12 (2010): e95–e96.

Stahl, S. M. *Essential Psychopharmacology—Neuroscientific Basis and Practical Applications.* New York: Cambridge University Press, 2000.

Stroebel, C. F., and Glueck, B. C. "Passive Meditation: Subjective, Clinical and Electrographic Comparison with Biofeedback." In *Consciousness and Self-Regulation,* edited by G. E. Schwartz and D. Shapiros. New York: Plenum Press, 1978.

Travis, F., and Arenander, A. "Cross–sectional and Longitudinal Study of the Effects of Transcendental Meditation Practice on Interhemispheric Frontal Asymmetry and Frontal Coherence." *International Journal of Neuroscience* 116, no. 12 (2006): 1519–38.

Travis, F., Haaga, D. A., Hagelin, J., Tanner, M., Nidich, S., Gaylord-King, C. et al. "Effects of Transcendental Meditation Practice on Brain Functioning and Stress Reactivity in College Students." *International Journal of Psychophysiology* 71, no. 2 (2009): 170–76.

Wallace, R. K. "Physiological Effects of Transcendental Meditation." *Science* 167 (1970): 1751–54.

Wallace, R. K., Benson, H., and Wilson, A. F. "A Wakeful Metabolic Physiological State." *American Journal of Physiology* 221 (1971): 795–99.

SEVEN

Transcendental Meditation in the Treatment of Depression

James S. Brooks, M.D.

Depression remains one of the most common of the mental illnesses. In any given year, 6.7 percent of adults will experience a major depressive episode. Women are 70 percent more likely to develop major depression than men during their lifetime. Depression is an illness that often goes untreated. Only about 50 percent of individuals who develop depression receive treatment, and it is estimated that in one-third of these cases, this treatment is "minimally adequate."[1] According to the Centers for Disease Control, about 1 in 10 adults suffers from depression and most are between the ages of 45 and 64.[2] But depression is not only a problem for adults. According to the National Association of Mental Illness, 28 percent of adolescents who present for primary care treatment have a diagnosis of depression, and in any given year, 1 out of 5 teenagers is experiencing depression. The same organization notes that in studies of "point prevalence," about 2 percent of school-age children are experiencing major depression.[3]

A complicating factor in the identification and treatment of depression is that many individuals who suffer from this disorder do not even know that they have it. For example, depression can often take the form of physical symptoms and complaints which essentially mask the underlying causes of the real illness of depression. Individuals rarely come to their family physician and tell their doctor that they feel depressed. More commonly, physicians hear complaints such as these: I am exhausted all the time; I have no get up and go; I have no sex drive; I can't feel my emotions; I am numb; I don't sleep well at night; I can't concentrate at work; I'm so irritable all the time. These complaints are what are termed *neurovegetative* signs of depression and can occur with or without the feelings

137

of deep sadness that come to mind when one thinks of depression. Some clinicians call these symptoms "depressive equivalents."

During any six-month period, at least 9 million American adults are suffering from depression. Countless millions of others suffer from minor periods of sadness, low energy, and lack of motivation. Everyone experiences "the blues" at times, whether caused by external circumstances, internal conflicts and indecision, hormones, or by being overwhelmed, overworked, and fatigued. Feeling blue can be associated with mild or moderate depression or can be a normal expression of the stresses of life. Distinguishing the normal emotions of depression from an actual depressive illness is the job of a medical or mental health professional. Depression and depressive symptoms are often underreported or not reported at all in primary care settings because of the continued stigma of mental illness and misinformation about the disease of depression.

Although Western psychiatry has made significant progress toward treating and reducing the symptoms of depression, treatment continues to be difficult. Fully 30–40 percent of patients do not respond to antidepressant medications, and often multiple trials on several medications are needed. Augmentation strategies with two or more antidepressants prescribed concurrently or the addition of other psychiatric medications may be required in particularly difficult cases. Additionally, many patients experience what is known as "poop out" with their medications as the medications' clinical effects wear off after a period of time, leaving many patients feeling desperate, weary, and wary of future treatments for their illness.

Depression is a serious, chronic illness and is considered a mood disorder, characterized by recurrence and relapse. It is often a lifelong disorder. Depression is typically treated through pharmacotherapy and psychotherapy. On the positive side, many new medications to treat depression have been developed over the past two decades.[4] However, a number of these medications have strong, unpleasant side effects that reduce treatment compliance for the patient expected to take them. Many patients taking an antidepressant stop the medication without informing their doctor because of the side-effect profile. Moreover, depression is often accompanied by other comorbid psychiatric disorders, for example, anxiety disorders. Some studies indicate that this combination occurs in at least 50 percent of cases of depression. Other comorbid problems include alcohol abuse, drug abuse, and personality disorders.

Despite advances in the understanding of depression as an illness and a search for its etiology, Western medicine has formulated a number of theories but has not identified a definitive cause or causes for depression. Likewise, there are no proven ways in Western medicine to prevent the development of depression, although some progress is being made in this area[5] and current conventional treatments are of limited efficacy.[6]

The treatment of depression can become quite complex, especially when the depression is atypical, intractable, or poorly responsive to various treatments. Patients may receive one, two, or even three antidepressants concurrently. Augmentation strategies may involve the inclusion of an atypical antipsychotic medicine, such as apiprizole, or a mood stabilizer, such as lithium, to potentiate the effects of the antidepressant medication. Some patients may even be treated with psychostimulant medicines that are typically used to treat attention deficit hyperactivity disorder (ADHD). In severe cases, electro-convulsive therapy (ECT) can offer some help for severely depressed patients.

Much has been written about the conventional treatments for depression. In this chapter, Transcendental Meditation (TM®), a natural form of treatment for depression which has been shown to be very effective in many cases of this disorder, and which is without side effects, will be considered. TM is a treatment modality that does not involve taking a medication. Rather, it is a *technique* which is simple, natural, and easy to learn and practice. Meditation is typically practiced twice daily for twenty minutes. There is a growing trend among mental health professionals worldwide to include TM in their treatment arsenal, and many have pursued professional training in learning to teach this technique.

Early research[7] has identified the positive effects of the use of TM in treating depression and other psychiatric disorders in an inpatient psychiatric setting. In one study,[8] significant decreases in depressive symptomatology were achieved within three months of the practice of TM, and at one year there was a 50 percent decrease in the symptoms of depression through the practice of TM alone. Although research on the use of TM to treat depression, either alone or in combination with conventional treatments, is in its preliminary stages, initial studies indicate significant promise in the application of this mental technique for this disorder.[9]

Some recent studies show the benefit of using TM to reduce symptoms of depression.[10] These studies included African Americans and native Hawaiians, fifty-five years and older, who were at risk for cardiovascular disease. Researchers placed participants randomly in a TM group or in a health education control group. Study members were then assessed using a standard test for depression called the Center for Epidemiologic Studies Depression Scale (CES-D). The study was over a twelve-month period. Results indicated clinically meaningful reductions in depressive symptoms.

TM originates in an ancient tradition of natural medicine from India termed *Ayurveda*. Ayurvedic texts date back 5,000 years.[11] More recently,

Maharishi Mahesh Yogi has rediscovered, reinterpreted, and presented these texts to the world. The resurgence of interest in Ayurveda brings a new perspective to the treatment of depression and a fresh wave of hope for millions of sufferers of depression. Ayurveda appears to offer a more complete understanding of the nature and causes of depression, suggests effective treatments that have no side effects, and shows indications that it can play a role in the prevention of depression, while research indicates it promotes higher levels of psychological health in general.[12]

In the following discussion, depression will be considered as it is understood in allopathic Western medicine, and then this position will be contrasted with the Vedic understanding of TM. It is my belief that the application of TM to the treatment of depression offers great hope to suffering individuals who are struggling to overcome depression with only conventional modalities. One of the reasons for this optimism is that TM works in a truly holistic fashion. The practice of this technique "treats" the person's entire physiology, psychology, and spirituality at the same time and enriches all these domains of a person's life.

THE WESTERN PERSPECTIVE ON THE STATE OF DEPRESSION

In the state of depression, life loses its charm. The sufferer feels that nothing in life matters, thinking becomes pessimistic, and feelings of hopelessness and helplessness creep into one's mind. The future seems to be nothing but bleak. The sufferer of depression reports low energy, indecisiveness, and problems with concentrating and making even very simple decisions in day-to-day living. From a perceptual angle, life looks flat, static, and gray, and the sufferer of depression may even forget what it was like to feel non-depressed.

The following is a list of the most frequent symptoms of major depression.

- persistent, sad, or empty mood
- loss of interest in friends and usual activities
- insomnia, early morning awakening, or oversleeping
- anxiety, irritability, restlessness
- low energy, fatigue, "can't get going"
- poor appetite and weight loss or, at times, overeating and weight gain
- difficulty concentrating and making decisions
- decreased sex drive
- feelings of worthlessness and guilt
- feelings of hopelessness and helplessness

- frequent crying spells
- suicidal thoughts and even suicidal urges, plans, impulses, and behaviors

The severity and frequency of the above symptoms can vary from mild or moderate to profound, severe, and, ultimately, disabling.

THE PUTATIVE CAUSES OF DEPRESSION

Although the etiology of depression as an illness remains unknown, there are several theories and ideas about how it comes about. The first is external. A high degree of stress, such as the death of someone close, serious financial problems, or a prolonged stressful situation that seems inescapable or unresolvable (for example, a bad marriage, a tyrannical parent, an abusive spouse, parent, or relative) can contribute to depression. These external causes often lead to feelings of hopelessness and the feeling and idea that there is "no way out" of the problem.

A second domain in the consideration of the causes of depression is biological. A genetic predisposition to depression is apparently passed from one generation to the next, just as the tendency to develop a medical illness such as diabetes is passed on. This may explain why some individuals become depressed "out of the blue" with no obvious, external reason to stimulate a depressive episode. This is a common scenario in young adults in their twenties and thirties who develop depression for no apparent external reason.

A third contributory factor is psychological. An early psychoanalytic maxim for depression was that it is "anger turned inward." Although there is little or no research to back up this observation, the idea is that if a person is frustrated and angry for a prolonged period of time and does not express it, the anger may be turned back on the self, and the retroflexed feelings of anger and hatred will turn inward and contribute to the development of depression. Other psychological theories on the causes of depression (e.g., cognitive-behavioral therapy) focus on the role of dysfunctional thoughts, beliefs, and attitudes that are *depressogenic* and both predispose an individual to developing depression and worsen when the person is in a depressive state. Theorists from humanistic to existential backgrounds, as well as transpersonal or psychospiritual schools of thought, emphasize that a lack of purpose in life or the lack of a connection to a sense of spirituality can be a contributory factor in the development of depression. From a practical perspective, there is probably no single cause of depression. Depression is most likely a combination of all the factors considered above.

Whatever the causes of depression, one of the first lines of treatment is the use of psychotropic medications to correct an imbalance in the neurophysiology. This is the approach used by both Western medicine and natural therapies, although through different means.

TYPES OF DEPRESSION

The Diagnostic and Statistical Manual of Psychiatry–V reports three major types of depression.[13]

1. Adjustment Reaction—This type of depression can last weeks to months and usually follows some specific stressful event in one's life, such as divorce, job loss, or the death of a loved one. With time, the person usually recovers spontaneously. Psychotherapy utilized to facilitate self-understanding and provide emotional support, ventilation, and release, or the temporary use of antidepressant medications, can be helpful in relieving these symptoms, preventing their recurrence, and accelerating the healing process.
2. Dysthymic Disorder—This is a chronic form of depression with moderate symptoms which may linger for long periods of time, even for years. Individuals suffering from this kind of depression live in a kind of emotional desert: as the months and the years of depression drag on, they experience little pleasure in life, typically report very low energy, and feel genuine feelings of hopelessness concerning their future.
3. Major Depression—This form of depression is characterized by comparatively more severe symptoms than the above disorders, including dark moods, sleep disturbances, appetite disturbances, feelings of hopelessness, and often suicidal thoughts and impulses. Major depression is typically preceded by a prolonged period of stress. Biochemical and genetic factors are also frequently involved in the development of this disorder.

STANDARD TREATMENTS FOR DEPRESSION— BENEFITS AND LIMITATIONS

The first type of depression mentioned, adjustment reaction, frequently occurs spontaneously. It can respond positively to psychotherapy or behavioral therapy. Research shows the cognitive-behavioral approaches work particularly well for this type of depression. However, psychotherapy alone is rarely sufficient to treat major depression because biochemical imbalances in the brain must be addressed, so other treatments are generally required. There are several theories as to what these imbalances are, and the majority of the theories focus on a deficiency in various neurotransmitters in the brain, especially serotonin, norepinephrine, and dopamine.

The major approaches of Western psychiatric treatment for major depression are

1. Antidepressant medications—These often very strong medications are thought to act upon either of two neurotransmitter systems of the brain, norepinephrine and serotonin, and in some cases dopamine, when there is some deficiency or dysregulation in the synthesis or availability of these neurotransmitters.
2. Electro-convulsive therapy (ECT; known as "shock treatment" in the past)—This has enjoyed a recent resurgence in use and interest in research on its effects, and it can be very helpful in certain types of depression.

THE DRAWBACKS OF
CONVENTIONAL DEPRESSION TREATMENTS

Individuals who take psychiatric medications frequently suffer significant side effects. These can include dry mouth, tachycardia, jitteriness, constipation, sexual dysfunction (impotence, erectile dysfunction, lack of orgasm), dizziness, blurred vision, memory impairment, and weight gain. The memory loss often associated with ECT is frequently so severe that memory of the entire period surrounding the shock treatment is wiped out completely, and clinical experience has shown that many patients complain of more subtle, sustained memory impairments.

Even when psychotropic medications for depression successfully alleviate or eliminate depressive symptoms in the short run—which they frequently do accomplish—at least 50 percent of major depressions recur. In other words, the medications developed by allopathic medicine are effective for temporary relief of symptoms, but a long-range, enduring program to maintain mental and physical balance and minimize recurrence or relapse of a depressive episode is at present unknown.

This observation has led some psychiatrists and other physicians to advocate that individuals who have been treated for major depression remain on antidepressant medication continuously, even lifelong, even though they may have to endure unpleasant side effects throughout the treatment. Millions of individuals with depressions ranging from mild to severe are taking antidepressant medications on a daily basis and consequently have to deal with this dilemma. Natural herbal and nutritional treatments for depression are available, and in some instances, patients report benefit from these supplements, especially for milder forms of depression. Research into the benefit of these approaches continues.[14]

All the treatments for depression mentioned so far aim to restore people to their baseline, or premorbid, level of functioning prior to their development of the depressive illness. Western medicine has barely considered, much less pursued, approaches that assist the individual with depression to grow and develop to higher levels of happiness and functioning in contrast to returning to premorbid functioning. In most cases, such a goal is not seen as an option, and current methods to foster it are lacking.

Similarly, no effective, meaningful help is available for the depression and dysphoria experienced by tens of millions who are considered normal, healthy individuals. Most individuals experience minor depressive symptoms, or even a milder form of clinical depression, from time to time in their lives. These less-severe forms of depression have received little attention in the field of psychiatry. They may be dismissed as not serious enough to be addressed since they are not critical problems. However, even minor depression and depressive episodes can be very disabling. Symptoms such as insomnia, irritability, lack of energy, and other unpleasant symptoms associated with depression can seriously and adversely affect one's quality of life and work.

Likewise, even if an individual is aware that because of their family history, they are prone to developing depression, little can be done to prevent the manifestation of a depressive episode. The unfortunate truth is that modern medicine is still in its infancy in this regard. In the field of psychology in recent years, humanistic psychologists and others have realized that healthy lifestyles and practices can have a positive effect upon mental health in general, and interest is growing in the field of health psychology in applying the principles of preventive medicine to mental health, although this is in its early stages.

THE AYURVEDIC UNDERSTANDING OF DEPRESSION

Ayurveda is a source of immense knowledge of methods to treat depression in a natural, holistic way. Ayurvedic diagnostic procedures, such as a specialized way to palpate the radial pulse, along with a physical inspection of the body and mental-status examination in the hands of an Ayurvedic physician (*vaidya*), can be effective in determining which of the components of an individual's physiological and psychological makeup contain imbalances that can be addressed through Ayurvedic treatment methods.

In traditional Ayurvedic knowledge, there are three components or expressions of an individual physiology.

- *vata*—This is an aspect of the physiology responsible for movement and flow in the various systems in the body.
- *pita*—This component is associated with the metabolic processes in the body.
- *kapha*—This component is responsible for maintaining physiological and physical structure and fluid balance in the body.

Through Ayurvedic diagnostic methods, including those mentioned above, a physician trained in Ayurveda can determine which of these systems is out of balance and in what way. Ancient Ayurvedic medical textbooks, such as the *Charaka Samhita*, describe how these three components, or doshas, cause symptoms and diseases if imbalances in these systems are present; and in this case, they describe how these components relate to the development of depression. Individuals with a vata type of depression often show symptoms of agitation and anxiety with their depressive illness. Pita-related depression is characterized by marked irritability. A kapha type of depression is characterized by symptoms such as lethargy, sluggishness, and weight gain.

Ayurveda provides a wide array of effective treatment options for those suffering from depression as adjuncts to conventional approaches, or in some cases, alternative approaches to allopathic medical approaches to depression. Imbalances in the physiology, or the doshas, can be corrected by specific diets and recommendations for daily routines that promote balance in the physiology and the mind. There is extensive scientific research demonstrating that Ayurvedic treatment methods are effective in the treatment of depression.[14]

TRANSCENDENTAL MEDITATION

The most effective natural treatment among the many options available through Ayurveda is TM, an ancient form of meditation. Maharishi Mahesh Yogi restored this style of meditation and made it available to millions throughout the world nearly fifty years ago. Maharishi trained thousands of teachers of the TM technique in nearly every country in the world, making it easily available to learn worldwide.

The practice of TM is easy to learn from a qualified teacher (see chapter 2, this volume). In short, it involves simply closing the eyes and practicing a simple mental technique that results in the mind settling down to a very calm state while at the same time, paradoxically, remaining fully alert. This state of what has been termed "restful alertness" results in deep physiological relaxation throughout the body. This state of peaceful rest has been researched heavily, and studies have found that the rest achieved during a session of TM can be twice as deep as the rest an individual will get at the deepest point of sleep in the night. This deep rest is key to the effectiveness of TM. It leads to a release of deep stresses and fatigues that can include emotional as well as physical traumas and stresses that could be contributory to the development of depression and a multitude of other physical and mental illnesses. As noted by other authors in this book, there are more than six hundred published studies on the effect of TM on the mind and body and its induction of the state of restful alertness leading to improved mental, physical, and even societal health.[15]

As the research citations noted previously indicate, a number of scientific studies show that TM is very effective in the treatment of depression and other forms of psychopathology. The practice of TM results in a host of physiological changes in the neurohormonal systems of the body, which include improved levels and availability of serotonin, norepinephrine, and dopamine[16] and regulation and balance of the hypothalamic-pituitary-adrenocortical (HPA) axis, as well as a high degree of brain-wave coherence, indicating a balanced, integrated state of brain functioning.[17] These and other striking physiological changes that occur during the practice of TM can help explain why this particular meditation technique, in many cases, is as effective and in some instances even more effective than antidepressant medications and other allopathic treatments while being at the same time devoid of the negative side effects associated with these treatments.[18]

A VEDIC EXPLANATION OF THE EFFECTIVENESS OF TM

The scientific evidence for the use of TM in treating a wide variety of illnesses, including mental illnesses such as depression, is robust and is covered in other chapters in this volume. Although rarely discussed in the field of psychiatry, there is a role for the treatment of depression from a psychospiritual perspective. In this section, the Vedic concept of the nature of the Self is considered along with the usefulness of TM in building and restoring a healthy expression of the Self.

From the Vedic perspective, the Self is one's innermost spiritual center, and it is experienced during the practice of TM. The experience is characterized by deep feelings of inner peace, contentment, and joy often characterized as "bliss." When the individual's attention is directed exclusively outward to the objects of experience without the experience of meditation, one can easily lose touch with this inner, unbounded awareness and bliss of the Self. The experience of most individuals is that awareness, consciousness, and attention are directed outward toward the objects of perception. This outward orientation of awareness is described in the Vedic texts as "object referral." Conversely, the turning inward of consciousness during meditation to experience the Self is called "self-referral."

Self-referral is an experience and not an intellectual exercise or type of psychological introspection. When a depressed person looks within his or her mind, the experience may be nothing but darkness and hopeless thoughts and feelings. The inward turning of consciousness referred to in the Vedic system is not one of introspection or contemplation. Rather, it involves the transcendence of thoughts, feelings, and perceptions to experience what is known as the state of pure consciousness, which is the source of and underlies all thoughts, feelings, and perceptions. It is characterized by an experience of quietness or silence, a state known as "pure being." This state is said to be characterized by a sense of unboundedness and expansion.

The importance of the experience of the Self achieved during the practice of TM is extremely important and fundamental because ultimately all happiness comes from within. This statement may not be intuitively obvious and may seem extreme. An individual may ask, "What about my wife? What about my husband? What about the beauty of nature? What about my new house? What about my children? I derive great happiness from them." However, during the experience of a depressive episode, none of these outer experiences can alleviate depression and bring happiness. The fragile nature of these sources of happiness is exposed during a depressive episode. Happiness, joy, and bliss evade the sufferer of depression. It is also important to note that all of the sources of external happiness noted above are experienced internally. That is, they are metabolized through the mind of the individual. Without an inner awareness, there can be no perception or experience of happiness.

Family members and friends often experience great frustration in attempting to assist the depressed individual, asking them to consider the blessings that they have in life or other sources of happiness. It is as if the depressed individual is wearing a pair of darkened glasses and hence sees nothing but darkness everywhere, internally and externally. Nothing external can affect or change this basic, internal state of distorted darkness.

From the Vedic perspective, depression is an extreme form of object referral in which one completely loses touch with the inner experience and hence the bliss and happiness of the Self. It is as if during depression, the doors to a bank are locked and one is doomed to poverty due to the inaccessibility of the riches that lie therein. In desperation, the depressed person often goes to extremes to find some type of comfort outside his or her Self. These can include addictive behaviors such as substance abuse, sex abuse, gambling, alcohol abuse, and other activities designed to alter one's state of consciousness. These desperate attempts to seek an outer source of gratification can provide at least a temporary relief, and some of them do. However, all of them lead to increased problems that ultimately complicate the expression, course, and treatment of the depressive illness.

According to the Vedic perspective, the more one loses touch with the joy and freedom of the inner Self, the more one is bound to feel frustrated and unhappy. However, if the experience of the inner Self which accompanies the practice of TM is introduced, one has the opportunity to gain readmission into the inner dimension of the Self and all its fullness, and consequently, unhappiness begins to diminish and eventually disappear.

This principle is similar to that of the basic premise of the new field of positive psychology: To treat unhappiness, one increases happiness. From the Vedic perspective, darkness is diminished or eliminated by introducing or increasing light. An effective technique for this process is essential. TM is a simple but profound and very effective way of treating depression by introducing happiness, which can displace unhappiness and other symptoms of a depressive illness.

The following is an extended case study designed to personalize and humanize all the material presented in this chapter. This case study could be considered representative of the experiences of hundreds of patients who have learned TM to treat a depressive illness.

HEALING DEPRESSION WITH SELF-REFERRAL—A CASE HISTORY

When Mary first came for evaluation, she described herself as "a wreck." She hesitated to go to treatment but finally forced herself to seek help. Mary was a successful attorney with a good income, and she enjoyed being a lawyer. She had endured severe depression for months before she made an appointment with a psychiatrist. Her persistent feelings of darkness, helplessness, and despair had become unbearable and intolerable. She reported, "My life and my future seem empty." She went on to say, "I can barely force myself to go to work, even though I know I have to—I have children to support. I seem to have totally lost my appetite and I've lost about fifteen pounds. I toss and turn for hours before I fall asleep and I can't seem to make up my mind about anything." In addition, she reported frequent crying spells and a great deal of difficulty concentrating and functioning in her work environment.

Frightening memories from her childhood prompted Mary to attempt to harm herself, first by cutting herself with a knife, then by trying to drive off a bridge. These feelings became more powerful, and it was dangerous for her to be left alone with these impulses and ideas very active in her mind. She had to be psychiatrically hospitalized in a locked unit. She had 24-hour supervision. She received intensive individual and group psychotherapy in the hospital environment, but she reported that those experiences actually intensified her suicidal thoughts and the perceived severity of her depression.

In a clinical case of such profound, disabling depression with a patient such as Mary, Western psychiatry currently has two basic alternatives: antidepressant medications alone or in combination with adjunctive medications, or ECT. Mary refused ECT. Several medications from the various groups of antidepressants were attempted, but she proved to be extremely sensitive to them and experienced such uncomfortable side effects that she was unable to take clinically effective doses to diminish her symptoms of depression.

After several attempts with various pharmacotherapies, Mary's doctor decided it would be an appropriate time to discuss alternative or unconventional forms of treatment with Mary. Her physician, who had been trained in Ayurveda, told her that a central reason for her depression was a lack of contact with a deep aspect of her inner Self. He described this internal experience as a feeling of happiness and fullness and explained to her that she lacked access to and experience of this. This is the experience of self-referral. Mary was very receptive to this line of thinking, especially since the allopathic alternatives she received were less and less an option for her at this point in her illness. Despite her severely depressed state, she was able to appreciate that opening up to that part of her inner Self might be precisely what was needed to heal her life. She felt particularly drawn to meditation. Because she was so disgusted with the side effects of the medications she had taken, a natural approach which she could utilize by herself without drugs or a therapist and one which would be easy, effortless, and comfortable to perform seemed like a nearly miraculous, wonderful, and welcome change.

Mary was taught TM. She immediately enjoyed a deep experience of pure consciousness, a very quiet, peaceful level of awareness that meditators report, and she described the feeling as one of being "filled with light and happiness." Her meditation experience left her with such an intense degree of inner fullness that the experience and transformation startled her. Likewise, the nurses, doctors, and other mental health professionals of the psychiatric unit also appeared startled and surprised.

Within a few days—literally—most of her symptoms had disappeared. Her appearance was almost immediately brighter, and everyone could see her mood was significantly improved. She reported, "My appetite is back and I can concentrate better." Most importantly, she felt a strong desire to live. She saw many wonderful possibilities for her life, and the future did not look bleak but rather hopeful and exciting. From the darkness of suicidal despair, her outlook had become positive and hopeful in a brief period of time through the practice of this mental technique.

The magnitude and rapidity of the changes Mary experienced surprised even her psychiatrist. He wondered if the sudden transformation might be due to what is known as the placebo effect. Did the expectation that she would be helped by an alternative treatment trigger a merely temporary state of improvement? He kept her in the hospital for a few more days just to be certain. But the changes lasted and appeared genuine. Moreover, Mary continued to improve every day. She was compliant with and immensely enjoyed her twice-daily meditation sessions.

While she was in the hospital, Mary's transformation was measured biochemically using the dexamethasone suppression test, which at the time of her hospitalization was an accepted way to determine the degree of depression in some patients. High levels of cortisol are often correlated with high levels of stress, anxiety, and depression. The normal range in a non-depressed person is a serum cortisol level under 5. Before learning TM, Mary had measured as high as 41. Three weeks after learning TM and being released from the hospital, her serum cortisol level had dropped to 7. Her test scores on another commonly used measure of depression, the Hamilton Depression Rating Scale (HAM-D), also dropped significantly from a profound level of depression down into the normal range for mood. This occurred within a three-week period.

After hospitalization, with continued regular meditation combined with individual psychotherapy, Mary made more rapid progress. At twelve months, she was functioning extremely well, and she was working and continuing to feel better and better every day. The depression did not return. She appeared to be a different person, being much more self-reliant, independent, settled, trusting of others, and deeply appreciative of her meditation and the contribution it was making and had made to her life.

RESTORING SELF-REFERRAL

If this story sounds extreme (it is accurate except for a name change), consider hypothetically something that *might* have happened to Mary. When she finally sought help, she felt hopeless and trapped and she saw herself, as she said, "getting older, with no hope for happiness anywhere on the horizon." Her marriage had fallen apart months earlier, and she was lonely and struggling to maintain a good life for herself and her children.

Now suppose that by chance, she met a warm, loving, and responsible man, fell in love, and was loved in return. How would she feel? Her inner world would suddenly be so much brighter. The weight of hopelessness would fall away. Imagine the sense of joy and freedom she would feel, the almost intoxicating release from restricting boundaries. Now anything would seem possible.

But it would all be dependent upon the change in her outer circumstances. And that could change again, as is often the case in rebound relationships. The sense of freedom and blossoming possibilities gained from the experience of the inner Self is analogous to our hypothetical romance, with one added advantage: It is entirely one's own. It is not dependent upon a new romance or a new job. Mary did not have to rely on a change of outer circumstances. Inner happiness and joy bubbled up spontaneously, so depression began to dissolve. Life and progress again felt possible and desirable.

If meditation could turn around a depression as serious as Mary's, it can certainly shine light into the far less severe blue moods many people go through from time to time. That is why I always recommend meditation for depression (for those who are open to the idea of a natural approach), and indeed to everyone who wants to alleviate any form of mental or emotional distress.

I think it is important to mention that while some patients with depression may respond fully with TM as the primary method of treatment, others, in my experience, require a combination of medication and psychotherapy, along with TM. Sometimes other forms of natural medicine, such as diet, routine, exercise, herbs, and acupuncture, can help as well.

OTHER MOOD DISORDERS—BIPOLAR DISORDER

Most of the research and clinical experience with TM has focused on major depression. Recently several studies have indicated that individuals with bipolar disorder can benefit greatly from the addition of TM to their treatment regimen. Two such studies researched the use of TM for bipolar patients in a psychiatric hospital setting, and the subjects were patients with severe psychiatric illnesses, including schizophrenia and bipolar disorder.[19] Results indicated significant symptom reduction with the addition of TM to other conventional treatments for these extremely ill patients.

It is my experience in over thirty-five years of psychiatric practice that for patients who have had a diagnosis of bipolar disorder, the inclusion of TM can be a highly effective treatment adjunctive to medication in the comprehensive approach to the clinical management of bipolar illness. The main benefits of the addition of TM seem to be a better quality of life, more happiness, and more vitality and energy when the patient is experiencing a depressive episode. Another advantage of TM is greater balance in the physiology so that the frequency and severity of mood swings, particularly when triggered and exacerbated by stress, are diminished.

Similar experiences and results have been found with bipolar II patients. However, care must be taken when a patient is experiencing a florid, full-blown manic episode. It would be nearly impossible to teach TM to a patient during such a period because of their instability, erratic behavior, irrational thinking, and other symptoms associated with mania. However, once the manic episode is controlled with appropriate medications and the patient becomes stable and coherent, TM can be introduced and the patient can learn it properly and in an organized fashion.

In a small study by Rosenthal[20] with patients suffering from depression and bipolar disorder, eleven patients received immediate TM training, while fourteen were placed on a waiting list. Both groups continued with their previous medical treatments. A few from the TM group reported a drop in manic symptoms. However, the patient reports stated that depressive symptoms were especially relieved, and when Rosenthal inspected the results of TM, he noted, "Several patients reported increased calmness, improved focus, and improved ability to stay organized and set priorities—no surprise given TM's known effects on the prefrontal cortex."

TM helped bipolar patients improve their executive function just as it has done for people with anxiety disorders and attention deficit hyperactivity disorder. "All in all," reported Rosenthal, "our study suggests that TM might be very helpful for bipolar patients. In fact, all the clinicians who worked on the study are now referring certain of their bipolar patients, particularly those with residual depression, for TM training along with their other treatments."

CONCLUSION

I believe it is important to mention perhaps the most ground-breaking implications of the use of TM in the treatment of depression and other mental illnesses: prevention and promotion of mental health. Research studies and clinical experience have demonstrated that when practiced regularly, this meditation technique serves to prevent mental illnesses, including depression, from developing in the first place. This approach is referred to as *primary prevention*, and in my opinion, it should be the direction for modern medicine and psychiatry in the future.

The cost of mental illness and of depression in particular is staggering. The mental pain is incalculable. One out of seven patients with recurring depression commits suicide. Seventy percent of suicides have major depressive illness, and there are 30,000–35,000 suicides per year. The cost to society is also great, including family dysfunction, work absenteeism, decreased productivity, job-related injury, and reduced quality control in the workplace, among many other costs.

Finally, the idea that consciousness can be purified, can expand, develop, and grow to what are known as higher states of consciousness should also become a part of the treatment of mental health and medical illnesses.[21] Perhaps it should be a standard treatment and used to guide mental health workers in their training and work. These higher states of consciousness culminate in what has traditionally been termed *enlightenment*. They are real, they are concrete, and they are being increasingly documented by researchers (see chapter 2, this volume).

Epidemiologically, making TM available to the population at large would be a powerful, effective, preventive approach for the reduction of mental illness. It is a proven methodology for bringing higher levels of inner peace, joy, mental alertness, and clarity to all groups of people. This clearly has broad implications for the health of society (see chapter 11, this volume) and, even beyond that, cooperation, harmony, and peace among the peoples of the world.

NOTES

1. R. C. Kessler et al., "Lifetime Morbid Risk of Anxiety and Mood Disorders in the U.S.," *International Journal of Psychiatric Methods in Research* 21, no. 3 (2012): 164–86.

2. Center for Disease Control, www.cdc.gov./features/depression.

3. www.nami.org.

4. S. Stahl, *Essential Psychopharmacology-Neuroscientific Basis and Practical Applications* (New York: Cambridge University, 2013).

5. P. Cuijpers et al., "Preventing Depression: A Global Priority," *Journal of the American Medical Association* 307, no. 10 (2012): 1033–34.

6. G. Andrews et al., "Utilizing Survey Data to Inform Public Policy: Comparison of the Effectiveness of Treatment of 10 Mental Disorders," *British Journal of Psychiatry* 184 (2004): 526–33.

7. T. Candelent et al., "Teaching Transcendental Meditation in a Psychiatric Setting," *Hospital and Community Psychiatry* 26 (1975): 156–59.

8. L. F. Fergusson, A. J. Bonshek, and J. M. Bodigues, "Personality and Health Characteristics of Cambodian Undergraduates: A Case for Student Development," *Journal of Instructional Psychology* 22 (1995): 308–19.

9. C. N. Alexander et al., "Effects of the Transcendental Meditation Program on Stress Reduction: Health and Employee Development," *Stress, Anxiety and Coping* 6 (1993): 245–62.

10. S. Nidich and M. Toomey. "Transcendental Meditation, Reduced Symptoms of Depression, Randomized Controlled Mind-Body Intervention Trials," presented at the 31st Annual Meeting of the Society of Behavioral Medicine, Seattle, WA, April 9, 2010.

11. R. K. Sharma. *Charaka Samhita* (New Delhi, India: Ministry of Health and Family Planning, 2011).

12. H. S. Kasture et al., "Improvements in Mental Health with the Maharishi Ayurveda Panchkarma Program," presented at the 8th World Congress of the International College of Psychosomatic Medicine, Chicago, IL, September, 1985.

13. American Psychiatric Association, *Diagnostic and Statistical Manual of Mental Disorders—5th Edition* (Washington, DC: American Psychiatric Association Press, 2013).

14. J. S. Brooks and P. Anselmo, *Ayurvedic Secrets to Longevity and Total Health* (New York: Prentice Hall, 1995).

15. R. Chalmers and G. Clements, *Scientific Research on Maharishi's Transcendental Meditation and TM/Sidhi Program: Collected Papers, Volumes 2–4* (Vlodrop, The Netherlands: Maharishi Ayurveda University Press, 1989).

16. M. Bujatti and P. Reiderer, "Serotonin, Noradrenaline and Dopamine Metabolites in the Transcendental Meditation Technique," *Journal of Neural Transmission* 39 (1976): 257–67.

17. P. H. Levine, J. R. Hebert, C. T. Haynes, and U. Strobel, "EEG Coherence During the Transcendental Technique" (Psychophysiological Laboratory, Centre for the Study of Higher States of Consciousness, Maharishi European Research University, 1976).

18. J. S. Brooks and T. Scarano, "Transcendental Meditation in the Treatment of Post–Viet Nam Adjustment," *Journal of Counseling and Development* 64 (1985): 212–14.

19. N. E. Rosenthal, *Transcendence: Healing and Transformation through Transcendental Meditation* (New York: Tarcher-Penguin, 2011).

20. Ibid.

21. M. M. Maharishi Yogi, *Mahesh Yogi on the Bhagavad Gita* (New York: Penguin, 1988).

BIBLIOGRAPHY

Alexander, C. N. et al. "Effects of the Transcendental Meditation Program on Stress Reduction, Health and Employee Development." *Stress, Anxiety and Coping* 6 (1993): 245–62.

American Psychiatric Association. *Diagnostic and Statistical Manual of Mental Disorders—5th Edition.* Washington, DC: American Psychiatric Association Press, 2013.

Andrews, G. et al. "Utilizing Survey Data to Inform Public Policy: Comparison of the Effectiveness of Treatment of 10 Mental Disorders." *British Journal of Psychiatry* 184 (2004): 526–33.

Brooks, J. S., and Scarano, T. "Transcendental Meditation in the Treatment of Post–Viet Nam Adjustment." *Journal of Counseling and Development* 64 (1985): 212–14.

Brooks, J. S., and Anselmo, P. *Ayurvedic Secrets to Longevity and Total Health.* New York: Prentice Hall, 1985.

Bujatti, M., and Reiderer, P. "Serotonin, Noradrenaline and Dopamine Metabolites in the Transcendental Meditation Technique." *Journal of Neural Transmission* 39 (1976): 257–67.

Candelent, T. et al. "Teaching Transcendental Meditation in a Psychiatric Setting." *Hospital and Community Psychiatry* 26 (1975): 156–59.

Chalmers, R., and Clements, G. Scientific *Research on Maharishi's Transcendental Meditation Program and the TM/Sidhi: Collected Papers Volumes 2–4.* Vlodrop, Netherlands: Maharishi Ayurveda University Press, 1989.

Cuijpers, P., Aartjan, J., Beekman, T. F., and Reynolds, C. F. "Preventing Depression: A Global Priority." *Journal of the American Medical Association* 307, no. 10 (2012): 1033–34.

Fergusson, L. F., Bonshek, A. J., and Bodigues, J. M. "Personality and Health Characteristics of Cambodian Undergraduates: A Case for Student Development." *Journal of Instructional Psychology* 22 (1995): 308–19.

Kasture, H. S., Rothenberg, S., Averbach, R., and Wallace, R. K. "Improvements in Mental and Physical Health with Maharishi Ayurveda Panchakarma." Presented at the 8th World Congress of the International College of Psychosomatic Medicine, Chicago, IL, 1985.

Kessler, R. C. et al. "Lifetime Morbid Risk of Anxiety and Mood Disorders in the U.S." *International Journal of Psychiatric Methods in Research* 3 (2012): 164–68.

Levine, P. H., Hebert, J. R., Haynes, C. T., and Strobel, U. "EEG Coherence During the Transcendental Meditation Technique." Psychophysiological Laboratory, Centre for the study of Higher States of Consciousness, Maharishi European Research University, 1976.

Mahesh Yogi, M. *Maharishi Mahesh Yogi on the Bhagavad Gita.* New York: Penguin, 1988.

Nidich, S., and Toomey, M. "Transcendental Meditation Reduced Symptoms of Depression, Randomized Controlled Mind-Body Intervention Trials." Presented at the 31st Annual Meeting of the Society of Behavioral Medicine, Seattle, WA, 2010.

Rosenthal, N. E. *Transcendence: Healing and Transformation through Transcendental Meditation.* New York: Tarcher-Penguin, 2011.

Sharma, R. K. *Charaka Samhita.* New Delhi, India: Ministry of Health and Family Planning, 2011.

Stahl, S. *Essential Psychopharmacology: Neuroscientific Basis and Practical Applications.* New York: Cambridge University Press, 2013.

Waraich, P., Goldner, E. M., Somers, J. M., and Hso, L. "Revised Prevalence of Incidence Studies of Mood Disorders." *Canadian Journal of Psychiatry* 49, no. 2 (2004): 124–38.

EIGHT

The Use of Transcendental Meditation Practice in Promoting Recovery and Preventing Relapse for Addictive Diseases

David F. O'Connell, Ph.D., M.S., CFC, DABPS, and Alarik Arenander, Ph.D.

This chapter focuses on the practice of Transcendental Meditation (TM®) to treat addictions. A review of the major studies on TM and addiction is included. The psychological, physiological, neuropsychological, and social changes imparted by TM are considered, and a presentation of the putative mechanisms of action that underlie TM is given. Guidelines for the use of TM in clinical practice are considered, along with the implications of TM and addiction research results for the management and treatment of addictive diseases.

Alcoholism, other chemical dependencies, and behavioral addictions (e.g., sex, shopping, smoking, gambling, working, eating) continue to present a formidable clinical challenge to healthcare professionals. Recent research indicates that an estimated 22.5 million Americans (8.7 percent of the American population) age twelve and older use illicit drugs. Nearly 15 million Americans age twelve and older report binge drinking and heavy alcohol consumption,[1] and the annual cost of the impact of drug and alcohol abuse is $600 billion.[2]

Rates of drug and alcohol abuse or dependence in the general population, rates of relapse to active addiction, and the number of individuals receiving treatment for an addiction have remained essentially unchanged or have increased over the past decade, despite the development of an ever-growing array of prevention and treatment programs and clinical approaches for these disorders.[3] Up to 20 percent of patients seeking primary medical care have a chemical dependency disorder,[4] and nearly 50 percent presenting for psychiatric care have a comorbid addictions disorder.[5,6] This continued clinical challenge is no doubt related to the complexity and intractability of the addictive process and the multidimensional

157

nature of its causes, as well as its psychological, physical, social, and spiritual signs, symptoms, behaviors, and disparate clinical expressions.[6]

Among the varied clinical approaches devised and tested to treat addictions, the practice of TM has emerged—based on research and clinical experience—as a very effective and, in some cases, superior program to arrest this often chronic illness and to promote continuous recovery maintenance.

RESEARCH ON TM AND ADDICTION TREATMENT

A recent statistical meta-analysis[7] published in the *Harvard Review of Psychiatry* on several meditation techniques used to treat addiction and other psychiatric disorders indicates that meditation techniques, including TM, can have a significant impact on the course and treatment of addictive diseases. The authors of the study hypothesize that the following bring about the positive effects of meditation.

- Meditation may attenuate compulsive and fixed drug-taking behaviors.
- Meditation results in an improved ability to attend to and monitor thoughts and feeling states (self-awareness).
- Mediation results in greater self-regulation of moods, impulses, and behaviors.

Specific research results of the positive impact of TM on drug-abuse behaviors[8] suggest that TM induces the following neurophysiological, psychological, and perceptual changes thought to underlie the reduction in addictive behaviors.

- A reorganization of bi-hemispheric brain activity in the frontal lobes, enhancing executive ego functioning. This neuropsychological refinement also results in enhanced, healthy decision-making behaviors.
- Brain changes that dampen the emotional salience of cues for drug-abusing behaviors.

TM cultivates greater flexibility and adaptability in the functioning of the nervous system, allowing drug-abusing patients to experience greater inner freedom and choice in using these skills to negotiate abstaining and recovery-serving behaviors. This improved neuropsychological balance and integration helps to neutralize formerly dangerous perceptual associations to the "people, places, and things" (to employ a phrase from Alcoholics Anonymous [AA]) of active addictive behavior. TM also leads to increased inner awareness of thoughts, ideas, feelings, and impulses in daily activity that assist in freeing the addict of maladaptive, deeply embedded, inflexible drug-seeking thoughts, impulses, and behaviors. This allows for greater stability and regulation of moods and affective states, again helping free the addict from compulsive, impulsive, and destructive drug-use behaviors. The result is a healthier life-supporting plan that can counteract negative, addictive behaviors.

In addition, all the above changes induced by TM work synergistically with recovery processes, including addictions counseling, 12-step group involvement, AA sponsorship, and drug-free recreational activities. This allows the addict to make greater use of a comprehensive addictions-recovery program.

Two research reviews and meta-analyses, including a large statistical meta-analysis of nineteen studies using TM to treat addictions of all kinds,[9,10] demonstrated that overall, the practice of TM alone was 1.6 to 9 times more effective than other meditation/relaxation approaches and other conventional programs used to treat addictions. These effects were measures of rates of reduction of substance use, abstinence, psychological health, physiological stability and balance, quality of social relations, and stress resistance. More specifically, relative to controls, the effect sizes for TM were significantly greater in addressing the many dimensions of addiction. These results are summarized here.

- Improvements in psychological functioning in substance abusers practicing TM were approximately twice as large as those produced by other forms of meditation and relaxation.
- For alcohol, the effects of TM were 1.5 to 8 times larger than those of other treatment approaches.
- For tobacco dependence (smoking), the effects of TM were 2 to 5 times larger than those of other treatments.
- For illicit drug use, the effects of TM were 1.5 to 6 times larger than those of other treatments.
- In contrast to standard treatments, where success rates generally decrease over time, the effects of TM either increased or remained stable over time.
- The impact of TM could not be attributed to nonspecific treatment or placebo effects, such as expectancy, attention from trainer, quality of social support, or the patient's motivation to change.

TM has demonstrated effectiveness in treating and reducing relapse with one of the most difficult to treat patient populations: severe, chronic, transient, low-resource alcoholics (so-called skid-row alcoholics). An experiment[11] with 118 male, primarily African American, patients at the

Rehabilitation Center for Alcoholics and the District of Columbia Veterans Home in Occoquan, Virginia, revealed that patients practicing the TM program (as well as a group practicing EMG biofeedback) for eighteen months showed significantly more non-drinking days (up to 39 percent) than other groups, including patients receiving EEG neurotherapy and conventional counseling with an addictions therapist. The authors concluded that the addition of TM to AA attendance and conventional addictions counseling demonstrates that TM can increase the effectiveness of these therapeutic approaches, as well as provide hope and effective treatment for a typically treatment-refractory population.

More recent research demonstrates that TM can significantly contribute to the management of serious, growing drug- and alcohol-abusing behaviors on college and university campuses.[12] TM has been shown to reduce alcohol abuse significantly among male college students. A recent comprehensive review of the research on evidence-based, alternative, adjunctive medical treatments indicates that TM is effective in treating substance abuse.[13] A comprehensive review of the research literature on the impact of TM with prison inmates indicates that TM can be profoundly effective in reducing and eliminating prisoner anxiety and substance abuse in the very stressful environment of a correctional facility.[14,15] TM has also been found to be effective in addressing intervention and prevention in adolescent substance misuse.[16]

The unique advantages of TM for treatment of addictions include the following.

- TM is done by the patient independently after a brief period of instruction and guidance: no therapist, group, or additional programs are needed.
- The effects of TM are unidirectional and cumulative over time and result in a dramatic shift in neuropsychological functioning to one of lasting serenity, stability, happiness, and well-being.
- TM can serve as a spiritual program by itself, fulfilling the need for the "spiritual awakening" thought by AA and other 12-step groups to be the sine qua non of recovery.
- TM simultaneously reduces psychiatric symptoms common with addictive individuals (dual diagnosis, or psychiatric comorbidity).
- TM alters the distorted neurophysiological functioning of the practitioner to one of coherence.
- TM is enjoyable, simple, effortless, and natural, and it requires no effortful *working* of any particular recovery program.
- Countless authors have shown that TM can have positive healing effects on many physical disease states and can help reverse the physiological damage produced by alcohol and other neurotoxic drugs.

• The regular practice of TM can refine, purify, expand, and balance consciousness toward a permanent state of functioning characterized by happiness and psychological well-being, which counterbalances and blocks addictive tendencies.

RELATED TM RESEARCH RESULTS

Embedded in the disease of addiction are a host of psychological, physiological, social, environmental, and spiritual factors that are comorbid with and contributory to addiction's etiology, severity, expression, and course of treatment. A large body of research indicates that TM results in a host of positive changes in many domains of human functioning for both addicts and non-addicts. In the following sections, we consider these important effects of TM.

Psychological Effects of TM

TM reduces impulsive and rebellious behavior in prison inmates, as measured by reduced aggression, reduced rule infractions, and substantially reduced recidivism up to six years after release from prison.[16–18] Likewise, TM results in reduced impulsivity, hostility, and aggression in the normal population.[19] Additional psychological benefits from TM include enhanced positive social behaviors, including improved academic performance and job productivity.[20]

The toxic neurocognitive/neurodegenerative effects of alcohol and drug addiction are solidly documented, especially for alcohol, inhalants, and methamphetamine.[21,22] Associated with structural damage from substance abuse are a variety of psychological and neurocognitive decrements, including decreased executive ego functioning manifested in cognitive disorganization, poor decision making, poor planning, lower response times, and decreased visuo-spatial abilities. A number of longitudinal studies have shown growth in fluid intelligence in TM practitioners compared with matched controls.[23] Other cognitive skills enhanced by TM include improved cognitive flexibility, reaction time, learning and memory, creativity, and moral reasoning.[24,25]

Affective dysfunction and deregulation are known effects of substance abuse. Addicts turn to drugs for their positive, albeit brief, mood-altering effects. But the impact of drug abuse often results in severe depression, mood instability, and disabling anxiety states following intoxication. Long-established research and millions of first-hand accounts of TM's effects indicate that the practice increases positive affect, happiness, intimacy, emotional acceptance, and emotional stability when compared with other forms of meditation and relaxation.[26] In fact, it can provide an antidote to the negative mood symptoms associated with drug abuse and addiction.

Extensive research indicates that TM alters moods in a natural fashion, both immediately and long term, reducing negative effects, increasing positive emotions, and promoting mood stability.[27] A random assignment study over a three-month period found TM to be more effective than psychotherapy in decreasing anxiety, depression, and affective flattening and numbness in Vietnam veterans suffering from post-traumatic stress disorder (PTSD).[28]

Addicts typically suffer from low self-esteem and poor self-concept as a result of addiction and possibly prior to its onset as well. Research shows that TM practitioners experience significant improvements in these psychological processes as measured by instruments such as the Tennessee Self-Concept Scale, The Netherlands Personality Inventory, and the Repertory Grid.[29]

Self-actualization is a term for the highest level of human functioning and development, characterized by the realization of one's potential and feelings of high self-esteem, as well as high levels of ego integration, creativity, moral vision, and respect for others.[30] Results of research on TM, as measured by a comprehensive meta-analysis, has shown that compared with other methods that had only a slight influence on the development of self-actualization, TM produced a marked effect (increase of 30 percent) on self-actualization, even in a three-month period, as measured by the Personal Orientation Inventory (POI). Moreover, over longer periods, TM resulted in larger effect sizes compared with other methods of promoting self-actualization.[31]

TM and Personality Disorders

Although not focused on personality problems as psychiatric disorders, extensive research on TM and positive changes in personality, as measured by psychological tests, and the impact of TM on antisocial and other dysfunctional behaviors found in studies on prison inmates indicates that TM can have a dramatic effect on healing character issues. AA considers character defects as one expression of the disease of alcoholism. Personality disorders have been found to be frequent in addicted populations,[32] and some researchers have argued for the presence of a substance-abuse-induced personality disorder that can result directly from addiction itself.[33] A study of two hundred patients in drug- and alcohol-dependency treatment found that 60 percent presented with a personality disorder.[34] The presence of a personality disorder with substance abuse in patients in addictions treatment has solidly predicted post-treatment relapse.[35] Other research has indicated a strong positive correlation between the diagnosis of a personality disorder and a tendency toward an inability to remain abstinent. TM has been shown consistently to reduce negative personality characteristics and poor personality functioning, which may be very useful in the overall treatment of addicitions.[36,37]

The impact of TM on prison inmates is particularly noteworthy. Alexander[38] reported on a longitudinal study on TM and self-development with maximum-security-prison inmates with known histories of drug abuse. This group has significant antisocial personality traits and behaviors and is highly resistant to any efforts at increasing personality functioning. Results indicate that TM leads to significant ego development and psychological maturity in this population. TM was compared with wait-list controls and four other inmate programs. The TM-group paroles also showed a one-third-lower criminal relapse rate over a five-year period compared with random samples from four other prison rehabilitation programs. This research is highly significant because it demonstrates that this simple meditation practice can result in pervasive and lasting positive changes in the severe, maladaptive behaviors of addicts who are highly treatment-resistant or treatment-refractory (also see chapter 11, this volume).

Physiological Factors and TM

Chronic stress of all kinds—psychological, interpersonal, health, environmental—has been found to contribute to some forms of addictive diseases[39] (see chapter 3, this volume). A persisting state of autonomic over-arousal can lead to anxiety and other aversive affective states, which in turn can lead to drug and alcohol abuse to mitigate emotional, psychological, and physical discomfort. These effects are short lived, and painful states inevitably return, often at a greater level of severity as the psychoactive effects of the drugs of abuse wear off. Tolerance to the drugs' effects complicates matters further, as increasing levels of such substances are needed to achieve amelioration of negative states. A chronic state of physiological imbalance ensues, resulting in the depletion and deregulation of key neurotransmitters such as serotonin, norepinephrine, and dopamine, all of which are essential to mental and emotional physical homeostasis and equilibrium. At the same time, stress hormones, such as cortisol, are overproduced and can cause significant physiological damage, leading to a further addiction-related downward spiral for the drug abuser.[40] TM has also been shown to increase production of dopamine at the nucleus accumbens in the reward center of the brain, which may account, in part, for its pleasurable experience and the decreased interest in drug highs for the addict.[41] TM leads to a lasting decrease in cortisol production and ongoing higher levels of serotonin in the brain, indicating its stress-inoculating effects.[42]

Research has found that GABA (gamma-aminobutyric acid) mediates anxiety, and low/deregulated effects of this neurotransmitter are associated with pathological levels and experiences of anxiety. Researchers have found that TM increases the "GABAergic tone,"[43,44] which contributes to lowered levels of autonomic arousal and anxiety. Some addicts use alcohol and drugs to mitigate (self-medicate) strong feelings of anxiety, but TM can result in greater GABA balance, thus reducing the need to control anxiety with drugs.

Research has shown that TM is an effective antidote to the deleterious effects of the cycle of addiction. TM leads to increased levels of serotonin and dopamine even as it produces lowered cortisol levels. A statistical meta-analysis of thirty-one physiological studies indicated that during TM, there was a significantly greater reduction in autonomic arousal, including lower respiration rate, skin conductance level, and plasma lactate levels, compared with eyes-closed resting controls.[45] The lowered baseline arousal levels in meditating subjects continued after meditation practice, suggesting a lasting, cumulative effect of TM.

Brain-Wave Coherence

EEG coherence is a brain state of cortical connectivity characterized by orderliness of brain functioning, and high coherence is associated with a number of positive experiences and skills, including increased feelings of bliss and happiness, creativity, intelligence, and cognitive flexibility. EEG coherence is an indication of a high level of communication among all brain areas.[46] By contrast, low EEG coherence is characteristic of decreased cerebral blood flow, depression, schizophrenia, and normal aging.

A large body of research[47,48] demonstrates that TM leads to permanent EEG changes characterized by increased EEG amplitude and coherence across all frequencies and cortical areas compared with controls. EEG coherence increases bilaterally between both hemispheres in frontal cortical areas and between anterior and posterior brain regions during TM.[49]

There is no research specifically on EEG coherence and TM with addicts. However, there is no reason to believe that addiction, or any mental disorder, would nullify or block the effect of increased EEG coherence with this patient population. The enhanced brain coherence cultured by TM has obvious benefits for chemically dependent patients and may partly explain the effectiveness of TM in reducing or eliminating addictions. TM produces states of happiness and bliss, something desperately sought but transient or absent during an active addictive-disease process. The increase in creativity and cognitive flexibility, including better decision making, from improved brain coherence could assist the addict with dealing more adaptively with problems and stressors, which may lead to better psychological functioning and offer a buffer against a relapse to drug use.

Spiritual Factors and TM

Addicts often describe themselves as "spiritually bankrupt" due to their addiction.[50] A significant body of research over the past three decades reveals that one's sense of spirituality and spiritual practices—prayer, contemplation, meditation—can have profound healing effects for a wide range of mental and medical diseases. For example, recovery from surgery was more rapid in patient groups that practiced prayer and had a strong religious sense. Reduced morbidity and mortality were found for a number of diseases in studies that assessed patient health outcomes.[51]

Dr. Evan Finkelstein of Maharishi University of Management has posited[52] that the experience of transcendence, or pure consciousness, is the key ingredient in the effectiveness of spiritual practices. TM leads most directly to the experience of pure consciousness and may account for its effectiveness in culturing spirituality for ill and convalescing patients. TM has been found to deepen spiritual growth, largely through cultivating so-called higher states of awareness characterized by profound bliss, deep intimacy with others and the world, self-sufficiency, and inner contentment.[53] For many recovering patients, TM fulfills the role of a spiritual program in the recovery process and meets in particular the goals of the 11th step of AA, which encourages individuals to practice prayer and meditation to help them work through their sobriety because they increase feelings of surrender and acceptance. Patrick Gresham Williams organized Vedic knowledge and the practice of TM and related techniques in an integrated, comprehensive program to culture and refine addiction-recovery programs as outlined in his book for patients, *The Spiritual Recovery Manual: Vedic Knowledge and Yogic Techniques to Accelerate Recovery*.[54]

The practice of meditation, and of TM in particular, has been strongly recommended and promoted for all recovering patients and should be part of a structured, daily approach to addiction recovery.[55]

Social and Environmental Factors and TM

Social milieu can have a great impact on individual functioning.[56] Adverse social contacts, such as poverty, poor family cohesion, lack of social support, negative peer pressure, a chaotic, hostile environment, and other negative factors can all contribute to maladaptive psychological adjustment, poor self-concept, antisocial behavior, substance abuse, and dependency. Chemically dependent individuals who come from a stressful background often perform poorly in addiction-treatment programs compared with patients who have a more auspicious life situation.

TM studies show that this practice improves the capacity for warm social relationships, appreciation of others, and greater sociability. These in turn are associated with enhanced job satisfaction and work adjustment behaviors, as well as increased marital satisfaction.[57,58] Due to the reciprocal relationship between the individual and his or her social environment, when an individual is profoundly nourished from within through TM, a natural basis for better social relationships is created as the individual heals.

Since individual consciousness is considered a factor in a field phenomenon and embedded in the collective consciousness of society (see chapter 1, this volume), when individuals practice TM, research has demonstrated that there is a positive influence on the social environment (see chapter 11, this volume) characterized by significantly decreased negative social trends and a corresponding increase in quality of life for society. These significant societal changes include reduced substance abuse and reductions in crime, auto accidents, homicides, suicides, and political violence.[59]

CONCLUSION

Research has shown that applying the practice of TM to treat addictions of all kinds, alone or in conjunction with other treatments, is an effective approach to address these addictions. It offers a host of advantages over other treatment techniques. It is an enjoyable, easy, and pleasurable technique with immediate and ongoing availability, and it is backed by widespread education and support. It offers permanent neurophysiological effects to reduce and prevent relapse to active addiction with simultaneously profound, positive effects on comorbid mental and medical disorders. And it is an effective spiritual-recovery program, providing reduction and elimination of stress and a conscious-expanding, positive experience that can supplant substance abuse. Further, it can be implemented easily in primary medical care settings and psychiatric treatment settings.

Primary Care and Mental Healthcare Settings: Recommendations

1. Provide education and information on the benefits of TM and local resources for TM instruction.
2. Provide patients with informative literature on TM research and health.
3. Discuss how TM can have healing effects for specific disorders, including substance abuse, anxiety, depression, ADHD, PTSD, person-

ality (character) disorders, hypertension, diabetes, cardiovascular disease, obesity, and pain.

4. Prescribe TM as a part of patients' treatment plan.
5. Recommend that patients attend ongoing, free, meditation checking and lectures on meditation at a local TM center.

Research on how TM applies to the treatment of chemical dependency shows that this ancient mental technique is highly effective at arresting this complex disorder and should be considered a routine treatment and "standard of care," or "best practice," for addressing addictive diseases. Further, research is needed on the use of this mental technique to combat addictive diseases, especially in conjunction with conventional treatment approaches. As the neurobiology of both addictions and the effects of TM become better understood, the role of TM in addiction treatment will become clearer. For example, research on the epigenetics of TM, its unique impact on the brain's reward system, and its effect on maximizing decision-making processes and creativity through increased brain coherence is burgeoning.[60,61] Despite the impressive data presented in this chapter, research on the potential of TM to alter addictive and other destructive psychological conditions has barely begun.

NOTES

1. Substance Abuse Mental Health Services Administration, Center for Behavioral Health and Quality, "Results from the National Survey on Drug Abuse and Health: Summary of National Findings," http://store.samhsa.gov/home.

2. National Institute on Drug Abuse, www.drugabuse.gov/.

3. Ibid.

4. D. G. Buchsbaum, R. G. Buchanon, R. M. Poses, S. H. Schnoll, and M. J. Lawton, "Physician Detection of Drinking Problems in Patients Attending a General Medical Practice," *Journal of General Internal Medicine* 7 (1992): 517–21.

5. R. C. Kessler and K. R. Merikangas, "The National Co-morbidity Survey Replication (NCR-R): Background and Aims," *International Journal of Methods in Psychiatry Research* 13 (2004): 60–68.

6. R. C. Kessler et al., "The Epidemiology of Co-occurring Mental Disorders: Implications for Prevention and Service Utilization," *American Journal of Orthopsychiatry* 66, no. 10 (1996): 17–30.

7. L. E. Dakwar, "The Emerging Role of Meditation in Addressing Psychiatric Illness," *Harvard Review of Psychiatry* 17 (2009): 254–67.

8. F. T. Travis et al., "Patterns of EEG Coherence, Power and Contingent Negative Variation Characterize the Integration of Transcendental and Waking States," *Biological Psychology* 61 (2002): 293–319.

9. C. N. Alexander et al., "Treating and Preventing Alcohol, Nicotine and Drug Abuse through Transcendental Meditation: A Review and Statistical Meta-analysis,"

in *Self Recovery: Treating Addictions using Transcendental Meditation and Maharishi Ayurveda*, ed. D. F. O'Connell et al. (New York: Harrington Park Press, 1994).

10. P. Gelderloos et al., "Effectiveness of the Transcendental Meditation Program in Preventing and Treating Substance Misuse: A Review," *International Journal of the Addictions* 26 (1991): 293–95.

11. E. Taub et al., "Effectiveness of Broad-Spectrum Approaches to Relapse in Severe Alcoholism: A Long-Term, Randomized, Controlled Trial of Transcendental Meditation, EMG Biofeedback and Electronic Neurotherapy," in *Self-Recovery: Treating Addictions Using Transcendental Meditation and Maharishi Ayurveda*, ed. D. F. O'Connell et al. (New York: Harrington Park Press, 1994).

12. D. A. Haaga et al., "Effects of the Transcendental Meditation Program on Substance Abuse among University Students," *Cardiology Review and Practice* 10 (2011).

13. W. O. Donohue and N. Cummings, *Evidence-Based Adjuvant Treatments* (New York: Academic Press, 2008).

14. M. A Hawkins, "Effectiveness of the Transcendental Meditation Program in Criminal Rehabilitation and Substance Abuse Recovery: A Review of the Research," *Journal of Offender Rehabilitation* 36 (2006): 47–66.

15. R. F. Fergusson, "A Self-Report Evaluation of the Effects of the Transcendental Meditation Program at Massachusetts Correctional Institution Walmpole: A Follow Up," In *Scientific Research on Maharishi's Transcendental Meditation Program and TM/Sidhi Program: Collected Papers* 2, ed. R. A. Chalmers, F. Clements, H. Schenkluhn, and M. Weinless (Vlodrop, The Netherlands: Maharishi Vedic University Press, 1989).

16. A. I. Abrams and L. M Siegel, "The Transcendental Meditation Program and Rehabilitation at Folsom State Prison: A Cross-Validation Study," *Criminal Justice and Behavior* 5 (1978): 3–20.

17. C. N Alexander, "Ego Development, Personality, and Behavioral Change in Inmates Practicing the Transcendental Meditation Technique or Participating in Other Programs: A Cross-Sectional Longitudinal Study," *Dissertation Abstracts International* 43, no. 2 (1982): 59B.

18. C. R. Bleick and A. I. Abrams, "The Transcendental Meditation Program and Criminal Recidivism in California," *Journal of Criminal Justice* 15 (1987): 211–30.

19. W. J. Penner et al., "Does an In-depth Transcendental Meditation Course Effect Change in the Personalities of the Participants?" *Western Psychologist* 4 (1974): 104–11.

20. C. N. Alexander, M. V. Rainforth, T. W. Carlisle, and C. Todd, "The Effects of the Transcendental Meditation Program on Stress Reduction, Job Performance and Health in Two Business Settings," presentation at the National Conference for the Center for Management and Research, Maharishi International University, Fairfield, IA, March, 1987.

21. National Institute on Drug Abuse and Alcoholism, "Ninth Report to the U.S. Congress on Alcohol and Health" (Bethesda, MD: National Institute on Alcohol Abuse and Alcoholism, 1997), NIH pub. 97-4017.

22. B. Thrash et al., "Neurotoxic Effects of Methamphetamine," *Neurochemical Research* 35 (2010): 171–79.

23. R. W. Cranson et al., "Transcendental Meditation and Performance on Intelligence Measures: A Longitudinal Study," *Personality and Individual Differences* 12 (1991): 1105–6.

24. F. T. Travis, "The Transcendental Meditation Technique and Creativity: A Longitudinal Study of Cornell University Undergraduates," *Journal of Creative Behaviors* 13 (1979): 169–80.

25. H. M. Chandler, "Transcendental Meditation and Awakening Wisdom: A Ten-Year Study of Self-Development," *Dissertation Abstracts International* 51, no. 106 (1991): 5048

26. K. Eppley, A. I. Abrams, and J. Shear, "Differential Effects of Relaxation on Trait Anxiety: A Meta-analysis," *Journal of Clinical Psychology* 45, no. 6 (1989): 957–74.

27. P. Gelderloos, H. J. Herman, H. H. Ahlstrom, and R. Jacoby, "Transcendence and Psychological Health: Studies with Long-Term Participants of the TM and TM/Sidhis Program," *Journal of Psychology* 124 (1990): 177–97.

28. J. Brooks and T. Scarano, "Transcendental Meditation in the Treatment of Post-Vietnam Adjustment," *Journal of Counseling and Development* 64 (1985): 212–14.

29. P. Gelderloos, H. J. Herman, H. H. Ahlstrom, and R. Jacoby, "Transcendence and Psychological Health: Studies of Long-Term Participants of the TM and TM/Sidhis Program," *Journal of Psychology* 124 (1990): 177–97.

30. A. H. Maslow, *Toward a Psychology of Being* (New York: Harper and Row, 1968).

31. C. N. Alexander, M. V. Rainforth, and P. Gelderloos, "Transcendental Meditation, Self-Actualization and Psychological Health: A Conceptual Overview and Statistical Meta-analysis," *Journal of Social Behavior and Personality* 6 (1991): 189–297.

32. M. Sadigh, "Disorders of Personality and Substance Abuse: An Exploration of Clinical and Empirical Findings," in *Managing the Dually Diagnosed Patient: Current Issues and Clinical Approaches*, ed. D. F. O'Connell and E. P. Beyer (New York: Routledge, 2002).

33. E. P. Nace, "Substance Abuse and Personality Disorders," in *Managing the Dually Diagnosed Patient: Current Issues and Clinical Approaches*, ed. D. F. O'Connell (New York: Haworth Press, 1990).

34. A. E. Skodola, J. M. Oldham, and P. E. Gallagher, "Axis II Comorbidity of Substance Abuse among Patients Referred for Treatment of Personality Disorders," *American Journal of Psychiatry* 136 (1999): 733–38.

35. H. M. Pettinati, J. D. Pierce, P. P. Belden, and K. Meyers, "The Relationship of Axis II Personality Disorders to Other Known Predictors of Addiction Treatment Outcome," *American Journal of the Addictions* 8 (1999): 136–47.

36. V. H. Thomas, T. P. Melchert and J. A. Banken, "Substance Dependence and Personality Disorders: Comorbidity and Treatment Outcome in an Inpatient Treatment Population," *Journal of Studies on Alcohol* 60 (1997): 271–77.

37. Y. Jackson, "Learning Disorders and the Transcendental Meditation Program: Retrospects and Prospects, A Preliminary Study with Economically Deprived Adolescents," *Dissertations Abstracts International* 38 (1977): 3351A.

38. C. Dixon et al., "Accelerated Cognitive and Self-Development: Longitudinal Studies with Preschool and Elementary School Children," *Journal of Social Behavior and Personality* 17 (2005): 65–91.

39. C. N. Alexander, "Ego Development, Personality, and Behavioral Change in Inmates Practicing the Transcendental Meditation Technique or Participating in Other Programs: A Cross-Sectional and Longitudinal Study," *Dissertation Abstracts International* 43, no. 2 (1982): 539B.

40. D. O'Connell and C. Alexander, eds., *Self-Recovery: Treating Addictions Using Transcendental Meditation and Maharishi Ayurveda* (New York: Harrington Park Press, 1994).

41. K. G. Walton and D. Levitsky, "A Neuroendocrine Mechanism for the Reduction of Drug Use and Addictions by Transcendental Meditation," *Alcoholism Treatment Quarterly* 11 (1994): 89–117.

42. M. Bujatti and P. Riederer, "Serotonin, Noradrenaline, and Dopamine Metabolites in Transcendental Meditation," *Journal of Neural Transmission* 39 (1976): 257–67.

43. K. G. Walton and D. K. Levitsky, "Effects of the Transcendental Meditation Program on Neuroendocrine Abnormalities Associated with Aggression and Crime," *Journal of Offender Rehabilitation* 36 (2003): 67–88.

44. A. N. Elias and A. F. Wilson, "Serum Hormonal Concentrations Following Transcendental Meditation: A Potential Role of Gamma-Aminobutyric Acid," *Medical Hypotheses* 44 (1995): 287–91.

45. A. N. Elias et al., "Ketosis with Enhanced GABAergic Tone Promotes Physiological Changes in Transcendental Meditation," *Medical Hypotheses* 54 (2000): 660–62.

46. M. C. Dillbeck and D. W. Orme-Johnson, "Physiological Differences between Transcendental Meditation and Rest," *American Psychologist* 42 (1987): 879–81.

47. F. T. Travis and D. W. Orme-Johnson, "Field Model of Consciousness: EEG Coherence Changes as Indicators of Field Effects," *International Journal of Neuroscience* 49 (1989): 203–11.

48. F. T. Travis, "Autonomic and EEG Patterns Distinguish Transcending from Other Experiences during Transcendental Meditation Practice," *International Journal of Psychophysiology* 42 (2001): 1–9.

49. F. T. Travis et al., "Patterns of EEG Coherence, Power and Contingent Negative Variation Characterize the Integration of Transcendental and Waking States," *Biological Psychology* 61 (2002): 293–319.

50. F. T. Travis and C. Pearson, "Pure Consciousness: Distinct Phenomenological and Physiological Correlates of 'Consciousness Itself,'" *International Journal of Neuroscience* 100 (2000): 77–89.

51. D. F. O'Connell, *Awakening the Spirit: Developing a Spiritual Program in Addictions Recovery* (Baltimore, MD: Publish America, 2004).

52. C. M. Pucaiski, "The Role of Spirituality in Healthcare," *Proceedings of Baylor University Medical Center* 14, no. 4 (2001): 352–57.

53. E. I. Finkelstein, "Universal Principles of Life Expressed in Maharishi Vedic Science and in the Scriptures and Writings of Judaism, Christianity and Islam," Ph.D. dissertation, Maharishi University of Management, Fairfield, IA, 2005.

54. D. O'Murchu, "Spirituality, Recovery and Transcendental Meditation," in *Self-Recovery: Treating Addictions Using Transcendental Meditation and Maharishi Ayurveda,* ed. D. F. O'Connell and C. N. Alexander (New York: Harrington Park Press, 1994).

55. P. G. Williams, *The Spiritual Recovery Manual: Vedic Knowledge and Yogic Techniques to Accelerate Recovery* (Palo Alto, CA: Incandescent Press, 2002).

56. D. F. O'Connell and D. L. Bevvino, *Managing Your Recovery from Addictions: A Guide for Senior Managers, Executives and Other Professionals* (New York: Routledge, 2007).

57. B. Lakey, T. A. Tardiff, and J. Brittain Drew, "Negative Social Interactions: Assessment and Relations to Social Support, Cognition and Psychological Distress," *Journal of Social and Clinical Psychology* 13, no. 1 (1994): 42–62.

58. M. E. Chen, "A Comparative Study of Dimensions of Healthy Functioning between Families Practicing the TM Program for 5 Years or Less Than a Year," *Journal of Holistic Nursing* 5 (1987): 6–10.

59. C. N. Alexander, M. V. Rainforth, and P. Gelderloos, "Transcendental Meditation, Self-Actualization and Psychological Health: A Conceptual Overview and Statistical Meta-analysis," *Journal of Social Behavior and Personality* 6 (1991): 189–297.

60. M. C. Dillbeck, "Test of a Field Theory of Consciousness and Social Change: Time Series Analysis of Participation in the TM/Sidhi Program and Reduction of Violent Death in the U.S.," *Social Indicators Research* 22 (1990): 399–41.

61. A. Arenander, "No One Wants to Be an Addict: The Brain Science Behind Addiction and How Transcendental Meditation Can Effectively Help Prevent Addiction and Facilitate Recovery," unpublished manuscript (Fairfield, IA, 2014).

BIBLIOGRAPHY

Abrams, A. I., and Siegel, L. M. "The Transcendental Meditation Program and Rehabilitation at Folsom State Prison: A Cross-Validation Study." *Criminal Justice and Behavior* 50 (1978): 3–20.

Alexander, C. N. "Ego Development, Personality, and Behavioral Change in Inmates Practicing the Transcendental Meditation Technique or Participating in Other Programs: A Cross-Sectional Longitudinal Study." *Dissertation Abstracts International* 43, no. 2 (1989): 59B.

Alexander, C. N., Rainforth, M. V., Carlisle, T. W., and Todd, C. "The Effects of the Transcendental Meditation Program on Stress Reduction, Job Performance and Health in Two Business Settings." Presentation at the National Conference for the Center of Management, Maharishi International University, Fairfield, IA, 1987.

Alexander, C. N., Rainforth, M. V., and Gelderloos, P. "Transcendental Meditation, Self-Actualization and Psychological Health: A Conceptual Overview and Statistical Meta-analysis." *Journal of Social Behavior and Personality* 6 (1991): 189–297.

Alexander, C. N., Robinson, P., and Rainforth, M. "Treating and Preventing Alcohol, Nicotine and Drug Abuse through Transcendental Meditation." In *Self-Recovery: Treating Addictions Using Transcendental Meditation and Maharishi*

Ayurveda. Edited by D. F. O'Connell and C. N. Alexander. New York: Harrington Park Press, 1994.

Arenander, A. "No One Wants to Be an Addict: The Brain Science Behind Addiction and How Transcendental Meditation can Effectively Prevent Addiction and Facilitate Recovery." Unpublished manuscript, Fairfield, IA, 2014.

Bleick, C. R., and Abrams, A. I. "The Transcendental Meditation Program and Criminal Recidivism in California." *Journal of Criminal Justice* 15 (1987): 211–30.

Brooks, J., and Scarano, T. "Transcendental Meditation in the Treatment of Post-Vietnam Adjustment." *Journal of Counseling and Development* 64 (1985): 212–14.

Bujatti, M., and Riederer, P. "Serotonin, Noradrenaline, and Dopamine Metabolites in Transcendental Meditation." *Journal of Neural Transmission* 39 (1976): 257–67.

Buschsbaum, D. G., Buchanon, R. G., Poses, R. M., Schnoll, S. H., and Lawton, M. J. "Physician Detection of Drinking Problems in Patients Attending a General Medical Practice." *Journal of General Internal Medicine* 7 (1992): 517–21.

Chandler, H. M. "Transcendental Meditation and Awakening Wisdom: A Ten-Year Study of Self-Development." *Dissertation Abstracts International* 51, no. 106 (1991): 5048.

Chen, M. E. "A Comparative Study of Dimensions of Healthy Functioning between Families Practicing the TM Program for 5 Years or Less Than a Year." *Journal of Holistic Nursing* 5 (1987) 6–10.

Cranson, R. W., Orme-Johnson, D. W., Gackenbach, J., Dillbeck, M. C., Jones, C. H., and Alexander, C. N. "Transcendental Meditation and Performance on Intelligence Measures." *Personality and Individual Differences* 12 (1991): 1105–06.

Dakwar, L. E. "The Emerging Role of Meditation in Addressing Psychatric Illness." *Harvard Review of Psychiatry* 17 (2009): 254–67.

Dillbeck, M. C. "Test of a Field Theory of Consciousness and Social Change: Time Series Analysis of Participation in the TM/Sidhi Program and Reduction of Violent Death in the U.S. *Social Indicators Research* 22 (1990): 399–41.

Dillbeck, M. C., and Orme-Johnson, D. W. "Physiological Differences between Transcendental Meditation and Rest." *American Psychologist* 42 (1987): 879–81.

Dixon, C. et al. "Accelerated Cognitive and Self Development: Longitudinal Studies with Preschool and Elementary School Children." *Journal of Social Behavior and Personality* 17 (2005): 65–91.

Elias, A. N. et al. "Ketosis with Enhanced GABAergic Tone Promotes Physiological Changes in Transcendental Meditation." *Medical Hypotheses* 54 (2000): 660–62.

Elias, A. N., and Wilson, A. F. "Serum Hormonal Concentrations Following Transcendental Meditation: A Potential Role of Gamma-Aminobutyric Acid." *Medical Hypotheses* 44 (1995) 287–91.

Eppley, K., Abrams, A. I., and Shears, J. "Differential Effects of Relaxation on Trait Anxiety: A Meta-analysis." *Journal of Clinical Psychology* 45, no. 6 (1989): 957–74.

Fergusson, R. F. "A Self-Report Evaluation of the Effects of the Transcendental Meditation Program at Massachusetts Correctional Institution Walmpole." In *Scientific Research on Maharishi's Transcendental Meditation Program and TM/Sidhi Program: Collected Papers, Volume 2.* Edited by R. A. Chalmers, G. Clements, H. Schenkluhn, and M. Weinless. Vlodrop, The Netherlands: Maharishi Vedic University Press, 1989.

Fergusson, D. M., Lynskey, M. T., and Horwood, L. J. "Alcohol Misuse and Juvenile Offending in Adolescence." *Addictions* 91, no. 4 (1996): 483–94.

Finkelstein, E .I. "Universal Principles of Life Expressed in Maharishi Vedic Science and in the Scriptures and Writings of Judaism, Christianity and Islam." Doctoral dissertation, Maharishi University of Management, Fairfield, IA, 2005.

Gelderloos, P., Herman, H. J., Ahlstrom, H. H., and Jacoby, R. "Transcendence and Psychological Health: Studies with Long-Term Participants of the TM and TM/Sidhis Program." *Journal of Psychology* 124 (1990): 177–97.

Gelderloos, P., Walton, K. G., Orme-Johnson, D. W., and Alexander, C. N. "Effectiveness of the Transcendental Meditation Program in Preventing and Treating Substance Misuse: A Review." *International Journal of the Addictions* 26 (1991): 293–325.

Haaga, D. A., Grosswald, S., Gaylord-King, C., Rainforth, M. V., Tanner, M., Nidich, S., and Schneider, R. "Effects of the Transcendental Meditation Program on Substance Abuse among University Students." *Cardiology Review and Practice* 10 (2011), DOI: 10.4061.

Hawkins, M. A. "Effectiveness of the Transcendental Meditation Program in Criminal Rehabilitation and Substance Abuse Recovery: A Review of the Research." *Journal of Offender Rehabilitation* 36 (2006): 47–66.

Jackson, Y. "Learning Disorders and the Transcendental Meditation Program: Retrospects and Prospects, A Preliminary Study with Economically Deprived Adolescents." *Dissertations Abstracts International* 38 (1977): 3351A.

Kessler, R. C., Nelson, C. B., McGonagle, K. A., Edlund, M. J., Frank, R. J., and Leaf, P. J. "The Epidemiology of Co-occurring Mental Disorders: Implications for Prevention and Service Utilization." *American Journal of Orthopsychiatry* 66, no. 10 (1996): 17–30.

Lakey, B., Tardiff, T. A., and Drew, J. B. "Negative Social Interactions: Assessment and Relations to Social Support, Cognition and Psychological Distress." *Journal of Social and Clinical Psychology* 13, no. 1 (1994): 42–62.

Maslow, A. H. *Toward a Psychology of Being*. New York: Harper and Row, 1968.

Nace, E. P. "Substance Abuse and Personality Disorders." In *Managing the Dually Diagnosed Patient: Current Issues and Clinical Approaches*. Edited by D. F. O'Connell. New York: Haworth Press, 1990.

National Institute on Drug Abuse and Alcoholism. "Ninth Report to the U.S. Congress on Alcohol and Health." NIH Publication no. 97-4017. Bethesda MD: National Institute on Alcohol Abuse and Alcoholism, 1997.

O'Connell, D. F. *Awakening the Spirit: Developing a Spiritual Recovery Program in Addictions Recovery*. Baltimore, MD: Publish America, 2004.

———. *Dual Disorders: Essentials for Assessment and Treatment*. New York: Haworth Press, 1997.

O'Connell, D. F. and Bevvino, D. L. *Managing Your Recovery from Addiction: A Guide for Senior Managers, Executives and Other Professionals*. New York: Routledge, 2007.

O'Connell, D. F. and Beyer, E. *Managing the Dually Diagnosed Patient: Current Issues and Clinical Approaches*. New York: Haworth Press, 2002.

O'Connell, D. F. and Alexander, C. *Self-Recovery: Treating Addictions Using Transcendental and Maharishi Ayurveda*. New York: Harrington Park Press, 1994.

O'Donohue, W. and Cummings, N. *Evidence-Based Adjuvant Treatments*. New York: Academic Press, 2008.

O'Murchu, D. "Spirituality, Recovery and Transcendental Meditation." In *Self-Recovery: Treating Addictions Using Transcendental Meditation and Maharishi Ayurveda*. Edited by D. F. O'Connell and C. N. Alexander, 169–86. New York: Harrington Park Press, 1994.

Penner, W. J., Zingle, H. W., Dyck, R., and Truch, S. "Does an In-depth Transcendental Meditation Course Effect Change in the Personalities of the Participants?" *Western Psychologist* 4 (1974): 104–11.

Pettinatti, H. M., Pierce, J. D., Belden, P. P., and Meyes, K. "The Relationship of Axis II Personality Disorders to Other Known Predictors of Addiction Treatment Outcome." *American Journal of the Addictions* 8 (1999): 136–47.

Pucaiski, C. M. "The Role of Spirituality in Healthcare." *Proceedings of Baylor University Medical Center* 14, no. 4 (2001): 352–57.

Sadigh, M. "Disorders of Personality and Substance Abuse: An Exploration of Empirical and Clinical Findings." In *Managing the Dually Diagnosed Patient: Current issues and Clinical approaches*. Edited by D. F. O'Connell and E. P. Beyer, 317–36. New York, Routledge, 2002.

Skodola, A. E., Oldham, J. M., and Gallagher, P. E. "Axis II Comorbidity of Substance Abuse among Patients Referred for Treatment of Personality Disorders." *American Journal of Psychiatry* 136 (1999): 733–38.

Substance Abuse Mental Health Services Administration, Center for Behavioral Health and Quality. "Results from the National Survey on Drug Abuse and Health: Summary of National Findings." http://store.samhsa.gov.home.

Taub, E., Weingarten, S., and Walton, E. "Effectiveness of Broad-Spectrum Approaches to Relapse in Severe Alcoholism: A Long-Term, Randomized, Controlled Trial of Transcendental Meditation, EMG Biofeedback and Electronic Neurotherapy." In *Self-Recovery: Treating Addictions with Transcendental Meditation and Maharishi Ayurveda*. Edited by D. F. O'Connell and C. N. Alexander, 187–220. New York: Harrington Park Press, 1994.

Thrash, B., Karuppagounder, S. S., Uthayathas, S., Suppiramaniam, V., and Dhanasekaran, M. "Neurotoxic Effects of Methamphetamine." *Neurochemical Research* 35 (2010): 171–79.

Thomas, V. H., Melchert, T. P., and Banken, J. A. "Substance Dependence and Personality Disorders: Comorbidity and Treatment Outcome in an Inpatient Treatment Population." *Journal of Studies on Alcohol* 60 (1997): 271–77.

Travis, F. T. "Autonomic and EEG Patterns Distinguish Transcending from Other Experiences During Transcendental Meditation Practice." *International Journal of Psychophysiology* 42 (2001): 1–9.

Travis, F. T. and Orme-Johnson, D. W. "Field Model of Consciousness: EEG Coherence Changes as Indicators of Field Effects." *International Journal of Neuroscience* 49 (1989): 203–11.

Travis, F. T. and Pearson, C. "Pure Consciousness: Distinct Phenomenological and Physiological Correlates of 'Consciousness Itself.'" *International Journal of Neuroscience* 100 (2000): 77–89.

Travis, F. T., Teece, J., Arenander, A., and Wallace, R. K. "Patterns of EEG Coherence, Power and Contingent Negative Variation Characterize the Integration of Transcendental and Waking States." *Biological Psychology* 61 (2002): 293–319.

Walton, K. and Levitsky, D. "A Neuroendocrine Mechanism for the Reduction of Drug Use and Addictions by Transcendental Meditation." *Alcoholism Treatment Quarterly* 11 (1994): 89–117.

Walton, K. G., and Levitsky, D. K. "Effects of the Transcendental Meditation Program on Neuroendocrine Abnormalities Associated with Aggression and Crime." *Journal of Offender Rehabilitation* 36 (2003): 66–88.

Williams, P. G. *The Spiritual Recovery Manual: Vedic Knowledge and Yogic Techniques to Accelerate Recovery.* Palo Alto, CA: Incandescent Press, 2002.

NINE

Transcendental Meditation and the Treatment of Childhood Disorders

William R. Stixrud, Ph.D., and Sarina Grosswald, Ed.D.

INTRODUCTION: THE CRISIS OF STRESS-RELATED DISORDERS IN YOUTH

There is evidence that the practice of Transcendental Meditation (TM®) in young children and elementary-school students enhances normal child development and is associated with high levels of academic achievement and creativity. However, most research conducted on meditating young people has been done with students from middle-school age through college. This chapter will thus focus on TM as a tool for supporting the development of adolescents (including college students, who are at the later end of adolescent brain development), and on preventing and treating the problems faced by increasing numbers of young people.

TIRED, WIRED, AND STRESSED

Although adolescence is a period of tremendous developmental power and potential,[1] extensive research suggests that contemporary teens are at particularly high risk for a wide range of learning and mental health problems. Studies comparing responses to the adult and adolescent versions of the Minnesota Multiphasic Personality Inventory (MMPI) across generations have suggested that contemporary adolescents and young adults are five to eight times more likely to experience psychopathology, including anxiety and depression, than their counterparts fifty to seventy years ago, even those living at the height of the Great Depression.[2] A recent face-to-face survey of 10,123 adolescents in the continental

United States found that more than 45 percent of the teens surveyed were diagnosed with at least one type of anxiety or mood disorder, and that 49.5 percent of the total sample suffered from at least one mental health disorder during adolescence—including anxiety or mood disorders, behavioral disorders, substance-use disorders, or eating disorders.[3] Furthermore, 40 percent of the teens who were diagnosed with one class of disorder also met criteria for another disorder. Recent estimates suggest that the yearly economic burden of mental disorders on American youth and their families is nearly $250 billion.[4]

Evidence is also emerging showing substantial escalations in the incidence of learning and attention disorders and autism spectrum disorders, which may be caused partially by, and are unquestionably exacerbated by, stress, anxiety, and other mental health problems.[5] Furthermore, current research raises strong concerns about stress-related challenges to moral and character development in children and teens. For example, the majority of high school students admit to engaging in "serious cheating" and plagiarizing from the Internet,[6] and studies have found that contemporary high school and college students report the lowest levels of empathy in thirty years.[7]

The mental health picture does not appear to improve when adolescents enter college, as college freshman presently report the highest levels of stress and the lowest overall mental health levels in twenty-five years.[8] Although depression and anxiety are still the most common referral problems for college counseling centers, growing numbers of students are presenting with stress-related eating disorders, substance abuse, and self-injury.[9] Furthermore, almost half of college students report regular binge drinking.[10]

The heightened vulnerability to learning, attention, and mental health disorders experienced by contemporary youth is presumably related, in significant part, to the culture of stress and fatigue in which they are growing up. Stress and insufficient rest have serious detrimental effects on learning, mental health, and brain development.[11] Many factors may be contributing to the high stress levels of contemporary young people, including genetic vulnerability, chronic sleep insufficiency, rising academic pressures, the decline of play, stressed and overextended parents, financial insecurity, and the increased social isolation of families.[12] It is also important to note that evidence is rapidly accumulating to suggest that extensive technology use and multitasking raise stress hormone levels, and that technology overload appears to be contributing directly to unprecedented levels of sleep deprivation, as well as to the development of physical health problems, psychological disorders, attention deficits, and behavioral problems.[13] Concern has further been voiced about the fact that excessive engagement in technology is significantly limiting young people's experience of "downtime" and periods of self-reflection, which are important for stimulating the brain's default mode network and for the development of a strong sense of self.[14]

THE EFFECTS OF STRESS ON DEVELOPMENT

The high incidence of stress-related problems in young people is of particularly great concern in light of the fact that (1) the brain continues to develop well into young adulthood, (2) experience shapes brain development, and (3) the developing brain is more profoundly influenced by chemicals, including stress hormones, alcohol, and recreational drugs, than a fully mature brain.[15] Just as eating disorders can have profound effects on developing bodies, chronic stress, sleep deprivation, and chemical use shape brain development in ways that can predispose young people to cognitive difficulties and to life-long problems related to anxiety, mood disturbance, sleep disruption, and chemical abuse—partly through their effect on gene expression.[16] It is said, for example, that depression in adolescence "scars" the brain, making it vulnerable to recurring depression.[17]

The negative effects of stress on child and adolescent development are evident across the social and economic spectrum. For example, recent research has documented the harmful effects of chronic stress on brain function and cognition in children who are raised in poverty,[18] while numerous studies have found children of affluent families to be at higher risk for anxiety and mood disorders, substance abuse, and self-injury than poor children.[19]

Moreover, chronic stress over a prolonged period has been shown to shrink the hippocampus and the prefrontal cortex, with resulting impairment in memory, judgment, and executive functions.[20] Additionally, chronic stress increases the size and reactivity of the amygdala, making already stressed young people even more vulnerable to stress, anxiety, and mood-related problems.[21] This is particularly worrisome in light of the fact that effective stress regulation and impulse control are hugely predictive of academic, career, and relationship success.[22]

THE ROLE OF TM IN SUPPORTING HEALTHY
DEVELOPMENT AND HEALING DISORDERS

With the exception of two studies on middle-school students with ADHD discussed later in this chapter, no studies have been conducted to date on children or adolescents with diagnosed emotional, behavioral, or learning disorders. However, there is extensive research on the effects of TM on middle school, high school, and college age students that has very promising implications for (1) preventing and treating stress-related social/emotional problems in young people; (2) improving cognitive functioning, learning, and school achievement, and helping students with cognitive and learning disorders; (3) offsetting the mind-racing, mind-scattering, and mind-numbing effects of technology overload; and (4) promoting growth of self-awareness, self-regulation, self-esteem, and creativity.

The focus of this chapter will be on the ways in which TM can help to both prevent and treat a wide range of disorders affecting children and adolescents. The first section reviews the evidence that supports the use of TM in preventing and treating mental health problems, including anxiety disorders, mood disorders, substance-use disorders, and self-injury. Autism will also be discussed in this section due to the high incidence of anxiety disorders and stress-related challenges experienced by young people with autism spectrum disorders. The second section focuses on TM's potential for addressing school-related problems of learning and behavior, including the (to date) virtually unsolvable educational problems associated with poverty. The third section focuses on the logistics of getting children, teens, and adults to meditate regularly—including the inclusion of TM in school programs—and on the benefits children derive when their parents meditate.

WHY TM IS EFFECTIVE IN ADDRESSING A WIDE RANGE OF PROBLEMS

Two Key Mechanisms

While the extensive research on TM implies a number of potential mechanisms for its wide-ranging effects, the two primary mechanisms appear to be (1) inducing a state of restful alertness that leads to lowered stress levels and decreased stress reactivity, and (2) promoting more orderly and better organized brain functioning, as reflected by increased coherence in the electrical activity of the brain (EEG coherence).

As is discussed in other chapters in this volume, hundreds of studies have found that TM produces a state of restful alertness that is distinct from sleep, typical rest, and other forms of meditation.[23] An early meta-analytic study found that the level of rest during the practice of TM was, in some important respects, twice as great as that of ordinary rest.[24] Extensive evidence indicates that deep rest is highly beneficial for both the mind and body, presumably, in part, because it allows the nervous system to recover from the negative effects of stress and fatigue.[25]

Extensive research has documented the "de-stressing" effects of TM, including several studies that found decreased cortisol levels both during and outside of TM.[26] In a study funded by the National Institutes of Health (NIH),[27] forty-eight students were randomly assigned to a TM group or a control group. In the group practicing TM, basal cortisol levels and average cortisol levels across stress sessions decreased, while cortisol responsiveness to stressors increased. The findings suggest that the regular practice of TM reverses the effects of chronic stress and causes the stress response to become more efficient, i.e., responding sharply and adaptively to stressors but "turning off" quickly. With a more efficient stress response, young people are able to "let things go" and recover faster, in some studies twice as fast as controls, thereby increasing stress tolerance and resilience, which are powerful predictors of academic, career, and life success.[28] A more recent study of fifty college students found faster electrodermal habituation to a stressful stimulus in meditating students compared to wait-list controls,[29] reflecting the quicker recovery from stressors found in other studies. Furthermore, a study by Barnes et al. found that twice-daily TM practice by African American adolescents with high blood pressure led to significant decreases in resting blood pressure, heart rate, and sympathetic nervous system activity during two stress activities.[30] Other studies have similarly found a significant lowering of blood pressure in at-risk high school and college students,[31] providing additional evidence for the de-stressing effects of TM.

Lowering basal stress levels and improving the efficiency of the stress response would be expected to contribute importantly to the prevention and treatment of mental health problems because anxiety, depression, substance abuse, eating disorders, self-injury, and problems related to anger and aggression all involve dysregulation of the stress response.[32] For example, a hyper-reactive amygdala is the most common brain marker of depression and anxiety disorders in both adolescents and adults.[33] Severe and/or chronic moderate stress plays an extremely important role in triggering and maintaining mental health problems, suggesting that a significant portion of the suffering caused by these disorders could be prevented or minimized by lowering stress levels and improving stress regulation. It should also be noted that, as is discussed in more detail below, by decreasing levels of stress hormones and allowing more optimal reactivity to stressors, TM could be expected to improve all aspects of cognition since extensive research has documented the deleterious effects of even mild stress on cognitive function.[34]

In regard to brain functioning, studies since the early 1970s have consistently found a striking degree of brain-wave coherence across the hemispheres and between frontal and posterior brain regions both during and after TM.[35] Several studies have shown increased coherence and synchrony in the alpha frequency of EEGs,[36] which is associated with more-effective executive functioning,[37] greater creativity and stronger flexibility in concept learning, and improved abstract reasoning ability and leadership skill.[38] Alpha coherence is also negatively correlated with both trait and state anxiety and is positively related to increased emotional stability.[39]

TM AND MENTAL HEALTH

Anxiety Disorders

Perhaps the most obvious potential application of TM in mental health is in the prevention and treatment of anxiety disorders, which are common and appear early in life. In an extensive survey of American adolescents, Merikangas et al. found that almost one in three teens was or had been diagnosed with at least one type of anxiety disorder (e.g., generalized anxiety disorder, separation anxiety disorder, or a specific phobia), with the average age of onset being six.[40] The "load" of persistent anxiety in childhood and adolescence is associated with significant developmental and psychological complications. The vast majority of children and teens who develop anxiety disorders will experience the same or another anxiety disorder, mood disorder, or substance-use disorder over the course of their lifespan.[41] The evidence suggests that the development of depressive disorders is a particularly frequent complication across the whole range of anxiety disorders.[42]

Despite a very strong emphasis on early intervention in the treatment of anxiety, the majority of children, teens, and young adults who suffer from anxiety disorders (and other mental health problems) do not receive treatment.[43] Moreover, while there is evidence that treatments, including psychopharmacological therapy and cognitive behavioral therapy, can be beneficial, they are far from perfect and, in the case of medications, commonly have side effects that outweigh the benefits. Moreover, very few young people are given tools they can use on a daily basis for healing the effects of stress and reshaping their brains to be less reactive to stress and thus more resilient.

Although no studies have been done on meditating adolescents with diagnosed anxiety disorders, there is extensive research documenting TM's ability to significantly reduce stress and anxiety, particularly trait anxiety, in young people. Beginning with middle school students, a study of academic achievement in at-risk adolescents in an urban middle school found decreased trait anxiety in sixth- and seventh-grade students.[44] Similarly, a qualitative analysis of the self-reports of seventh-grade African American students found greater self-reported relaxation, patience, and adaptability, along with reduced emotional reactivity.[45] Also, a series of three randomized studies conducted with 362 adolescents, including both junior and senior high-school students, from both public and private schools in Taiwan found that the twice-daily practice of TM for 15–20 minutes produced significant decreases in both state and trait anxiety compared to students who napped or performed another form of meditation.[46] Additionally, a pilot study of middle school students with ADHD, which is discussed in more detail below, found significant reductions in self-reported stress and anxiety.[47]

The findings from studies of middle school students are comparable to those from studies of high school and college students. For example, an early study of African American college students found greater reductions in self-reported anxiety and neuroticism after practicing TM for one year compared to controls.[48] The results of a more recent study of racial and ethnic minority secondary students also found significant reductions in overall psychological distress and trait anxiety compared to controls.[49] Furthermore, a recent study of college students reported statistically significant reductions in self-reported psychological stress and trait anxiety.[50] Finally, a recent meta-analysis which included sixteen studies and 1,295 participants found TM to be better for reducing severe trait anxiety than psychotherapy or other relaxation techniques.[51]

Mood Disorders

According to the World Health Organization, depression is the leading cause of disability worldwide for American men and women ages 15 to 44. The previously mentioned epidemiological survey[52] found that more than 14 percent of adolescents were diagnosed with a mood disorder, with the average age of onset being thirteen. Some scientists argue that the prevalence of depression is increasing rapidly,[53] that it is affecting people at younger and younger ages, and that for an adolescent diagnosed with depression, it takes increasingly less stress to trigger subsequent depressions.[54]

At particularly high risk are post-pubertal females. In fact, data from the 2008–2010 National Survey on Drug Use and Health indicate that between the ages of 12 and 15, the percentage of girls experiencing a major depression triples (from 5 percent to 15 percent).[55] Depression takes a child's or adolescent's development off course, and it contributes greatly to the global burden of disease due to its high lifetime prevalence, early age of onset, high level of chronicity, and significant impairment of social and professional life.[56]

There is considerable empirical evidence that the regular practice of TM improves mood. A recent study by Burns et al. found that college freshman practicing TM twice daily for two semesters self-reported significantly lower levels of depressive symptoms.[57] Also, the previously-mentioned study of college students by Nidich et al. reported a 40 percent reduction in psychological distress, which included symptoms of depression, as well as stress and anxiety.[58] Regarding younger adolescents, studies of 60 sixth graders at two middle schools found that four months of TM practice produced positive effects on emotional development, with higher scores seen on measures of affectivity, self-esteem, and emotional competence.[59] Furthermore, a previously mentioned qualitative study found that meditating African American middle school students were happier, handled stress better, reported higher self-esteem, and had better peer relations than non-meditating students.[60]

It is additionally important to note that there is evidence that TM contributes to improved regulation of anger, which is commonly seen as an expression of mood disorders in children and teenagers.[61] Also, there is extensive evidence indicating improvement in psychological mechanisms related to depression, including increased internal locus control and improved self-esteem, mental flexibility, and coping skills.[62]

These findings are not surprising in light of the fact that depression is a disorder of stress regulation.[63] Stress hormones can trigger the onset of depression, in part by modifying the brain's ability to interpret situations, leading to more pessimistic perception.[64] The significant reduction in baseline stress levels and stress reactivity resulting from the practice of TM may thus be one mechanism for improved mood and decreased depressive symptoms. Another possible mechanism is the increase in serotonin levels reported in some studies of TM.[65] Improved sleep, a benefit of TM commonly reported by adolescents and college students, also contributes to mood elevation, For example, an early study found a 42 percent decrease in insomnia in veterans with PTSD.[66] Moreover, the recent study by Travis et al. discussed above found decreased sleepiness in college students practicing TM (in contrast to increased sleepiness in the control group),[67] and a recent meta-analysis by Orme-Johnson and Barnes reported evidence for decreased insomnia.[68] Finally, another mechanism that may help to account for reduced emotional pain and improved mood resulting from meditation is the effect of meditation on the brain's response to pain. A study of long-term TM meditators (thirty years) found a 40–50 percent reduction in the brain's reactivity to pain, particularly in the frontal cortex and the anterior cingulate.[69] After practicing TM for five months, the control group also demonstrated 40–50 percent decreased brain reactivity to pain. This may be relevant to mood disorders, particularly in light of the overlap of brain systems that mediate physical pain and social or psychological pain.[70]

Autism Spectrum Disorders

Evidence is emerging that TM may be a valuable tool in the treatment of the stress and anxiety symptoms seen in adolescents and young adults with autism spectrum disorders (ASDs). ASDs refer to a group of developmental abilities that are characterized by deficits in social interaction and communication, along with the presence of restricted and repetitive behaviors.[71] The prevalence of ASDs appears to be growing rapidly. Very recently, the Centers for Disease Control and Prevention (CDC) reported that 1 in 68 American children is believed to be on the spectrum,[72] a dramatic increase in incidence from the 1 in 88 reported just two years earlier.

Stress-related disorders involving anxiety and sleep disturbances are common in students with ASDs,[73] which is likely related to the fact that these students have particular difficulty managing the aspects of life that make it stressful, including new situations, transitions, and situations in which they experience a low sense of predictability and control.[74] Many students with ASDs have trouble coping with certain environmental stimuli such as crowds, bright lights, and loud sounds,[75] which can make the world "feel" more threatening to them than it does to most people. Not surprisingly, studies of individuals with ASDs have suggested that approximately 40 percent suffer from significant anxiety symptoms, although estimates have ranged as high as 84 percent.[76] Moreover, mothers of older adolescents with ASDs have been found to have cortisol levels that are comparable to those of soldiers in combat,[77] suggesting that stress reduction is equally important for these parents as for their children.

Presently, while there is some evidence for the effectiveness of cognitive-behavioral therapy in treating anxiety in young people with ASDs,[78] a recent review by White et al. concluded that there are no empirically supported treatments for the emotional and behavioral difficulties experienced by children and adolescents with ASDs, including anxiety.[79] Moreover, there presently are no medications with demonstrated efficacy in the reduction of anxiety in students with ASDs.[80] It is thus encouraging that there is currently one published case report of an adolescent with ASD that describes improved emotional regulation, self-regulation, and sleep resulting from the practice of TM.[81]

There is also an as-yet-unpublished, retrospective pilot study involving a case series on the effects of TM in adolescents and young adults with ASD conducted by David Black, Ph.D., an autism researcher at the National Institute of Mental Health (NIMH), and Norman Rosenthal, M.D., the discoverer of seasonal affective disorder (SAD) and an expert on TM.[82]

Drs. Black and Rosenthal studied six participants, ranging in age from 16 to 22 years. It was found that all participants were able to learn to meditate, and that five meditated consistently on a twice-daily basis (the sixth, who was away from home at college, reported meditating 8–10 times a week). All participants and their parents reported reductions in stress and anxiety, improved emotional and behavioral regulation, increased productivity, and greater capacity to cope with new situations and to make transitions. Additionally, the parents reported that since starting to practice meditation, their children were able to take on more responsibility, recovered faster following stressful experiences, and generally appeared more at ease.

Other reported benefits included improved concentration, decreased test anxiety, better sleep patterns, a reduction in tantrums, and fewer physiological symptoms of stress. The parents of some participants further reported a reduction in autism symptoms, including increased social motivation, improved eye contact, and greater flexibility. The evidence from these case studies has led to the funding for a controlled study scheduled to begin in March 2014 with thirty middle school students at an independent school serving children and adolescents with high-functioning autism.

Substance Abuse

Substance-abuse disorders typically begin in mid-adolescence and, according to the previously mentioned epidemiological survey, are diagnosed in over 10 percent of adolescents.[83] A primary risk factor for chemical addiction, as well as for other forms of addiction, is genetic vulnerability, including genes that regulate motivation/reward, emotional regulation, and inhibitory control.[84] Risk factors also include prenatal stress and inadequate care-giving in infancy, as well as severe or chronic stress during childhood; in fact, stress and associated increases in stress hormones at any stage of development can trigger an addictive process.[85] Stress hormones also compromise the functioning and development of brain systems that are crucial for the regulation of stress, including the amygdala, hippocampus, and prefrontal cortex.[86] A sensitive reward system, a dysregulated stress system, and lowered executive control contribute to repeated use and relapse. It is therefore suggested that anything that prevents or reduces stress will reduce the risk of substance abuse.[87]

Studies suggest that the adolescent brain is at particularly high risk for developing addictions due to the powerful effects that substances have on the developing brain.[88] There is also considerable evidence that life stresses in the teen years contribute to substance use and abuse.[89] The National Survey of American Attitudes on Substance Abuse VIII: Teens and Parents conducted by the National Center on Addiction and Substance Abuse (CASA) at Columbia University found that highly stressed teens are twice as likely as low-stress teens to smoke, drink, and use illegal drugs. Also, according to the 2007 Partnership Attitude Tracking Study of 6,511 teens (PATS Teens), seventy-three percent of the teens surveyed reported that school-related stress is the primary reason for drug use.[90]

The results of TM research in this area are encouraging. In an early analysis of twenty-four studies, Gelderloos et al. found TM to be strikingly effective in preventing and treating substance abuse.[91] The length of time a subject practiced TM was associated with a gradual decrease in alcohol and drug use. Also, in an early meta-analysis of nineteen studies on drug use, Alexander et al. found TM to lead to greater reduction in alcohol, cigarette, and drug use than other forms of meditation or relaxation techniques.[92] In fact, TM was twice as effective as conventional approaches in reducing alcoholism and substance abuse. More recently, a meta-analysis conducted by Orme-Johnson and Barnes found significantly decreased drug and alcohol use with TM,[93] and a recent study of college students practicing TM for three months reported significantly reduced alcohol use in males.[94]

Self-Injury

Self-injury, including self-cutting and self-burning, has become prevalent in young people. Estimates of prevalence vary, but studies imply that 13–25 percent of teens and young adults have at least some history of self-injury.[95] Similarly, a recent study of undergraduates at Cornell University and Princeton University found that 17 percent of the undergraduate students surveyed had a history of self-cutting or self-burning.[96] It is notable that most of the students at Cornell and Princeton did not have a formal psychiatric diagnosis and reported using self-injury as a tool for managing stress and negative emotions. There is evidence more generally that the primary purpose of self-cutting is to reduce stress and emotional pain.[97] While there are no direct studies of TM as a tool for preventing or treating self-injury, the evidence from the study of addictions suggests that TM may be a positive alternative for decreasing stress, neutralizing painful emotions, and increasing a sense of well-being.

Preventing Mental Health Problems

Given that mental health disorders in adults initially emerge in childhood or adolescence, mental health experts emphasize the importance of prevention, as well as treatment, of mental health problems.[98] In light of the fact that excessive stress and fatigue play a critical role in triggering the onset of mental disorders in adolescents, and as the regular practice of TM lowers stress levels, reduces anxiety, and improves mood and coping skills in young people, it is likely that TM could play an important role in the prevention—as well as the treatment—of emotional and behavioral disorders.

LEARNING, ATTENTION, AND BEHAVIOR DISORDERS

Stress and Learning

Perhaps the major conclusion drawn from neuroscience on education is that the optimal internal state for learning is "restful alertness,"[99] while the optimal environmental condition for learning is characterized by "high challenge and low threat."[100] These conclusions are based on findings from hundreds of studies showing that high levels of stress compromise virtually all important cognitive functions, including attention, memory, and executive functions such as inhibition, working memory, cognitive flexibility, planning, organization, and self-monitoring.[101] Arnsten has documented the toxic effects of stress on the prefrontal brain systems that mediate attention and executive functions, which she attributes to the fact that activation of the stress response results in the prefrontal cortex being flooded with dopamine and norepinephrine, following which it is unable to function effectively.[102] Also, Lupien and others have demonstrated the deleterious effects of stress on the hippocampus and associated impairments in learning and memory.[103] It is thus not surprising that by neutralizing stress and inducing a state of relaxed alertness, TM has been shown to produce improvements in numerous cognitive functions, including attention and the executive functions. For example, the series of studies on Taiwanese junior and senior high-school students conducted by So and Orme-Johnson found significant increases in creativity, practical intelligence (e.g., problem solving), field independence, and decision-making speed, as well is in creativity and fluid intelligence.[104] Additionally, the recent study of meditating college students found improvement on a brain integration scale on which higher scores are associated with greater breadth of planning, thinking, and perception of the environment.[105]

Attention Deficit Hyperactivity Disorder

One of the most common childhood disorders resulting from impaired executive function is attention deficit hyperactivity disorder (ADHD), which is believed to affect more than 10 percent of children and adolescents.[106] There is evidence that stress can play a causative role in ADHD. It is well known that early experiences of stress, including prenatal experiences, affect the level of responsiveness of the hypothalamic-pituitary-adrenal (HPA) axis and the autonomic nervous system.[107] Infants and young children exposed to chronic stress can become accustomed to dealing with high fear states and to tolerating high levels of stress hormones. Chronic stress and severe acute stress damage the body's ability to return to non-stress levels, leading to chronically elevated levels of cortisol, which is known to impair executive function, self-regulation, and letter knowledge in children with ADHD.[108] There is also evidence that children with ADHD may be particularly vulnerable to difficulty regulating stress. For example, Silk et al. has demonstrated dysfunction in the right prefrontal region in children with ADHD,[109] suggesting possible impairment in brain systems responsible for developing coping strategies, and thus influencing the ability to handle stress.

Dysregulation of the central noradrenergic pathways in the brain is believed to strongly underlie the pathophysiology of ADHD.[110] The noradrenergic system is associated with the modulation of attention, alertness, vigilance, and executive function. Specifically, dopamine is associated with behavior and impulse control, while norepinephrine is believed to mediate functions involving focusing, planning, and conceptual thinking, including concepts related to sequence and time. Abnormalities in the noradrenergetic systems are seen in students with ADHD, and most of the ADHD medication involves increasing the presence of dopamine and/or norepinephrine. As Arnsten has demonstrated, disruption of the noradrenergic function seen in the presence of the fight or flight response can, in itself, produce symptoms that are identical to those seen in individuals with ADHD (e.g., inattention, distractibility, impulsiveness, restlessness).[111]

In light of the above, there is good reason to think that TM should lead to improvement in ADHD symptomatology, in part because of its stress-reducing function, and in part because of its capacity for increasing coherence in brain functioning. Also, TM enlivens the prefrontal executive areas, which is associated with improved behavioral regulation in typically developing adolescents and young adults. For example, a study of TM using magnetoencephalography documented increased brain activation in frontal executive areas and the anterior cingulate attention areas,[112] and the results from a PET study found increased activation in frontal-parietal attention systems.[113]

Regarding the direct study of adolescents with ADHD, a pilot study of the effects of TM on middle school students with ADHD was conducted in 2009.[114] It found a 43 percent reduction in self-reported symptoms of stress and anxiety. There was also improvement in ADHD symptoms including behavioral regulation and emotional control after three months of daily practice of TM in school. Accompanying the improvements in stress, anxiety, and emotional control, were improvements in executive function, with 19 percent improvement in expressive attention and 13 percent improvement in executive planning and problem solving.[115]

A second study, a randomized controlled trial, explored the effects of TM on brain coherence and brain development in middle school students with ADHD.[116] It has been shown that the EEGs of students with ADHD are marked by decreased activation in parietal areas of the brain that weave sensory input into concrete perception, as well as higher density and amplitude of theta activity and lower density and amplitude of alpha and beta activity.[117] Theta is thought to block out irrelevant stimuli during memory processing, and it is believed that in students with ADHD, greater theta activity may block out relevant as well as irrelevant information. Theta/beta ratios are highly correlated with severity of ADHD symptoms.[118] It is also important to note that low EEG coherence is another brain marker of ADHD. In individuals with ADHD, coherence in all frequencies is lower, reflecting a reduced number and strength of connections between different brain areas.[119]

The Travis, Grosswald, and Stixrud study measured EEG coherence, theta/beta ratio, and executive function. Subjects were randomly assigned to a TM group or a delayed-start group. The delayed-start group served as controls for the first three months, then they also learned the TM technique. At the three-month post-test, theta/beta ratios increased in the delayed-start group, which is opposite of the desired effect, while the TM subjects moved closer to normal values. At the six-month post-test, after both groups were practicing TM, theta/beta ratios decreased in both groups. For the delayed-start group, theta/beta ratios also significantly decreased from the three-month to six-month post-test after three months practice of TM.

School-Based Meditation Programs

Several studies have examined the effects of TM in school on students' learning, behavior, and adjustment, hypothesizing that because high stress levels are associated with poor cognitive functioning and with behavioral and emotional dysregulation, lowering stress levels should improve cognition and behavior. For example, a study by Barnes et al. found that four months of TM practice by African American adolescents with high normal blood pressure led to significant reductions in days absent, rule violations, and suspensions from school, as well as reduced aggression and significantly decreased anger in girls.[120] Also, the previously mentioned qualitative study by Rosean and Benn found that TM leads to increased self-control (especially control of anger), as well as greater adaptability, patience, and tolerance in seventh-grade students.[121]

Based on the results of these and other studies, in 2007 the Center for Wellness and Achievement in Education (CWAE) launched the Quiet Time program in low-income, low-achieving public middle schools and high schools in San Francisco. The Quiet Time program is a whole-school intervention involving students and faculty that features two 15-minute restful periods during the school day. The great majority of students practice TM during the Quiet Time periods, while others rest, nap, or engage in silent reading. The goal of the program is transformation of the school climate by reducing stress, improving learning and academic performance, and lowering teacher burnout. Extensive research has been conducted—and continues to be conducted—on the effects of the Quiet Time program. Although much of the data is yet unpublished, it has led to articles extolling the program's benefits in the popular press and in educational publications. For example, David Kirp, a professor of public policy at the University of California at Berkeley, wrote in an online editorial that meditation "is transforming the roughest San Francisco schools."[122] According to Professor Kirp, "I've spent lots of time in urban schools and have never seen anything like it." He concluded by saying that while Quiet Time is not a panacea, "it's a game-changer for many students who otherwise might have become dropouts."

In an article written for school administrators, James Dierke, the principal of the first middle school to adopt the Quiet Time program, wrote that the meditation-based program in his school led to markedly reduced suspensions, increased attendance, and improved academic performance, with the greatest academic improvement seen in the lowest performing demographics.[123] Mr. Dierke reported that his school was transformed from having one of the highest suspension rates in San Francisco to having the second-lowest rate in the whole school district. He also stated that teacher absenteeism due to illness went down by 30 percent compared to the previous year and that the students in his school reported the highest level of happiness on the most recent California Healthy Kids Survey. As Dierke noted, this would not be expected in neighborhoods in which there were forty-one murders between 2005 and 2007. Dierke concluded, "By reducing the individual and collective stress and fostering a positive school climate, [the Quiet Time program] creates a foundation for all of our other school initiatives to be more successful." Based on its apparent success, the Quiet Time program has been adopted in other San Francisco public schools and in several schools across the country.

There are presently four published studies on the Quiet Time program, three reporting outcomes for students and one for school faculty. In his initial pilot study, Nidich et al. reported on 189 low-achieving middle school children, most of whom were racial and ethnic minority students, who practiced TM in school twice daily.[124] It was concluded that after three months of practice, the Quiet Time program lead to significant improvement in math and English scores on the California Standards Test compared to matched controls. A second study, discussed above,[125] found significantly reduced psychological distress and anxiety, with significant reduction in trait anxiety and symptoms of emotional problems more generally in racial and ethnic minority secondary students who practiced TM for four months as part of the Quiet Time program. In a third study, by Colbert et al.,[126] seniors in an East Coast urban high school who practiced TM for four months showed increased on-time graduation rates (especially for low-GPA students), dramatically lower dropout rates, and increased college acceptances compared to matched controls.

The most recent study of the Quiet Time program reported the effects of four months of TM on the psychological well-being of faculty at a residential therapeutic school in Vermont.[127] Compared to wait-list controls, the meditating teachers reported significantly lower levels of perceived stress, depressive symptoms, and overall burnout.

Extensive and as-yet-unpublished data collected by the Center for Wellness and Achievement in Education (CWAE) and the San Francisco Unified School District have additionally documented improvements in students' attendance, school behavior, psychological health, sleep, and achievement test scores. The data have also shown lower psychological stress levels in teachers and improvement in teachers' emotional intelligence, brain functioning, energy, and resilience. The findings from these studies are available through CWAE (www.cwae.org).

IDEAS ABOUT IMPLEMENTATION

The findings discussed above suggest that by lowering stress levels and increasing the orderliness of brain functioning, regular practice of TM can improve the cognitive, academic, and social/emotional functioning of adolescents and young adults, including adolescents living in poverty and attending low-achieving urban schools. The school-based meditation programs appear to be particularly powerful because at least five days a week, the students meditate twice every day as part of a group.

Because of the enormous importance of peer approval and support for adolescents, the support of meditating peers is highly valuable. In our experience, many adolescents and young adults will meditate on their own, especially if they see meditation as a tool that can alleviate their physical and/or emotional pain, or if it is part of the daily routine of their parents or whole family. However, they are more likely to meditate regularly with the support and approval of other young people.

For medical or mental health practitioners, we recommend that teens be introduced to TM and invited to learn, as long as they are willing to give meditation a good try, which we suggest means meditating every day for three months, usually twice a day. We do not recommend that teens be coerced into meditation but rather that the benefits be presented to them in an engaging format (including the many videos available through the

David Lynch Foundation). We also suggest helping teens think through how TM could be incorporated into their schedule (e.g., during a study hall or right before dinner) and that attempts be made to gain their "buy in" before starting a good meditation trial. Additionally, helping them to recognize benefits they are experiencing and to talk about changes they have noticed themselves (e.g., better grades, getting in trouble less) helps them take ownership of the practice and encourages them to maintain regular daily meditation.

Finally, it is important to note that children and teens benefit when their parents can, to a large extent, serve as a "non-anxious presence" within their families,[128] which means remaining calm and not becoming overly fearful or reactive in response to the ups and downs in their own—and their children's—lives. There is also evidence that many children's greatest wish for their parents is not that they spend more time with their children—but rather that they be happier and less stressed.[129] We thus recommend TM to parents of children and teenagers who are struggling, even if the children themselves do not want to meditate.

CASE STUDIES

Elizabeth, a nineteen-year-old college student, presented for neuropsychological testing after experiencing marked academic failure in her first year of college. She reported a history of anxiety and depression that started following the traumatic death of her father two years previously. She acknowledged that mild depression, frequent marijuana use, and difficulty sleeping contributed to her significant trouble "making herself" attend her college classes and study on a regular basis. In the course of discussion during the neuropsychological assessment, it was suggested that Elizabeth consider TM as an alternative to marijuana use, as meditation would likely help to quiet her mind, improve her sleep and, over time, heal the emotional pain associated with her loss and her academic failure—without any of the negative effects of smoking pot.

Elizabeth agreed to try. She stopped smoking marijuana for fifteen days (a prerequisite for learning TM) and started to practice meditation regularly. She quickly noticed that she felt calmer inside without self-medicating and that she was able to sleep better. Within several weeks, she also noticed that she was feeling happier and was experiencing a strong desire to pursue her true passion—visual art. She continued to refrain from marijuana use, and her pot-smoking friends commented on the "natural high" Elizabeth seemed to get from meditation. As she began to feel better, she started taking community college courses to reestablish her academic record and volunteered as a teaching assistant at a local art school. She urged her mother to learn TM to help with her own grief, and she considered becoming a TM teacher so that she could teach other young people to meditate. Elizabeth eventually decided, though, to transfer to a major university with an excellent visual arts program, and she is currently pursuing her education and training with great energy and enthusiasm. Based on the changes she observed in her daughter, Elizabeth's mother began to practice TM and also found it to be an extremely beneficial tool for healing and emotional growth.

Zachary, a fourteen-year-old boy, was diagnosed with ADHD inattentive type and language-based learning disorders. He had few if any friends at school, interacted very little with others, tended to sit alone, and did not participate with peers at lunch or gym period but instead sat alone reading during non-class time. He learned TM as part of research study in his school, where students meditated twice daily as part of the school schedule. After less than three months of meditating, Zachary was reported by the head of the school as being much more engaged in school activities and he had, in fact, presented a plan to her for student leadership. One year later, follow-up with Zachary's parents revealed that he had developed a group of friends and seemed happy. In his senior year of high school, he was student government president. An interview with him at age twenty-one revealed that he was happy, was involved in student government in a local college, had a part-time store-management job, was still doing TM, and credited the technique as a contributor to his development.

Oscar is an eleventh-grade student in an urban San Francisco high school. He started the Quiet Time program in middle school but, as a ninth grader, he stopped meditating and started hanging out with the "stoner" crowd. He began resisting authority and encouragement from his teachers and school administrators, and he was absent from school for weeks as a time. Early in his tenth-grade year, Quiet Time staff invested extra time in Oscar, trying to help him see his potential and encouraging him to resume meditating during Quiet Time. The investment paid off, as the twice-daily practice of TM appeared to have a transformative effect. Oscar began attending school every day, and by midyear he was seeking out leadership opportunities in an elective called Peer Resources. By the end of the year, he had undergone a major turnaround.

This year, Oscar is a high-functioning student who, according to Quiet Time staff, never misses a meditation session, a day of school, or an opportunity to make a difference. He is interested in political and social change and has taken internships with the San Francisco Mayor's office. He is determined to go to college, and he has maintained grades that are good enough for California State and University of California schools. Deeply reflective and interested in growth, Oscar has signed up for an elective class offered next year by Quiet Time staff called Social and Emotional Intelligence. He has also applied for membership in the Advanced Meditator Club, through which he will encourage ninth-grade students to foster their own development through the Quiet Time program.

NOTES

1. Spear, L., *The Behavioral Neuroscience of Adolescence* (New York: W. W. Norton, 2010); Daniel J. Siegel, *Brainstorm: The Power and Purpose of the Teenage Brain* (New York: Penguin, 2014).

2. Twenge, J., "Generational Differences in Mental Health: Are Children and Adolescents Suffering More or Less?" *American Journal of Orthopsychiatry* 81 (2011): 469–72, DOI:10.1111/j.1939-0025.2011.01115.x; J. Twenge, B. Gentile, C. N. DeWall, D. Ma, K. Lacefield, and D. R. Schurtz, "Birth Cohort Increases in Psychopathology among Young Americans, 1938–2007: A Cross-temporal Meta-analysis of the MMPI," *Clinical Psychology Review* 30, no. 2 (March 2010): 145–54, DOI:10.1016/j.cpr.2009.10.005.

3. Merikangas, K. et al., "Lifetime Prevalence of Mental Disorders in U.S. Adolescents: Results from the National Comorbidity Survey Replication–Adolescent Supplement (NCS-A)," *Journal of the American Academy of Child and Adolescent Psychiatry* 49, no. 10 (October 2010): 980–89.

4. National Research Council, *Preventing Mental, Emotional, and Behavioral Disorders Among Young People: Progress and Possibilities*, ed. Mary Ellen O'Connell, Thomas Boat, and Kenneth E. Warner (Washington, DC: National Academies Press, 2009).

5. Kinney, D. K. et al., "Prenatal Stress and Risk for Autism," *Neuroscience Biobehavioral Review* 32, no. 8 (October 2008): 1519–32, DOI:10.1016/j.neubio rev.2008.06.004.

6. Slobogin, K., "Survey: Many Students Say Cheating's OK," CNN Edition: Student News, http://edition.cnn.com/2002/fyi/teachers.ednews/04/05/high school.cheating/.

7. Konrath, S. H. et al., "Changes in Dispositional Empathy in American College Students over Time: A Meta-analysis," *Personality and Social Psychology Review* 15, no. 2 (2011): 180–98, www.sitemaker.umich.edu/eob/files/konrathetal2011.pdf.

8. Pryor, J. H. et al., *The American Freshman: National Norms for Fall 2010* (Los Angeles: University of California Press Books, 2011).

9. Gallagher, R. P., "National Survey of Counseling Center Directors 2010" (Alexandria, VA: International Association of Counseling Services), http://iacsinc .org/NSCCD%202010.pdf.

10. Wechsler, H., and T. F. Nelson, "What We Have Learned from the Harvard School of Public Health College Alcohol Study: Focusing Attention on College Student Alcohol Consumption and the Environmental Conditions that Promote It," *Journal of Studies on Alcohol and Drugs* 69 (2008): 481–90.

11. Arnsten, A. F. T., "Stress Signaling Pathways that Impair Prefrontal Cortex Structure and Function," *Nature Reviews Neuroscience* 10, no. 6 (June 2009), DOI:

10.1038/nrn2648; Megan Gunnar and Karina Quevedo, "The Neurobiology of Stress and Development," *Annual Review of Psychology* 58 (2007): 145–73, DOI: 10.1146/annurev.psych.58.110405.08560; R. Stickgold, "Sleep-Dependent Memory Consolidation," *Nature* 437, no. 27 (October 2005): 1272, DOI:10.1038/nature04286.

12. Gray, P., "The Decline of Play and the Rise of Psychopathology in Children and Adolescents," *American Journal of Play* 3, no. 4 (2011); Robert D. Putnam, *Bowling Alone, The Collapse and Revival of American Community* (New York: Simon & Schuster, 2000); Christopher Munsey, "The Kids Aren't All Right," *Monitor on Psychology* 41, no. 1 (2010): 22.

13. Sigman, A., "Time for a View on Screen Time," *Archives of Disease in Childhood* 97, no. 11 (2012): 935–42.

14. Immordino-Yang, M. H. et al., "Rest Is Not Idleness: Implications of the Brain's Default Mode for Human Development and Education," *Perspectives on Psychological Science* 7, no. 4 (2012).

15. Spear, L., "The Adolescent Brain and the College Drinker: Biological Basis of Propensity to Use and Misuse Alcohol," *Journal of Studies on Alcohol* (2002), suppl. 14; S. R. Sumpter et al., "Age and Puberty Differences in Stress Responses During Public Speaking Task: Do Adolescents Grow More Sensitive to Social Evaluation?" *Psychoneurobiology* 35 (2010): 1510–16.

16. Przybycien-Szymanska, M. N. et al., "Binge-Pattern Alcohol Exposure During Puberty Induces Long-Term Changes in HPA Axis Reactivity," *PLOS ONE* 6, no. 4 (2011): 1–7, DOI:10.1371/journal.pone.0018350.

17. Tsankova, N. M. et al., "Sustained Hippocampal Chromatin Regulation in a Mouse Model of Depression and Antidepressant Action," *Nature Neuroscience* 9, no. 4 (2006): 419–525.

18. Kishiyama, M. M., and R. T. Knight, "Poverty, Stress, and Cognitive Functioning," AccessScience, www.accessscience.com/content/poverty-stress-and-cognitive-functioning/YB100070.

19. Luther, S. S., "The Culture of Affluence: Psychological Costs of Material Wealth," *Child Development* 74, no. 16 (2003): 1581–93; Madeline Levine, *The Price of Privilege: How Parental Pressure and Material Advantage Are Creating a Generation of Disconnected and Unhappy Kids* (New York: Harper Perennial, 2008).

20. Ansell, E. B. et al., "Cumulative Adversity and Smaller Gray Matter Volume in Medial Prefrontal, Anterior Cingulate, and Insula Regions," *Biological Psychiatry* 72, no. 1 (2012): 57–64, DOI:10.1016/j.biopsych.2011.11.022; Sonia J. Lupien et al., "Stress Hormones and Human Memory Function across the Lifespan," *Psychoneuroendocrinology* 30 (2005): 225–42.

21. Amy Arnsten et al., "This Is Your Brain in Meltdown," *Scientific American* 306 (2012): 48–53, DOI:10.1038/scientificamerican0412-48; Robert M. Sapolsky, "How to Relieve Stress," *Greater Good E-Newsletter* (March 22, 2012), http://greatergood.berkeley.edu/article/item/how_to_relieve_stress.

22. Diamond, A., and K. Lee, "Interventions Shown to Aid Executive Function Development in Children 4 to 12 Years Old," *Science* 19, vol. 333, no. 6045 (August 2011), DOI:10.1126/science.1204529.

23. Orme-Johnson, D. W., "Autonomic Stability and Transcendental Meditation," *Psychosomatic Medicine* 35, no. 4 (July–August 1973), 341–49; L. I. Mason et al., "Electrophysiological Correlates of Higher States of Consciousness During

Sleep in Long-Term Practitioners of the Transcendental Meditation Program," *Sleep* 20, no. 2 (February 1997): 102–10, www.ncbi.nlm.nih.gov/pubmed/9143069.

24. Dillbeck, M. C., and D. W. Orme-Johnson, "Physiological Differences between Transcendental Meditation and Rest," *American Psychologist* 42, no. 9 (September 1987): 879–81, DOI:10.1037/0003-066X.42.9.879.

25. McEwen, B. S., "Sleep Deprivation as a Neurobiologic and Physiologic Stressor: Allostasis and Allostatic Load," *Metabolism* 55, no. 10, suppl. 2 (October 2006): S20–S23, www.ncbi.nlm.nih.gov/pubmed/16979422.

26. Jevning, R. et al., "Adrenocortical Activity During Meditation," *Hormonal Behavior* 10, no. 1 (February 1978): 54–60, www.ncbi.nlm.nih.gov/pubmed/350747.

27. MacLean, C. R. et al., "Effects of the Transcendental Meditation Program on Adaptive Mechanisms: Changes in Hormone Levels and Responses to Stress after 4 Months of Practice," *Psychoneuroendocrinology* 22, no. 4 (May 1997): 277–95, www.ncbi.nlm.nih.gov/pubmed/9226731.

28. Orme-Johnson, D. W., "Autonomic Stability and Transcendental Meditation," *Psychosomatic Medicine* 35, no. 4 (July–August 1973): 341–49; Cohn, M. A. et al., "Happiness Unpacked: Positive Emotions Increase Life Satisfaction by Building Resilience," *Emotion* 9, no. 3 (2009): 361–68, DOI:10.1037/a0015952.

29. Travis, F. et al, "Effects of Transcendental Meditation Practice on Brain Functioning and Stress Reactivity in College Students," *International Journal of Psychophysiology* 71, no. 2 (February 2009): 170–76, DOI:10.1016/j.ijpsycho.2008.09.007.

30. Barnes, V.A. et al., "Impact of Transcendental Meditation on Cardiovascular Function at Rest and During Acute Stress in Adolescents with High Normal Blood Pressure," *Journal of Psychosomatic Research* 51, no. 4 (October 2001): 597–605.

31. Barnes, V. A. et al., "Impact of Stress Reduction on Ambulatory Blood Pressure in African American Adolescents," *American Journal of Hypertension* 17, no. 4 (2004): 366–69; S. I. Nidich et al., "A Randomized Controlled Trial on Effects of the Transcendental Meditation Program on Blood Pressure, Psychological Distress, and Coping in Young Adults," *American Journal of Hypertension* 22, no. 12 (December 2009): 1326–31.

32. Pennington, B. *The Development of Psychopathology: Nature and Nurture* (London: Taylor & Francis Books, 2002).

33. Yang, T. et al., "Adolescents with Major Depression Demonstrate Increased Amygdala Activation," *Journal of the American Academy of Child Adolescent Psychiatry* 49, no. 1 (January 2010): 42–51.

34. Arnsten, A. F. T. "Stress-Signalling Pathways That Impair Prefrontal Cortex Structure and Function," *Nature Reviews Neuroscience* 10, no. 6 (2009): 410–22; "Lupien, Stress Hormones."

35. Dillbeck, M. and E. C. Bronson, "Short-Term Longitudinal Effects of the Transcendental Meditation Technique on EEG Power and Coherence," *International Journal of Neuroscience* 14, nos. 3–4 (1981): 147–51.

36. Travis, F., "Development Along an Integration Scale: Longitudinal Transformation in Brain Dynamics with Regular Transcendental Meditation Practice," *Psychophysiology* 39 (2002): S81; Frederick Travis et al., "Patterns of EEG Coherence, Power, and Contingent Negative Variation Characterize the Integration of Transcendental and Waking States," *Biological Psychology* 61, no. 3 (November 2002): 293–319.

37. Travis, F. et al., "ADHD, Brain Functioning, and Transcendental Meditation Practice," *Mind & Brain, The Journal of Psychiatry* 2, no. 1 (July 2011), www.rencapp .com/travis-adhd_brain_functioning_and_transcendental_meditation_practice.pdf.

38. Dillbeck, M. C. et al., "Frontal EEG Coherence, H-Reflex Recovery, Concept Learning, and the TM-Sidhi Program," *International Journal of Neuroscience* 15, no. 3 (1981): 151–57, www.ncbi.nlm.nih.gov/pubmed/7031000.

39. Orme-Johnson, D. W. and V. A. Barnes, "Effects of the Transcendental Technique on Trait Anxiety: A Meta-analysis of Randomized Controlled Trials, *Journal of Alternative Complement Medicine* 19, no. 10 (2013): 1–12, http://online .liebertpub.com/doi/abs/10.1089/acm.2013.0204.

40. Merikangas, *Lifetime Prevalence*.

41. Beesdo, K. et al., "Anxiety and Anxiety Disorders in Children and Adolescents," *Psychiatric Clinics of North America* 32, no. 3 (September 2009): 483–524, DOI:10.1016/j.psc.2009.06.002.

42. Woodward, L. J. and D. M. Fergusson, "Life Course Outcomes of Young People with Anxiety Disorders in Adolescence," *Journal of American Academy of Child Adolescence Psychiatry* 40, no. 9 (September 2001): 1086–93, www.ncbi.nlm .nih.gov/pubmed/11556633.

43. Merikangas, *Lifetime Prevalence*.

44. Nidich, S. et al., "Academic Achievement and Transcendental Meditation: A Study with At-Risk Middle School Students," *Education* 131, no. 3 (2011): 556–65.

45. Rosean, B., and R. Benn, "The Experience of Transcendental Meditation in Middle School Students," *Journal of Science and Healing* 2, no. 5 (2006): 422–25.

46. So, K., and D. W. Orme-Johnson, "Three Randomized Experiments on the Longitudinal Effects of the Transcendental Meditation Technique on Cognition," *Intelligence* 29 (2001): 419–40.

47. Grosswald, S. J. et al., "Use of the Transcendental Meditation Technique to Reduce Symptoms of Attention Deficit Hyperactivity Disorder (ADHD) by Reducing Stress and Anxiety: An Exploratory Study," *Current Issues in Education* 10, no. 2 (December 2008), http://cie.ed.asu.edu/volume10/number2/.

48. Gaylord, C. et al., "Effects of Transcendental Meditation Technique and Progressive Muscular Relaxation on EEG Coherence, Stress Reactivity, and Mental Health in Black Adults," *International Journal of Neuroscience* 46, nos. 1–2 (1989): 77–86.

49. Elder, C., "Reduced Psychological Distress in Racial and Ethnic Minority Students Practicing the Transcendental Meditation Program," *Journal of Instructional Psychology* 38, no. 2 (June 2011).

50. *Nidich, Randomized Controlled Trial, Blood Pressure.*

51. Orme-Johnson, *Trait Anxiety*.

52. Merikangas, *Lifetime Prevalence*.

53. Seligman, M., "Why Is There So Much Depression Today?" *Contemporary Psychological Approaches to Depression*, ed. R. E. Ingram (New York: Plenum Press, 1990): 1–9.

54. Pennington, *Nature and Nurture*.

55. "Depression Triples Between Ages 12 and 15 in Girls in U.S.," *Medical New*, HealthDay News (July 31, 2012): 17, www.empr.com/depression-triples-between -ages-12-and-15-in-girls-in-us/article/252579/.

56. Alloy, L. B., and L. Y. Abramson, "The Adolescent Surge in Depression and Emergence of Gender Differences: A Biocognitive Vulnerability-Stress Model in Developmental Context," in *Adolescent Psychopathology and the Developing Brain: Integrating Brain and Prevention Sciences* (New York: Oxford University Press, 2007), 284.

57. Burns, J., "The Effect of Meditation on Self-Reported Stress, Anxiety, Depression, and Perfectionism in a College Population," *Journal of College Student Psychotherapy* 25 (2011): 132–44.

58. Nidich, *Randomized Controlled Trial, Blood Pressure.*

59. Benn, R., Ph.D., director of the Complementary and Alternative Medicine Center at the University of Michigan, presenter of TM research at the NIH International Center for Integration of Health and Spirituality in Bethesda, Maryland, April 2003, and at the International Symposium for Complementary Health Care in London, November 2003.

60. Rosean, *Experience of TM in Middle School.*

61. Nidich, S. et al., "A Randomized Controlled Trial on Effects of the Transcendental Meditation on Quality of Life in Older Breast Cancer Patients," *American Journal of Hypertension* 22, no. 12 (December 2009): 1326–31; Rosean, *Experience of TM in Middle School;* V. A. Barnes et al., "Impact of Stress Reduction on Negative School Behavior in Adolescents," *Health and Quality of Life Outcomes* 1, no. 10 (April 2003), DOI:10.1186/1477-7525-1-10.

62. So, *Longitudinal Effects of TM Technique.*

63. Pennington, *Nature and Nurture.*

64. Sapolsky, *Greater Good.*

65. Bujatli, M. and P. Riederer, "Serotonin, Noradrenaline, Dopamine Metabolites in Transcendental Meditation Technique," *Journal of Neural Transmission* 39, no. 3 (1976): 257–67, www.ncbi.nlm.nih.gov/pubmed/789821.

66. Brooks, J. S., "Transcendental Meditation in the Treatment of Post-Vietnam Adjustment," *Journal of Counseling & Development* 64 (1985): 212–15.

67. Travis, *Effects of TM Practice on Brain Functioning.*

68. Orme-Johnson, *Trait Anxiety.*

69. Orme-Johnson, D. W. et al., "Neuroimaging of Meditation's Effect on Brain Reactivity to Pain," *NeuroReport* 17, no. 12 (August 21, 2006).

70. Eisenberger, N. I. et al., "Does Rejection Hurt? An MRI Study of Social Exclusion," *Science* 302, no. 5643 (October 2003): 290–92, www.scn.ucla.edu/pdf/Cyberball290.pdf.

71. American Psychiatric Association, *Diagnostic and Statistical Manual of Mental Disorders, Fifth Edition: DSM-5* (Arlington, VA: American Psychiatric Association, 2013).

72. Centers for Disease Control and Prevention, "CDC Estimates 1 in 68 Children Has Been Identified with Autism Spectrum Disorder," press release, March 27, 2014, www.cdc.gov/media/releases/2014/p0327-autism-spectrum-disorder.html.

73. White, S. W. et al., "Anxiety in Children and Adolescents with Autism Spectrum Disorders," *Clinical Psychology Review* 29 (2009): 216–29.

74. Lupien, S., *Well Stressed: Manage Stress Before It Turns Toxic* (John Wiley & Sons, 2012).

75. Corbett, B. A. et al., "Comparing Cortisol, Stress, and Sensory Sensitivity in Children with Autism," *Autism Research* 2, no. 1 (February 2009): 39–49.

76. White, *Anxiety in Children with Autism*.

77. Seltzer, M. M. et al., "Maternal Cortisol levels and Behavior Problems in Adolescents and Adults with ASD," *Journal of Autism and Developmental Disorders* (November 5, 2009), http://aging.wisc.edu/pdfs/2303.pdf.

78. Wood, J. J. et al., "Cognitive Behavioral Therapy for Anxiety in Children with Autism Spectrum Disorders: Randomized, Controlled Trial," *Journal of Child Psychology and Psychiatry* 50, no. 3 (2008): 224–34, www.ncbi.nlm.nih.gov/pubmed/19309326.

79. White, *Anxiety in Children With Autism*.

80. Farmer, C. et al., "Pharmacotherapy for the Core Symptoms in Autistic Disorder: Current Status of the Research," *Drugs* 73, no. 4 (March 2013): 303–14, DOI:10.1007/s40265-013-0021-7.

81. Kurtz, Y., "Adam, Asperger's Syndrome, and the Transcendental Meditation Program," *Autism Digest* (July–August 2011): 46–47, www.adhd-tm.org/pdf/Aspergers-JulAug2011.pdf.

82. Black, D. O., and N. Rosenthal, "Use of Transcendental Meditation to Treat Anxiety and Stress Among Adolescents with Autism Spectrum Disorders: A Case Study," unpublished manuscript.

83. Merikangas, *Lifetime Prevalence*.

84. Goodman, A., "The Neurobiological Development of Addiction," *Psychiatric Times* 26, no. 9 (August 28, 2009), www.psychiatrictimes.com/addiction/neurobiological-development-addiction.

85. Ibid.

86. Sapolsky, *Greater Good*.

87. Goodman, *Neurobiological Development of Addiction*.

88. Spear, *Adolescent Brain*.

89. CASAColumbia, "National Study Reveals: Teen Substance Use America's #1 Public Health Problem," (2011), www.casacolumbia.org/newsroom/press-releases/national-study-reveals-teen-substance-use-americas-1-public-health-problem.

90. Partnership for a Drug-Free America, "Partnership Attitude Tracking Study, PATS: Teens 2007 Report," (August 4, 2008), www.drugfree.org/wp-content/uploads/2011/04/PATS-Teens-2007-Full-Report.pdf.

91. Gelderloos, W. et al., "Effectiveness of the Transcendental Meditation Program in Preventing and Treating Substance Misuse: A Review," *International Journal of Addictions* 26, no. 3 (1991).

92. Alexander, C. N., P. Robinson, and M. Rainforth, "Treating and Preventing Alcohol Nicotine, and Drug Abuse through Transcendental Meditation: A Review and Statistical Meta-analysis," *Alcohol Treatment Quarterly* 11, nos. 1–2 (1994) 13–87.

93. Orme-Johnson, *Trait Anxiety*.

94. Hanga, D. A. F. et al., "Effects of the Transcendental Meditation Program on Substance Use among University Students," *Cardiology Research and Practice* 2911 (2011), article 537101, www.hindawi.com/journals/crp/2011/537101/.

95. Rodham, K., and K. Hawtong, "Epidemiology and Phenomenology of Non-suicidal Self-Injury," in *Understanding Non-suicidal Self-Injury: Origins, Assessment, and Treatment*, ed. M. K. Nock (Washington, DC: American Psychological Association, 2009): 37–62.

96. Whitlock, J. et al., "Self-Injurious Behaviors in a College Population," *Pediatrics* 117, no. 6 (2006): 1939–48, www.ncbi.nlm.nih.gov/pubmed/16740834.

97. Whitlock, J., "The Cutting Edge: Non-suicidal Self-Injury in Adolescence" (2009), Cornell University, Act for Youth Center of Excellence, www.actforyouth.net/resources/rf/rf_nssi_1209.pdf.

98. Merikangas, *Lifetime Prevalence*; Alloy, *Adolescent Surge*.

99. Cain, R. N. et al., *12 Brain/Mind Learning Principles in Action: Developing Executive Functions of the Human Brain* (Thousand Oaks, CA: Corwin Press, 2009).

100. Organization for Economic Cooperation and Development, *Understanding the Brain: Towards a New Learning Science* (Organization for Economic Cooperation and Development Publishing, 2002), DOI:10.1787/9789264174986-en.

101. Stixrud, W. R., "Why Stress Is Such a Big Deal," *Journal of Management Education* 36, no. 2 (April 2012): 135–42.

102. Arnsten, *Stress Signaling Pathways*.

103. Lupien, *Stress Hormones*.

104. So, *Longitudinal Effects of TM Technique*.

105. Travis, *Effects of TM Practice*.

106. Visser, S. N. et al., "Trends in the Parent-Report of Health Care Provider-Diagnosis and Medication Treatment for ADHD Disorder: United States, 2003–2011," *Journal of American Academy of Child & Adolescent Psychiatry* 53, no. 1 (January 2014): 34–46.e2, DOI:10.1016/j.jaac.2013.09.001.

107. Gunnar, M. R. and D. Vazquez, "Stress Neurobiology and Developmental Psychopathology," in *Developmental Psychopathology* 2, *Developmental Neuroscience,* ed. D. Cicchetti and D. Cohen, 2nd ed. (New York: John Wiley & Sons, 2006).

108. Silk, T. J. et al., "White-Matter Abnormalities in Attention Deficit Hyperactivity Disorder: A Diffusion Tensor Imaging Study," *Human Brain Mapping* 30, no. 9 (September 2009): 2757–65.

109. Silk, T., "Fronto-Parietal Activation in Attention-Deficit Hyperactivity Disorder, Combined Type: Functional Magnetic Resonance Imaging Study," *British Journal of Psychiatry* 187, no. 3 (September 2005): 282–83.

110. Biederman, J. and T. Spencer, "Attention-Deficit/Hyperactivity Disorder (ADHD) as a Noradrenergic Disorder," *Biological Psychiatry* 46, no. 9 (November 1999): 1234–42.

111. Arnsten, *Stress Signaling Pathways*.

112. Yamamoto, N., "Medical Prefrontal Cortex and Anterior Cingulate Cortex in the Generation of Alpha Activity Induced by Transcendental Meditation: A Magnetoencephalographic Study," *Acta Medicine Okayama* 60, no. 1 (2006): 51–58.

113. Newberg, A. B. et al., "Cerebral Glucose Metabolic Changes Associated with Transcendental Meditation Practice," paper presented at the meeting of the Society of Nuclear Medicine, San Diego, California, August 2006.

114. Grosswald, *Use of the Transcendental Meditation Technique*.

115. Grosswald, S. J., and F. Travis, "ADHD and Stress: The Role of Meditation to Reduce Stress, and Improve Brain Function and Behavior Regulation," *Current Directions in ADHD and Its Treatment*, ch. 10, ed. J. M. Norvilitis, www.intechopen.com/books/howtoreference/current-directions-in-adhd-and-its-treatment/adhd-and-stress-the-role-of-meditation-to-reduce-stress-and-improve-brain-function-and-behavior-regu.

116. Travis, *ADHD, Brain Functioning, and TM*.

117. Silk, *Fronto-Parietal*.

118. Di Michele, F. et al., "The Neurophysiology of Attention-Deficit/Hyperactivity Disorder," *International Journal of Psychophysiology* 58, no. 1 (October 2005): 81–93.

119. Janzen, T. et al., "Differences in Baseline EEG Measures for ADD and Normally Achieving Preadolescent Males, *Biofeedback Self Regulation* 20, no. 1 (March 1995): 65–82; Barry, R. J. et al., "A Review of Electrophysiology in Attention-Deficity/Hyperactivity Disorder: Qualitative and Quantitative Electroencephalography," *Clinical Neurophysiology* 114, no. 2 (February 2003): 171–83.

120. Barnes, *Impact of Stress Reduction*; Rosean, *Experience of TM*.

121. Ibid.

122. Kirp, D. L., "Meditation Transforms Roughest San Francisco Schools," SFGate (January 12, 2014), www.sfgate.com/opinion/openforum/article/Medi tation-transforms-roughest-San-Francisco-5136942.php.

123. Dierke, J. S. "A Quiet Transformation," *Leadership* 42, no. 1 (September–October 2012): 14, http://connection.ebscohost.com/c/articles/87052628/quiet -transformation.

124. Nidich, *Academic Achievement*.

125. Elder, C., S. Nidich, F. Moriarty, and R. Nidich, "Effect of Transcendental Meditation on Employee Stress, Depression, and Burnout: A Randomized Controlled Study," *Permanente Journal* 18, no. 1 (Winter 2014), DOI:10.7812/TPP/13-102.

126. Colbert, R. D., and S. Nidich, "Effect of the Transcendental Meditation Program on Graduation, College Acceptance and Dropout Rates for Students Attending an Urban Public High School," *Education* 133, no. 4 (2013): 495–501.

127. Elder, *Reduced Psychological Distress*.

128. Friedman, E. H., *A Failure of Nerve: Leadership in the Age of the Quick Fix* (New York: Seabury Books, 2007).

129. Galinsky, E., *Ask the Children: What America's Children Really Think About Working Parents* (New York: William Morrow, 1999).

Section III

APPLICATIONS

Ten

Transcendental Meditation as a Preventive Approach for Improving Healthcare Outcomes

Maxwell V. Rainforth, Ph.D., M.S., M.A., B.Sc (Hons), and Robert E. Herron, Ph.D., M.B.A., M.S.C.I., B.A.

Preventable disorders account for 70 percent of the burden of disease and the associated healthcare costs.[1] Moreover, preventable causes account for roughly 8 of 9 deaths in the United States.[2] Yet in the United States, less than 10 percent of total healthcare resources are spent on prevention and wellness.[3] Hence the U.S. healthcare system is really a disease-care system. However, disease care is prone to undesirable side effects and negative quality-of-life outcomes.[4] Moreover, neglect of prevention in favor of disease treatment is costly. Healthcare systems in developed countries face the challenge of aging populations and prices of healthcare services that are rising faster than inflation.[5,6] These factors underscore the current need to identify ways to prevent serious illnesses, to improve the cost-effectiveness of medical care, and to improve patient quality-of-life outcomes.

In 2013, the American Heart Association issued a scientific statement that recognized that Transcendental Meditation (TM®) may be beneficial for patients with elevated blood pressure and included evidence of its efficacy with cardiovascular disease patients.[7] In chapters 3–9 of this book, the clinical usefulness of TM is examined for specific types of medical conditions.

In this chapter, we examine the effects of TM in regard to a broad range of medical disorders and its potential to prevent disease and to promote overall good health and well-being. The first part of the chapter summarizes evidence regarding how TM affects healthcare outcomes. The second part of the chapter examines how TM can prevent stress and disease, and the mechanisms through which this occurs.

In part 1, we summarize the evidence regarding efficacy of TM with stress-related disorders. Evidence indicates that TM improves patient outcomes with several types of diseases. In fact, incidence rates across a broad range of medical conditions appear to be lower among long-term practitioners of TM.

If TM helps prevent disease and improves patient outcomes, then it should lead to lower medical-resource utilization and costs. Also, one would hope to see better patient outcomes translate into enhanced quality of life, reduced effects of aging, and greater life expectancy. Hence, part 1 also examines the reduced need for medical services and better long-term patient outcomes among those practicing TM, outcomes such as enhanced quality of life and longevity.

In part 2, we present a conceptual framework for TM in terms of primary, secondary, and tertiary prevention of stress and disease. This framework is based on the health effects of TM reviewed in part 1, as well as research regarding the profound and wide-ranging effects of TM, which simultaneously influences the neurophysiological, cognitive, emotional, and behavioral domains. The evidence indicates that TM is useful not only for stress-reduction, but also for enhancing resilience and adaptive capacity, hence, enabling patients to take more effective control of their own health.

PART 1: IMPACT ON HEALTHCARE OUTCOMES

Research on TM and Specific Disorders

In clinical practice, stress is a major factor for patient outcomes, and stress-related conditions account for 60–90 percent of visits to healthcare professionals.[8] The effect of high stress levels on annual medical costs, independent of other factors, is estimated to be at least double that of each of the major lifestyle risk factors—physical inactivity, excess body weight, current tobacco use, and hypertension.[9] Stress is known to be directly linked to a broad set of medical conditions, including hypertension, cardiovascular disease, decreased immune function, headaches and certain pain conditions, insomnia, and certain types of mental health disorders.[10,11]

In view of evidence that TM is effective in mitigating and dissolving harmful effects of acute and chronic stressors on mind and body, practicing TM is expected to be beneficial in a variety of stress-related disorders. Table 10.1 presents a brief summary of the extensive evidence regarding TM and specific health conditions. In this section, the emphasis is on the breadth and scope of the evidence. Note that the evidence included in table 10.1 is not an exhaustive list of the conditions that may accrue when patients learn TM; its purpose is to note and highlight con-

Table 10.1. Effects of TM on Stress-Related Health Conditions

Broad Medical Category	Specific Conditions	Research Findings on TM
Mental Health	Psychological Distress Emotional instability Sleep Disorders Substance-Abuse Disorders Psychiatric Disorders Other Behavioral Disorders	• Decreased anxiety, depression, anger • Decreased job stress and burnout • Reduced neuroticism • Reduced symptoms of insomnia, better sleep quality • Reduced consumption of cigarettes, alcohol, marijuana, narcotics, and non-prescribed drugs • Lower incidence of mental health disorders • Improved outcomes in psychiatric in-patients • Reduced symptoms of post-traumatic stress disorder • Reduced ADHD in children • More-effective rehabilitation of juvenile and adult offenders
Pain	Headaches Chronic Pain Disorders	• Reduced frequency of migraine headaches and other pain disorders • Decreased distress from pain sensation • Reduced use of pain-relieving medications
Inflammatory Diseases	Bronchial Asthma Allergies	• Improved airway conductance; reduced symptoms • Less eczema and fewer allergic reactions
Cardiovascular Disease (CVD) and Metabolic disorders	Elevated CVD Risk Factors Type-2 Diabetes Atherosclerosis Heart Disease Cardiovascular Events	• Reduced blood pressure levels in hypertensive patients • Decreased cholesterol levels in patients with hypercholesterolaemia • Decreased cigarette and alcohol consumption • Decreased insulin resistance • Decreased carotid intima-medial thickness • Reduced symptoms of myocardial ischemia • Decreased left ventricular hypertrophy • Increased functional capacity and improved quality of life in patients with congestive heart failure • Decreased rates of heart attacks, strokes, and deaths

ditions in regard to specific supporting evidence. In a later section, the strength of the evidence will be considered in terms of the methodologies used in research studies.

A large number of studies have reported improvements in psychological health outcomes due to practice of TM. These research findings imply benefits for patients with episodic or chronic stress and related health conditions that are frequently seen by primary healthcare providers. Randomized controlled studies and meta-analyses have shown reductions in mood disturbances, including anxiety, depression, and anger for TM compared to control conditions.[12-14] Several studies have shown reductions in job stress and employee burnout.[15,16] Numerous studies have reported lower neuroticism and hostility among TM practitioners compared to control subjects.[17,18] There is extensive evidence that TM promotes positive psychological health, as indicated by improvements in self-esteem, self-concept, and growth toward self-actualization.[19] A meta-analysis found that in regard to decreasing use of alcohol, cigarettes, and illicit drugs, TM is more effective than standard substance-abuse prevention and treatment programs.[20]

Pre-sleep arousal due to stressful experience is a major factor in insomnia.[21] Over 50 million Americans suffer from sleep deficits due to chronic insomnia and other sleep disorders, which have serious long-term health consequences, including increased incidence of cardiovascular disease and psychiatric disorders.[22] Reduced time to fall asleep and improved sleep quality have been reported in studies of subjects who learn TM.[23-26] This apparently leads to decreased reliance on sleep medications.[27-29]

Acute and chronic stress can lead to severe impacts on psychological health. Intense stressors may also trigger depressive illness or posttraumatic stress disorder (PTSD), depending on the type of stressor and predisposition of the individual to vulnerability.[30,31] Stress may also contribute to and trigger psychotic states.[32]

On the other hand, several studies have found lower incidence of mental health disorders among practitioners of TM and better outcomes among psychiatric patients and prison inmates. A survey by the Swedish National Health Board found that the rate of psychiatric admissions among 35,000 TM meditators was less than 1 percent of the general population.[33] In a qualitative case series, improved outcomes were observed for schizophrenia and bipolar and severe personality disorders.[34] A randomized study found improved outcomes among Vietnam veterans with PTSD who practiced TM, relative to a group who received individual psychotherapy.[35] Reductions in obsessive-compulsive tendencies have been measured in meditating prison inmates compared to controls.[36] Several studies have shown improved rehabilitation outcomes for criminal offenders, a population that has a high incidence of psychopathology.[37]

(Research indicating that TM is effective in rehabilitation of criminal offenders is reviewed in chapter 11 of this volume.)

Stress is known to worsen symptoms of attention deficit hyperactivity disorder (ADHD) in children because it interferes with self-regulation, attentional, and cognitive processes.[38,39] A pilot study in children with ADHD showed a reduction in ADHD symptoms and enhancement of higher-order brain functions.[40] Other studies have shown reduced behavioral problems in children and improved behavioral outcomes among juvenile offenders.[41,42]

Prolonged exposure to stress is known to depress immune system functioning and to aggravate inflammatory conditions, including asthma and skin rashes.[43] On the other hand, practice of TM enhances immune system responses to stress.[44] TM has been found to lessen symptoms of gingival inflammation, eczema, and allergic reactions.[45,46] A study of asthma patients reported improved airway conductance, as well as decreased symptoms as rated by physicians and patients.[47]

Stressful experiences may also exacerbate distress from physical pain and may increase incidence of headaches and back pain.[48] In addition, TM has been found longitudinally to decrease the brain's response to pain stimuli and reduce distress associated with pain experience.[49,50] TM is also associated with reduced reported frequency of headaches and pain-related disorders.[51,52] Individuals who practice TM also report decreased use of medications for pain relief.[53–55]

Cardiovascular disease affects one-third of American adults, and it is the cause of one-third of all deaths in the United States.[56] People under stress may fall into unhealthy lifestyle habits, leading to elevated risk factors for cardiovascular disease, including smoking, hypertension, and high cholesterol.[57] Repeated cardiovascular responses due to chronic stress can result in small tears in arterial walls, which the body repairs by forming arterial plaques, which in turn leads to atherosclerosis.[58] TM lowers blood pressure levels in hypertensive patients,[59] decreases cholesterol in patients with elevated cholesterol levels,[60] and leads to decreased cigarette consumption.[61] TM reverses atherosclerosis in the carotid artery, an indicator of the development of cardiovascular disease and of risk of strokes.[62] As noted in chapter 5, there is evidence that TM is useful in the prevention of diabetes,[63] a disease that overlaps with cardiovascular disease in terms of risk factors and disease pathways. In patients with myocardial ischemia, TM has been found to increase tolerance to exercise stress.[64] Efficacy of TM has been reported by studies on serious heart conditions, including left ventricular hypertrophy[65] and congestive heart failure.[66] In a randomized controlled trial with patients with preexisting coronary artery disease, rates of heart attacks, strokes, and death among the TM group were reduced by 48 percent relative to a health education

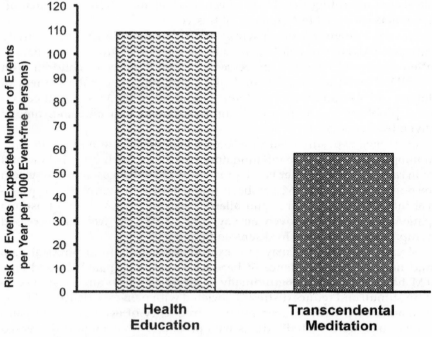

Figure 10.1.   Effects of the Transcendental Meditation program on mortality, myocardial infarction, and stroke.

Note: In a randomized controlled trial in subjects with coronary heart disease, there was a 48% lower rate in Transcendental Meditation group compared to a health education control group, over an average followup period of 5 years.

control group[67] (see figure 10.1; for a detailed review of research on TM and cardiovascular disease, see chapter 4, this volume).

TM and Healthcare Resource Utilization

The above research findings are encouraging in that they pertain to major stress-related health conditions. To scientifically investigate effects of each health condition is time- and resource-intensive, and each investigation requires a sufficient sample size of patients who are willing to participate in a research study. Hence to date, a finite number of health conditions have been investigated with controlled trials. However, the impact on a broader set of health categories has been examined in studies of large numbers of individuals practicing TM.

A study based on health insurance data provided further evidence that TM decreases incidence of a range of medical conditions.[68] David Orme-Johnson analyzed five years of data on more than 2,000 members of a health insurance plan offered by Blue Cross/Blue Shield who practiced TM regularly for at least six months. The TM group, which included adults and their dependent children over the age of ten, was spread throughout the United States, with 20 percent of members residing in Fairfield, Iowa. The TM group was compared to a normative group of over 600,000 other members of Blue Cross/Blue Shield plans. The age distributions of the two groups were similar overall. Table 10.2 compares rates of hospital admissions in fifteen medical categories for the TM group compared to the normative group. As shown in the table, admission rates were markedly lower for the TM group in all categories and 87 percent lower for cardiovascular diseases and for nervous system disorders. However, for childbirth and obstetric services, utilization rates for the TM group and the normative group were virtually identical, which suggested that lower hospitalization rates in other medical categories for the TM group were probably not due to a predisposition of TM patients against using conventional medical services.

Orme-Johnson also examined rates of inpatient and outpatient medical care utilization by age group (10–18, 19–39, and 40+).[69] Compared to the normative group, TM patients used outpatient services less frequently and had lower hospital admission rates in all age bands. Across all age groups, the rate per 1,000 members of outpatient visits was 45 percent lower in the TM group. Hospital admission rates across all

Table 10.2.   Impact of TM on Hospital Admissions

Medical Category	Admission Rate for TM Group Compared to Normative Group
Cardiovascular diseases	Lower by 87%
Nervous system disorders	Lower by 87%
Ill-defined conditions	Lower by 76%
Nose, throat, and lung diseases	Lower by 73%
Bone and muscle diseases	Lower by 68%
Metabolism diseases	Lower by 65%
Injuries	Lower by 63%
Tumors	Lower by 55%
Congenital diseases	Lower by 51%
Intestinal disorders	Lower by 49%
Genital and urinary diseases	Lower by 37%
Blood diseases	Lower by 33%
All mental disorders	Lower by 31%
Infectious diseases	Lower by 30%
Other diseases	Lower by 91%

disease categories and age groups were 53 percent lower in the TM group. The number of days per 1,000 members in which TM members were hospitalized was 61 percent lower compared to the normative group. Rates of inpatient and outpatient utilization for the TM group were markedly lower in both medical and surgical categories.

Results that were even stronger than those of Orme-Johnson's five-year study were reported by Orme-Johnson and Herron's study of 693 employees and dependents at Maharishi University of Management, all of whom regularly practiced TM and as an employee benefit were offered preventative healthcare based on Ayurveda.[70] This follow-up study tightly controlled for occupational grouping and demographics by making comparisons with an age- and gender-matched sample of 4,148 employees at private colleges in the same state. Both groups were covered by the same Blue Cross/Blue Shield health insurance plan. Data for a four-year period were analyzed. Relative to the control group, hospital admission rates were lower in the TM-Ayurveda group across all disease categories, with reductions of at least those reported by Orme-Johnson[71] (i.e., 92 percent for cardiovascular disorders, 74 percent for tumors, and 87 percent for mental health disorders/substance abuse). Rates of outpatient visits, in-hospital days, and total hospital expenditures per person were all substantially lower, with reductions similar to those observed in the previous study.

TM and Healthcare Costs

Reduction in healthcare resource utilization would be expected to translate into lower healthcare costs. In fact, among Orme-Johnson's nationwide sample of TM practitioners, lower rates of inpatient and outpatient utilization yielded an estimated total savings of $4.4 million in 2013 dollars based on the U.S. rate of inflation of medical services,[72,73] or approximately $2,000 per participant over a five-year period. In Orme-Johnson and Herron's follow-up study of TM plus Ayurveda, hospital expenditures per person for individuals under 45 were 60 percent lower in the intervention group compared to the matched controls.[74] Among the over-45 age range, even greater savings were realized for meditating employees compared to the controls, with an 84 percent reduction in hospital expenditures.

A series of studies by Herron et al. investigated the impact of TM on the payments to physicians in all specialties for treating patients in all settings (i.e., office, hospital, home, etc.).[75-78] The researchers compared 1,418 people in Quebec, Canada, who learned TM with 1,418 control subjects who were randomly selected to match the TM group in age, gender, and region. The average age of the sample was thirty-eight years. Physician payment data for 1981–1994 was obtained from the Quebec government and adjusted for inflation using the Canadian Consumer Price Index. During a seven-year pre-intervention period, there were similar rates of increase in inflation-adjusted medical costs in the TM group and the control group. During the six years after patients learned and practiced TM, their costs of physician services decreased by 1–2 percent per year, versus rates of increase of 8–14 percent in the control group—depending on the estimators used for comparison. Hence the TM group showed statistically significant reductions in rates of change in physician payments—a decrease of 9–14 percent relative to the non-meditating comparison group.[79]

As people age, they use disproportionately large amounts of medical care. In North America, people over age 65 comprise only 13 percent of the population, but they account for approximately one-third of all medical spending. To investigate whether TM could help reduce the medical expenditures of older people, Herron et al. focused on subjects in the dataset over age 65 to compare 163 older TM subjects with 163 matched controls. After five years of practicing meditation, there was a cumulative average reduction of 70 percent in annual payments to physicians of the people in the TM group relative to the non-TM controls.[80] This finding suggests that TM could help reduce the medical expenses of the elderly— a result that may be important because the elderly are the fastest-growing demographic category worldwide.

Another study by Herron[81] focused on a subset of high-cost patients among the same dataset as Herron's initial fourteen-year study. He followed patients in the upper 10 percent of physician payments, so that there were 142 patients in the TM group and the same number in the matched control group. Compared with the baseline (the year before TM practice commenced), medical costs in the TM group decreased by 11 percent in the first year and by 28 percent cumulatively over five years. In the untreated control group, medical costs were virtually level over the same five-year follow-up period (see figure 10.2).

This study has critical relevance because high-cost patients account for a disproportionately high percentage of all medical costs. In the United States, 60 percent of total U.S. medical expenditures are due to patients whose medical costs are in the top 10 percent compared to all patients.[81] Consistently high-cost patients are also prone to poor health, with multiple chronic conditions.[82,83]

Another important component of healthcare costs is the use of prescription medications. Based upon a randomized controlled trial with hypertensive patients, reductions of 10.7 mmHg in systolic blood pressure and 6.4 mmHg in diastolic blood pressure were achieved in patients assigned

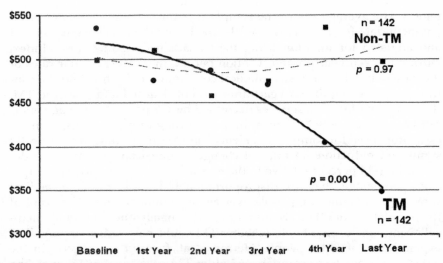

Figure 10.2. Reduced Medical Expenses for High-Cost Patients
Note: The graph shows mean annual total per capita payments to physicians for treating consistently high-cost patients. Over five years, the TM group's medical expenses decreased by 28%.

to the TM group relative to a lifestyle education control group.[84] In this study over a three-month intervention period, patients' medication prescriptions were kept unchanged by their physicians so that there would be no interference between starting TM and any changes in medication, as far as observing effects on blood pressure levels. In a further randomized controlled trial that evaluated the effect of TM on hypertension with a twelve-month intervention period, physicians changed medication levels as appropriate, and this study found significant reductions in medication levels in the TM group compared with the control subjects.[85] Herron et al. estimated that the decreased blood pressure levels in the TM group could translate into potential savings in medication costs.[86]

Thus there is evidence that savings to the healthcare system can be achieved through TM, savings resulting from decreased expenses for physicians, outpatient visits, in-hospital stays, and medications.

Quality of Life and TM

Of course healthcare professionals are not just concerned with providing effective and efficient medical services. Patient quality of life is a primary concern, especially in view of the fact that conventional treatment of chronic diseases can have serious adverse side effects. When individuals learn and practice TM, reductions in psychological distress and improvements in psychological well-being are reported.[87] Empirical evidence for this is mostly drawn from studies conducted with research participants who were generally in good health at study entry.[88]

More specifically, two randomized controlled trials of patients with chronic diseases have demonstrated improvements in quality of life and other health outcomes. In a clinical trial with 33 congestive heart failure patients, significant improvements were observed in functional capacity, as measured by the standard six-minute walk test and by scales for depression, emotional distress, and perceived stress.[89] In a study of 130 patients with breast cancer (stages II to IV),[90] the TM group showed significant improvement in social and spiritual well-being and in emotional, functional, and overall quality of life. In this study, there was also a 75 percent risk-reduction in death rate, although this difference did not reach statistical significance because the overall number of deaths was relatively small.

Successful Aging and TM

Effective healthcare should ideally promote the maintenance of good health into old age. Unfortunately, aging is typically associated with increasing morbidity risk, reflected in declines in physical health and cognitive function and increased incidence of chronic diseases. Due to burgeoning elderly populations, healthcare of the aged is a critical issue in Western countries.

Research on TM and aging is summarized in chapter 11 of this volume. Here, we briefly note that this research indicates that TM slows or even reverses changes in physiological and cognitive parameters associated with aging. In a randomized controlled trial of residents of homes for the elderly, TM was shown to increase cognitive flexibility and enhance survival compared to the active and untreated comparison groups in the study.[91] Research has shown substantially reduced mortality rates among older persons who learn TM compared to control groups.[92]

Aging should be accompanied not only by good health, but also by the growth of wisdom. These studies and other research indicate that TM helps to maintain mental acuity into old age, while enhancing both quality of life and longevity.

TM and Vulnerable Populations

As discussed above, TM has shown improved health outcomes with the elderly and patients with certain types of chronic diseases—both of whom are at risk for poor health outcomes. Studies of TM have reported improvements in cardiovascular health outcomes among minority populations who are subject to health disparities—for example, African Americans and Native Hawaiians.[93,94]

How Strong Is the Evidence?

The critical "bottom line" for any prevention strategy is whether it achieves objectives for improvements in patient outcomes (e.g., restoration of health) and in system-level performance (e.g., achieving economies in medical-resource utilization). Viewed as a whole, the evidence presents a cohesive picture regarding the impact of TM on healthcare outcomes. Some of this evidence is based upon the gold standard of clinical research: the randomized controlled trial. However, in some of the studies it was not feasible to randomly assign patients to treatment and control groups. Reasons for this included feasibility of recruiting the large samples that would have been required and difficulty gaining patient consent to be randomized to an intervention or control group over a period of several years. Based on the different kinds of research conducted with varying degrees of methodological rigor, there is solid evidence that supports the usefulness of TM as a preventive approach.

Orme-Johnson's initial study of medical-resource utilization was based on cross-sectional comparisons between a population that had been practicing TM regularly for at least six months compared to a general population of patients insured under similar health plans. The age compositions of the two populations were similar. Orme-Johnson and Herron's follow-up study incorporated tighter matching of the meditating and non-mediating groups on demographic variables. These two studies were cross-sectional and did not assess change from a baseline level of utilization. However, Herron's studies on costs of physician services did assess longitudinal change relative to a long baseline period and also utilized matched control groups.

In meditation research, it is important to rule out alternative explanations that could be associated with any intervention or with any relaxation technique. Examples of such nonspecific treatment factors include attention from trainers, expectancies fostered by participating in an experiment, simple relaxation effects due to sitting while meditating, or novel deployment of attention. To control for such factors that presumably would have similar influences across different types of treatments, meta-analyses have compared effects of TM to effects of other forms of meditation, relaxation, and standardized intervention programs. These meta-analyses showed that TM yields substantially larger treatment effects in comparison to other treatments.[95] In regard to reducing trait anxiety and promoting psychological health, TM was associated with substantially larger treatment effects compared to other meditation and relaxation techniques.[96] Compared to standard substance-abuse prevention and treatment programs, TM was again more effective.[97] TM was found to significantly lower blood pressure, whereas stress-management approaches and biofeedback did not.[98]

At least twenty-seven randomized controlled trials of TM and health-related outcomes have been published in peer-reviewed journals. In these studies, research participants were randomly assigned to an intervention or control group.[99] This eliminates alternative explanations such as preexisting differences between the TM and control groups and justifies stronger conclusions regarding efficacy of TM. Several studies have included rigorous controls such as blind testing of research participants and structurally similar control conditions.[100]

For example, Robert Schneider et al. conducted a randomized controlled trial of TM compared to a health education control group over a nine-year follow-up period.[101] Participants in the comparison group had the same amount of contact with trainers and were also asked to practice what they learned at home so as to provide a research structure that paralleled the TM group. Collection of outcome data was performed by research staff who were blind to participants' treatment group status. The primary outcome was clinical events, which were based on hospital discharge summaries. The TM group showed a 48 percent reduction in the rate of heart attacks, strokes, and deaths, relative to the control group, and also reductions in blood pressure and anger. In this study, objective outcome measures were used which were not subject to self-reporting biases by research participants. The impact on clinical events in this randomized trial was consistent with the other studies that showed lower medical-resource utilization and costs.

A consideration in regard to plausibility of treatment efficacy is whether there is a dose-response relationship between patient outcomes and the intensity or length of the intervention. Correlations have been observed in several studies between the regularity of participants' practice of TM and the study outcomes.[102] For example, in one randomized trial, among participants in the TM group, the frequency of their TM practice was inversely associated with risk of heart attack, strokes, and deaths.[103] Other studies have observed larger improvements in health-related variables of TM in long-term meditators compared to short-term meditators, who in turn had better outcomes than non-meditating control groups.[104–106]

PART 2: HOW TM WORKS AS A PREVENTIVE APPROACH

Effectiveness as a Preventive Healthcare Strategy

The evidence presented in this chapter indicates that TM can be effective in the primary, secondary, and tertiary prevention of disease (see table 10.3 for definitions[107]). Below, we give examples of the use of TM to achieve each level of prevention; these are examples, not an exhaustive list.

Table 10.3.   Definitions of Primary, Secondary, and Tertiary Disease Prevention

Level of Disease Prevention	Goals
Primary Prevention	• Reduction of likelihood of illness • Elimination of causes of disease or enhancement of resistance to disease • Promotion of health and well-being on a general level, including healthy lifestyle habits
Secondary Prevention	• Interruption of the disease process before it can become symptomatic
Tertiary Prevention	• Stopping or slowing down progression of symptomatic disease • Prevention of complications, damage, and pain from the disease • Restoration or preservation of functional capacity

With regard to primary disease prevention, TM promotes overall health in that it has been found to promote physical and emotional well-being and reduce symptoms of stress. Research also suggests that TM lowers disease incidence rates, showing that TM enhances immune function[108] and reduces hospitalization rates across major categories of disease[109] (see table 10.2). As noted above, a Swedish survey found dramatically lower incidence rates of mental health disorders among TM practitioners compared to the general population.[110] TM provides primary prevention of cardiovascular disease by reducing risk factors such as elevated blood pressure and high cholesterol levels.[111]

Secondary disease prevention interrupts the disease process before it can become symptomatic. Decreased use on a casual basis of alcohol, cigarettes, and illicit drugs among adolescents and young adults practicing TM indicates secondary prevention of addictions to substance use.[112] Reduced insulin resistance due to TM practice indicates secondary prevention of diabetes.[113] TM has been found to halt or reverse the development of atherosclerosis, thereby providing secondary prevention of cardiovascular disease.[114]

Tertiary disease prevention limits the consequences of symptomatic disease. The goals of tertiary disease prevention are to slow down progression of the disease; to prevent complications, damage, and pain from the disease; and to restore or preserve functional capacity. Improved treatment outcomes in practitioners of TM have been found with war veterans with PTSD,[115] with psychiatric patients,[116] and with drug addicts in rehabilitation programs,[117] indicating tertiary prevention. Practicing TM was found to substantially lower incidence of clinical events and deaths in coronary disease patients, showing that complications and adverse consequences of cardiovascular disease decreased.[118] Consistent with the goals of tertiary prevention to restore quality of life in chronic-disease patients, in breast cancer patients who learned TM, quality of life improved.[119] Also, in patients with congestive heart failure, functional capacity and quality of life improved as a result of TM, again showing tertiary prevention.[120]

Why TM Is Effective for Prevention

It is easy to understand how meditation, as a form of mental relaxation, might calm the mind and relieve symptoms of stress. It is well understood that stress is a contributing cause of many health disorders, and there is abundant evidence that TM mitigates or neutralizes the effects of stress. However, stress reduction in terms of relaxation effects does not fully account for the extent to which TM is distinctively effective in preventing and treating stress-related disorders.

One might expect that all meditation techniques would produce some degree of relaxation and hence relieve stress. Yet TM is distinguishable from other meditation techniques with regard to the magnitude of treatment effects on reducing trait anxiety[121] and fostering growth of self-actualization.[122] Why then might TM be so effective in regard to its health effects?

An effective stress-intervention program should neutralize or mitigate the effects of acute and chronic stress. However, to prevent recurrence of stress-related problems, it is not enough to alleviate psychological distress and repair or relieve neurophysiological damage after it has occurred. As shown in table 10.4, a prevention-oriented stress intervention should boost resilience or immunity to stress (level 1), as well as provide short-term and long-term stress reduction (levels 2 and 3).

Each of levels 1–3 in table 10.4 is applicable to primary, secondary, and tertiary prevention of illness. Increasing resilience to stress is obviously important for primary prevention of stress-related disorders. Relief from episodic stress is vital for secondary prevention of common stress-related conditions seen in primary care that have not progressed to chronic disorders. With chronic disorders, the need for long-term stress-reduction is obviously needed for tertiary prevention. Moreover, with chronic conditions, it is necessary to boost a patient's resilience to stress (level 1) so as to prevent continuing stress-related damage (tertiary prevention). With cardiovascular disease and other stress-related disorders, chronic stress contributes to risk factors and to the early stages of disease onset. Hence for primary disease prevention, reduction of effects of chronic stress (level 3) is necessary. Therefore, at each stage of disease prevention—primary, secondary, or tertiary—all three levels of stress intervention are pertinent and essential.

Table 10.4. Effects of TM on Neurophysiological, Cognitive/Emotional, and Behavioral Domains in Relation to Goals of Stress Intervention

Goals of Stress Intervention	Effects of TM		
	Neurophysiological	Cognitive/Emotional	Behavioral
Level 1: Stress prevention— Enhancement of immunity and resilience to stress	Greater adaptability, stability, and integration of the nervous system— Increased frontal EEG coherence, increased neurological efficiency, and more-rapid habituation of galvanic skin responses to repeated stressful stimuli	Increased problem-solving and coping abilities; greater happiness; growth of self-concept and self-esteem; improved emotional intelligence; enhanced ego development	Improved interpersonal relationships; improved job performance
Level 2: Short-term stress recovery— Relief from acute and episodic stress	Reduced psychosomatic arousal and lower stress-hormone levels from each meditation session	Improvements in mood states; decreased state anxiety	Reduced use of alcohol, cigarettes, caffeine, and prescription medications
Level 3: Long-term stress reduction— Release from cumulative effects of chronic stress; rehabilitation from trauma and stress-related psychological disorders	Fewer spontaneous galvanic skin responses; lower basal skin conductance	Decreased trait anxiety, neuroticism, and PTSD symptoms; improvements in psychiatric disorders; reduced cognitive distortion in prison inmates	Reduced anti-social behavior; successful rehabilitation of drug addicts and criminal offenders

Table 10.4 includes examples of how TM promotes adaptive capacity in the neurophysiological, cognitive/emotional, and behavioral domains (see also chapters 3 and 11, this volume). As shown in table 10.4, effects of TM in these domains indicate increased resilience and stress prevention (level 1), recovery from acute or episodic stress (level 2), and neutralization of effects of chronic stress (level 3). As shown in the columns of the table, TM produces holistic effects across domains, counteracting the effects of stress on body, mind, and behavior.

Research indicating increased resilience as a result of TM—which is briefly noted in table 10.4 (level 1)—will be summarized in the next two sections. Changes that counteract those during acute and short-term stress episodes are a result of TM: reduced physiological arousal,[123] improvements in mood states,[124] and reduced use of tranquillizers, sleeping pills, caffeine, and other substances often used to relieve emotional distress[125] (table 10.4, level 2). The cumulative impact of chronic stress is counteracted by regular practice of TM over the long term. This is indicated by decreased neuroticism, reduced depressive symptoms,[126] and effective rehabilitation of drug addicts[127] and criminal offenders[128] (table 10.4, level 3). A physiological indication of successful rehabilitation through regular TM practice is increased autonomic stability.[129] Emotionally unstable individuals tend to exhibit higher autonomic instability, which is detectable in skin conductance responses that occur spontaneously, independent of sensory stimuli.

TM and Resilience to Stress

Resilience refers to "the individual's adaptive or equilibrative capabilities under conditions of environmental stress, conflict, or disequilibrium."[130] The term is also used broadly in regard to our ability to "bounce back" from stress and disease and to recover adaptive capacity.[131] Several personality characteristics are correlated with a person's resilience. These include dimensions of positive psychological health, including positive affect and emotional intelligence.[132,133] Having a reserve of positive emotions is important to buffer against distressful feelings that may arise when dealing with challenges.[134] Adequate self-esteem and self-concept are key resilience factors, especially in children and adolescents.[135] Situations that involve interpersonal conflict or ambiguity require a person to maintain a healthy self-concept and to manage emotions appropriately. Other characteristics of resilient individuals include having an internal locus of control (i.e., attributing personal success or failure to one's own actions, rather than blaming others) and finding existential meaning in life.[136] Successful adaptation to challenging situations often requires deliberation and problem solving. Hence cognitive skills, including fluid intelligence, verbal skills, and cognitive flexibility, are also predictors of resilience.[137,138] Healthy relationships with family and friends are an essential basis for adequate social support as a buffer in times of stress or illness.[139]

TM has been shown to enhance cognitive abilities: intelligence, verbal ability, problem-solving ability, and cognitive flexibility.[140–142] On multiple dimensions of psychological health associated with resilience, improvements have been consistently seen in research studies after participants learn and practice TM—on measures of self-actualization, self-concept, self-esteem, internal locus of control, and various indicators of life satisfaction.[143] Enhanced behavioral and emotional coping ability and improved mood states as a result of TM were found in a randomized controlled trial of 298 university students.[144] Higher levels among TM practitioners compared to non-meditating controls have also been reported in emotional intelligence.[145] These competencies appear to translate into better work and personal relationships, which have been reported by investigators after study participants start to practice TM.[146]

Particularly noteworthy are the effects of TM on the brain and nervous system because of their role in stress responses (see chapters 2 and 11, this volume). Orme-Johnson conducted a seminal study which showed faster habituation of physiological responses to noxious stimuli, indicating increased resilience to stress.[147] The research participants were presented with a series of loud tones, each of which triggered a peak in skin conductance levels, an indicator of a stress response of the sympathetic nervous system. With repeated exposure to the stressors, the magnitude of reaction diminished over time in all subjects. However, in the TM group relative to the non-TM control subjects, less time was needed for the reaction to be extinguished. The results of this study were replicated in a study with prison inmates[148] and also in a randomized longitudinal study of college students.[149]

In a study of two U.S. automotive facilities' employees, improvements were seen on several predictors of resilience among subjects who learned TM and practiced it regularly.[150] Significant changes relative to the non-meditating control group included greater effectiveness on the job, higher job-satisfaction levels, and better work and personal relationships. Among the regular meditators, there were also larger improvements in stress variables, sleep quality, and self-reported general health, as well as greater reduction in consumption of hard liquor and cigarettes.

Development of Consciousness and Peak Levels of Resilience

Full rehabilitation from physical or mental illness should mean that a patient does not suffer a relapse. If resilience means bouncing back to one's previous state of well-being and health, then doing so may not be enough to ensure one does not succumb to the stress of severe problems or major life events that precipitated the illness. To ensure that patients do not relapse, they must increase in adaptive capacity so that they become stronger than the stresses they face. Leading researchers on successful aging, Prem Fry and Corey Keys, advocate proactively developing one's latent potentialities so as to attain high levels of resilience.[151] They state,

> What differentiates individuals who thrive from those who succumb to disease and stagnation is not merely toughness or ability to recover quickly from challenge and misfortune, but rather their adaptability and flexibility in reacting to stress.

Thriving health implies not merely absence of disease, but rather older adults' intensive search for positive trajectories and sources of internal strengths, and older adults' conscious pursuit of ways to attain improved levels of emotional, social, and cognitive functioning.

For business entrepreneurs, high levels of resilience are a "must have" for survival. Small business owners are often subject to high stress levels due to the never-ending business challenges they face every day. In an empirical qualitative study of twenty-one entrepreneurs who were long-term practitioners of TM, systematic thematic analysis identified several competencies that interviewees associated with their business survival and success which they felt had developed as a result of their TM practice.[152] These factors included greater mental clarity and purposefulness, enhanced interpersonal skills, more integrated functioning, and greater inner strength and stability. Other factors which respondents consistently said were important to surmount challenges included the ability for self-renewal and having an unshakeable self-identity in terms of an expanded level of inner self-awareness or consciousness.[153]

If business owners can develop the strengths needed to survive great challenges, what about other kinds of people confronted by seemingly insurmountable problems? In modern society, challenging situations typically require more-complex responses than a simple flight or fight reaction to an immediate threat. Typical situations may involve decision making under pressure, and resolving ambiguity and/or interpersonal conflict. Resolving such challenges requires cognitive flexibility, planning, moral reasoning, and self-regulation of thought and emotions—executive function competencies whose seat is the prefrontal cortex. Ironically, stressful experiences tend to inhibit and impair the same prefrontal cortical functions that are necessary for enabling a person to handle such situations effectively. Long-term regular practice of TM also promotes integrated prefrontal brain functioning during daily activity (see chapters 2 and 11, this volume), thus enhancing executive functions. Although the above findings on meditating entrepreneurs were based on in-depth interviews of a non-random sample rather than on a quantitative controlled study, the findings are nevertheless insightful and consistent with other research findings on TM, showing development of strong self-concept and psychological integrity. For example, several studies of individuals who practice TM reflect profound growth toward advanced levels of self-development. Development of the ego, or individual self, typically proceeds through a series of stages during childhood, but in most individuals, the ego stage remains fixed from early adulthood onward. Adults incarcerated in prisons or in long-term psychiatric care often are at very low levels of ego development, which are characterized by externalizing blame, low impulse control, little capacity for empathy, and unsophisticated verbal skills. At the highest stages of ego development, emotional intelligence competencies such as self-awareness and empathy are highly developed, and individuals have enriched abilities for communicating subtle nuances of thought and emotion and for resolving ambiguity, existential paradox, and conflicts. Advancement to higher stages of ego development brings increased inner strength, greater personal integrity, and maximum psychological resilience. In a ten-year prospective longitudinal study, university alumni practicing TM advanced, on average, by an entire ego stage, whereas non-meditating alumni of three other universities either showed virtually no change or actually decreased over the same period.[154] Less than 10 percent of the adult population progressed beyond the usual "conventional" level of ego development typical of adults.[155] However, among the alumni who practiced TM, 53 percent scored at post-conventional ego-development levels.[156] Other research has shown that indicators of greater psychological integration—higher levels of creativity, moral reasoning, and more-developed self-concept—are correlated with EEG measures of brain integration, and that these psychological measures are enhanced by regularly practicing TM.[157,158] High levels of brain integration are a characteristic feature of transcendence (or pure consciousness) during TM and the stabilization of pure consciousness during waking activity outside of meditation.[159,160] Fred Travis developed a brain integration scale, which he showed distinguishes world-class performing athletes, musicians, and managers from others in the same professions who perform at more mediocre levels.[161] The scale is comprised of three EEG measures taken during task performance. In a randomized longitudinal study, college students who learned TM improved significantly compared to non-meditating control subjects over a three-month period.[162] The meditation group also significantly decreased in sympathetic nervous-system reactivity compared to control subjects.[163] These findings suggest that TM helps develop a more optimal style of brain functioning that is characteristic of high-performance individuals and is consistent with growth toward high levels of physiological and psychological resilience.

CONCLUSION

The survey of evidence presented in this chapter reveals that Transcendental Meditation is beneficial for a broad range of medical conditions. Clinical studies show improvements in stress-related disorders. A series of randomized clinical trials has demonstrated blood pressure reductions among hypertensive patients and retardation of the progression of cardiovascular disease, which is the leading cause of death in the United States. This has been shown to translate into decreased rates of clinical events ending in death. Dramatically lower rates of hospital admissions across diagnosis-related categories have been found among meditators who practice TM regularly for several months or more. Lower incidence of disease evidently results in lower healthcare resource utilization and costs.

The research reviewed in this chapter indicates that regular practice of TM is effective in primary prevention of disease. This is indicated, for example, by lower hospitalization rates across categories of medical disorders. Moreover, it was noted that for some kinds of disorders (e.g., addictions and cardiovascular diseases), there is evidence indicating that TM appears to decrease risk factors that lead to the progression of several types of disease.

While stress reduction is an important mechanism that TM provides, its health benefits should not be attributed solely to symptomatic stress-relief. TM is a powerful tool not only to neutralize long-term effects of chronic stress on body and mind, but also as a means of stress prevention through increasing resilience. There is strong evidence that practicing TM optimizes adaptive functioning of the brain and other stress-response systems in the body, enabling a person to handle challenging situations more effectively and to achieve greater vocational success and life satisfaction. Hence TM can be helpful not only in neutralizing effects of stress, but also in enabling a person to cope with challenges more effectively, thereby preventing stressful situations and averting harmful effects of stress on mind and body.

The evidence indicates that TM is efficacious for primary, secondary, and tertiary prevention of health disorders. Moreover, research indicates that TM both extends longevity and improves quality of life. TM has been found to be particularly effective with high-risk populations, such as minorities and the elderly.

In light of its comprehensive range of health effects, TM merits inclusion as a standard option in healthcare along with conventional treatments. The result will be improved patient outcomes and reduction of the escalating medical costs that are burdening Western nations.

NOTES

1. J. F. Fries, C. E. Koop, C. E. Beadle, P. P. Cooper, M. J. England, R. F. Greaves, J. J. Sokolov, D. Wright, and the Health Project Consortium, "Reducing Health Care Costs by Reducing the Need and Demand for Medical Services," *New England Journal of Medicine* 329 (1993): 322.

2. Ibid.

3. G. Miller, C. Roehrig, P. Hughes-Cromwick, and C. Lake, "Quantifying National Spending on Wellness and Prevention," *Advances in Health Economics and Health Services Research* 19 (2008): 1.

4. B. Starfield, "Is U.S. Health Really the Best in the World?" *JAMA* 284, no. 4 (2000): 483, 484.

5. U.S. National Institute of Aging, "Global Health and Aging" (Bethesda, MD: National Institutes of Health, 2011), www.nia.nih.gov/research/publication/global-health-and-aging/humanitys-aging.

6. H. Komisar, "The Effects of Rising Health Care Costs on Middle-Class Economic Security," in *Insight on the Issues* (Washington, DC: AARP Public Policy Institute, 2013), 1, www.aarp.org/content/dam/aarp/research/public_policy_institute/security/2013/impact-of-rising-healthcare-costs-AARP-ppi-sec.pdf.

7. R. D. Brook, L. J. Appel, M. Rubenfire, G. Ogedegbe, J. D. Bisognano, W. J. Elliott, and F. D. Fuchs et al., "Beyond Medications and Diet: Alternative Approaches to Lowering Blood Pressure; A Scientific Statement from the American Heart Association," *Hypertension* 61, no. 6 (2013): 1365.

8. K. R. Pelletier and R. Lutz, "Healthy People—Healthy Business: A Critical Review of Stress Management Programs in the Workplace," *American Journal of Health Promotion* 2, no. 3 (1988): 5.

9. D. R. Anderson, W. Whitmer, R. Z. Goetzel, R. J. Ozminkowski, J. Wasserman, S. Serxner, and the Health Enhancement Research Organization, "The Relationship between Modifiable Health Risks and Group-Level Health Care Expenditures," *American Journal of Health Promotion* 15, no. 1 (2000): 50.

10. Pelletier and Lutz (1988): 6.

11. R. Contrada and A. Baum, eds. *The Handbook of Stress Science* (New York: Springer, 2011), 1, 213, 425.

12. S. I. Nidich, M. V. Rainforth, D. A. Haaga, J. S. Hagelin, J. W. Salerno, F. Travis, and M. Tanner et al., "A Randomized Controlled Trial on Effects of the Transcendental Meditation Program on Blood Pressure, Psychological Distress, and Coping in Young Adults," *American Journal of Hypertension* 22, no. 12 (2009): 1326.

13. K. R. Eppley, A. I. Abrams, and J. Shear, "Differential Effects of Relaxation Techniques on Trait Anxiety: A Meta-Analysis," *Journal of Clinical Psychology* 45, no. 6 (1989): 957.

14. W. Sheppard, F. Staggers, and L. John, "The Effects of a Stress Management Program in a High Security Government Agency," *Anxiety, Stress, and Coping* 10 (1997): 341.

15. C. N. Alexander, G. Swanson, M. Rainforth, T. Carlisle, C. Todd, and R. Oates, "Effects of the Transcendental Meditation Program on Stress Reduction, Health, and Employee Development: A Prospective Study in Two Occupational Settings," *Anxiety, Stress, and Coping* 6 (1993): 245

16. C. Elder, S. Nidich, F. Moriarty, and R. Nidich, "Effect of Transcendental Meditation on Employee Stress, Depression, and Burnout: A Randomized Controlled Study," *Permanente Journal* 18, no. 1 (2014): 19.

17. A. Tjoa, "Meditation, Neuroticism and Intelligence: A Follow-up," *Gedrag: Tijdschrift voor Psychologie* 3, no. 3 (1975): 167.

18. W. P. van den Berg and B. Mulder, "Psychological Research on the Effects of the Transcendental Meditation Technique on a Number of Personality Variables," *Gedrag: Tijdschrift voor Psychologie* 4 (1976): 206.

19. C. N. Alexander, M. Rainforth, and P. Gelderloos, "Transcendental Meditation, Self-Actualization, and Psychological Health: A Conceptual Overview and Statistical Meta-Analysis," *Journal of Social Behavior and Personality* 6, no. 5 (1991): 189.

20. C. N. Alexander, P. Robinson, and M. V. Rainforth, "Treating and Preventing Alcohol, Nicotine and Drug Abuse through Transcendental Meditation: A Review and Statistical Meta-Analysis," *Alcoholism Treatment Quarterly* 11, no. 1 (1994): 11.

21. P. G. Williams, T. W. Smith, H. E. Gunn, and B. N. Uchino, "Personality and Stress: Individual Differences in Exposure, Reactivity, Recovery, and Restoration," ch. 18 in *The Handbook of Stress Science*, edited by Richard Contrada and Andrew Baum (New York: Springer, 2011), 239.

22. H. R. Colten and B. M. Altevogt, eds. *Sleep Disorders and Sleep Deprivation: An Unmet Public Health Problem* (Washington, DC: National Academies Press, 2006), 55.

23. D. E. Miskiman, "Long-Term Effects of the Transcendental Meditation Program in the Treatment of Insomnia," in *Scientific Research on the Transcendental Meditation Program: Collected Papers*, vol. 1, edited by David W. Orme-Johnson and John T. Farrow (Fairfield, IA: Maharishi International University Press, 1977), 299.

24. D. A. Throll, "The Effects of the Transcendental Meditation Technique Upon Adolescent Personality," in *Scientific Research on Maharishi's Transcendental Meditation and TM-Sidhi Programme: Collected Papers*, vol. 2, edited by Roger Chalmers, Geoffrey Clements, Hartmut Schenkluhn, and Michael Weinless (Vlodrop, The Netherlands: Maharishi Vedic University Press, 1990), 1094.

25. L. Farinelli, "Possibilita Di Applicationi Della Technologia Della Conscienza in Aspetti Di Medicina Preventiva: Una Ricerca Pilota," in *Scientific Research on Maharishi's Transcendental Meditation and TM-Sidhi Programme: Collected Papers*, vol. 3, edited by Roger Chalmers, Geoffrey Clements, Hartmut Schenkluhn, and Michael Weinless (Vlodrop, The Netherlands: Maharishi Vedic University Press, 1990), 1830.

26. J. S. Brooks and T. Scarano, "Transcendental Meditation in the Treatment of Post-Vietnam Adjustment," *Journal of Counseling and Development* 64 (1985): 212.

27. Throll (1990), 1093.

28. Farinelli (1990), 1830.

29. R. J. Monahan, "Secondary Prevention of Drug Dependence through the Transcendental Meditation Program in Metropolitan Philadelphia," *International Journal of the Addictions* 12, no. 6 (1977): 729.

30. D. A. Gutman and C. B. Nemeroff, "Stress and Depression," ch. 25 in *The Handbook of Stress Science*, edited by Richard Contrada and Andrew Baum (New York: Springer, 2011), 345.

31. A. L. Dougall and J. N. Swanson, "Physical Heath Outcomes of Trauma," ch. 27 in *The Handbook of Stress Science*, edited by Richard Contrada and Andrew Baum (New York: Springer, 2011), 373.

32. D. A. Jauch and W. T. Carpenter Jr.," Reactive Psychosis: I. Does the Pre-DSM-III Concept Define a Third Psychosis?" *Journal of Nervous and Mental Disease* 176, no. 2 (1988): 72.

33. J. O. Ottoson, "Transcendental Meditation" (Stockholm: Socialstrytelsen, 1977).

34. R. Carter and J. E. Meyer, "The Use of the Transcendental Meditation Technique with Severely Disturbed Psychiatric Inpatients" in *Scientific Research on Maharishi's Transcendental Meditation and TM-Sidhi Programme: Collected Papers*, vol. 3, edited by Roger Chalmers, Geoffrey Clements, Hartmut Schenkluhn, and Michael Weinless (Vlodrop, The Netherlands: Maharishi Vedic University Press, 1990), 2112.

35. Brooks and Scarano (1985): 212.

36. D. W. Orme-Johnson, J. Kiehlbauch, R. Moore, and J. Bristol, "Personality and Autonomic Changes in Prisoners Practicing the Transcendental Meditation Technique," in *Scientific Research on the Transcendental Meditation Program: Collected Papers*, edited by David W. Orme-Johnson and John T. Farrow (Fairfield, IA: Maharishi International University Press, 1977), 556.

37. M. Rainforth, C. N. Alexander, and K. L. Cavanaugh, "The Transcendental Meditation Program and Criminal Recidivism in Folsom State Prisoners: A 15-Year Follow-up Study," *Journal of Offender Rehabilitation* 36 (2003): 181.

38. C. Blair, D. Granger and R. Peters Razza, "Cortisol Reactivity Is Positively Related to Executive Function in Preschool Children Attending Head Start Child Development," *Child Development* 76 (2005): 554.

39. S. J. Grosswald, W. R. Stixrud, F. Travis, and M. A. Bateh, "Use of the Transcendental Meditation Technique to Reduce Symptoms of Attention Deficit Hyperactivity Disorder (ADHD) by Reducing Stress and Anxiety: An Exploratory Study," *Current Issues in Education* 10, no. 2 (2008).

40. Ibid.

41. V. A. Barnes, L. B. Bauza, and F. A. Treiber, "Impact of Stress Reduction on Negative School Behavior in Adolescents," *Health and Quality of Life Outcomes* 1, no. 10 (2003).

42. A. Aron and E. N. Aron, "Rehabilitation of Juvenile Offenders through the Transcendental Meditation Program: A Controlled Study," in *Scientific Research on Maharishi's Transcendental Meditation and TM-Sidhi Programme: Collected Papers*, vol. 3, edited by Roger Chalmers, Geoffrey Clements, Hartmut Schenkluhn, and Michael Weinless (Vlodrop, The Netherlands: Maharishi Vedic University Press, 1990), 2163.

43. S. Cohen, D. Janicki-Deverts, W. J. Doyle, G. E. Miller, E. Frank, B. S. Rabin, and R. B. Turner, "Chronic Stress, Glucocorticoid Receptor Resistance, Inflammation, and Disease Risk," *PNAS* 109, no. 16 (2012): 5995.

44. K. S. Blasdell, "Acute Immunoreactivity, Transcendental Meditation, and Type A/B Behavior," abstract of Doctoral Dissertation, Department of Physiological and Biological Sciences," *Dissertation Abstracts International* 50, no. 10 (1990): 4806B.

45. Farinelli (1990), 1830.

46. Ian M. Klemons, "Changes in Inflammation in Persons Practicing the Transcendental Meditation Technique," in *Scientific Research on the Transcendental*

Meditation Program: Collected Papers, vol. 1, edited by David W. Orme-Johnson and John T. Farrow (Fairfield, IA: Maharishi International University Press, 1977), 287.

47. A. F. Wilson, R. W. Honsberger, John T. Chiu, and H. S. Novey, "Transcendental Meditation and Asthma," *Respiration* 32 (1975): 74.

48. Gutman and Nemeroff (2011), 345.

49. D. W. Orme-Johnson, R. H. Schneider, Y. D. Son, S. Nidich, and Z. -Hee Cho, "Neuroimaging of Meditation's Effect on Brain Reactivity to Pain," *NeuroReport* 17, no. 12 (2006): 1359.

50. W. W. Mills and J. T. Farrow, "The Transcendental Meditation Technique and Acute Experimental Pain," *Psychosomatic Medicine* 43 (1981): 157.

51. Orme-Johnson et al. (2006): 1359.

52. H. D. Lovell-Smith, "Transcendental Meditation and Three Cases of Migraine," *New Zealand Medical Journal* 98 (1985): 443.

53. Throll (1990), 1093.

54. Farinelli (1990), 1830.

55. Monahan (1977): 729.

56. U.S. Centers for Disease Control, "Heart Disease and Stroke Prevention: Addressing the Nation's Leading Killers," 2011.

57. R. Contrada and A. Baum, eds. *The Handbook of Stress Science* (New York: Springer, 2011).

58. N. S. Bekkouche, S. Holmes, K. S. Whittaker, and D. S. Krantz, "Stress and the Heart: Psychosocial Stress and Coronary Heart Disease," ch. 28 in *The Handbook of Stress Science*, edited by Richard Contrada and Andrew Baum (New York: Springer, 2011), 386.

59. M. V. Rainforth, R. H. Schneider, S. I. Nidich, C. Gaylord-King, J. W. Salerno, and J. W. Anderson, "Stress Reduction Programs in Patients with Elevated Blood Pressure: A Systematic Review and Meta-Analysis," *Current Hypertension Reports* 9, no. 6 (2007): 520.

60. M. J. Cooper and M. M. Aygen, "Transcendental Meditation in the Management of Hypercholesterolemia," *Journal of Human Stress* 5, no. 4 (1979): 24.

61. Alexander et al. (1994): 11.

62. A. Castillo-Richmond, R. H. Schneider, C. N. Alexander, R. Cook, H. Myers, S. Nidich, C. Haney, M. V. Rainforth, and J. W. Salerno, "Effects of Stress Reduction on Carotid Atherosclerosis in Hypertensive African Americans," *Stroke* 31 (2000): 568.

63. M. Paul-Labrador, D. Polk, J. H. Dwyer, I. Velasquez, S. Nidich, M. Rainforth, R. Schneider, and N. B. Merz, "Effects of Randomized Controlled Trial of Transcendental Meditation on Components of the Metabolic Syndrome in Subjects with Coronary Heart Disease," *Archives of Internal Medicine* 166 (2006): 1218.

64. J. W. Zamarra, R. H. Schneider, I. Besseghini, D. K. Robinson, and J. W. Salerno, "Usefulness of the Transcendental Meditation Program in the Treatment of Patients with Coronary Artery Disease," *American Journal of Cardiology* 77, no. 10 (1996): 867.

65. K. Kondwani, R. Schneider, C. N Alexander, C. Sledge, F. Staggers, B. M. Clayborne, and W. Sheppard et al., "Left Ventricular Mass Regression with the Transcendental Meditation Technique and a Health Education Program in Hypertensive African Americans," *Journal of Social Behavior and Personality* 17 (2005): 181.

66. R. Jayadevappa, J. C. Johnson, B. S. Bloom, S. Nidich, S. Desai, S. Chhatre, D. B. Raziano, and R. Schneider, "Effectiveness of Transcendental Meditation on Functional Capacity and Quality of Life of African Americans with Congestive Heart Failure: A Randomized Control Study," *Ethnicity and Disease* 17, no. 1 (2007): 72.

67. R. H. Schneider, C. E. Grim, M. V. Rainforth, T. Kotchen, S. I. Nidich, C. Gaylord-King, J. W. Salerno, J. Morley Kotchen, and C. N. Alexander, "Stress Reduction in the Secondary Prevention of Cardiovascular Disease: Randomized Controlled Trial of Transcendental Meditation and Health Education in Blacks," *Circulation: Cardiovascular Quality and Outcomes* 2, no. 5 (2012): 1.

68. D. W. Orme-Johnson, "Medical Care Utilization and the Transcendental Meditation Program," *Psychosomatic Medicine* 49 (1987): 493.

69. Orme-Johnson (1987): 498.

70. D. W. Orme-Johnson and R. E. Herron, "An Innovative Approach to Reducing Medical Care Utilization and Expenditures," *American Journal of Managed Care* 3, no. 1 (1997): 135.

71. Orme-Johnson (1987): 493.

72. Orme-Johnson (1987): 502.

73. U.S. Department of Labor, Bureau of Labor Statistics, "Economic Report of the President, Table B–60: Consumer Price Indexes for Major Expenditure Classes, 1969–2012," www.gpo.gov/fdsys/pkg/ERP-2013/pdf/ERP-2013-table60.pdf.

74. Orme-Johnson and Herron (1997): 137.

75. R. E. Herron, S. L. Hillis, J. V. Mandarino, D. W. Orme-Johnson, and K. G. Walton, "The Impact of the Transcendental Meditation Program on Government Payments to Physicians in Quebec," *American Journal of Health Promotion* 10, no. 3 (1996): 208.

76. R. E. Herron and S. L. Hillis, "The Impact of the Transcendental Meditation Program on Government Payments to Physicians in Quebec: An Update," *American Journal of Health Promotion* 14, no. 5 (2000): 284.

77. R. E. Herron and K. Cavanaugh, "Can the Transcendental Meditation Program Reduce the Medical Expenditures of Older People? A Longitudinal Cost Reduction Study in Canada," *Journal of Social Behavior and Personality* 17 (2005): 415.

78. R. E. Herron, "Changes in Physician Costs among High-Cost Transcendental Meditation Practitioners Compared with High-Cost Nonpractitioners over 5 Years," *American Journal of Health Promotion* 26, no. 1 (2011): 56

79. Herron et al. (2000): 288.

80. Herron and Cavanaugh (2005): 415.

81. Herron (2011): 56.

82. S. B. Cohen and F. Rohde, "The Concentration in Health Expenditures over a Two-Year Time Interval, Estimates for the U.S. Population, 2005–2006," in *Medical Expenditure Panel Survey: Statistical Briefs* (Rockville, MD: U.S. Agency for Healthcare Research and Quality, 2009).

83. J. D. Reschovsky, J. Hadley, C. B. Saiontz-Martinez, and E. R. Boukus, "Following the Money: Factors Associated with the Cost of Treating High-Cost Medicare Beneficiaries," *Health Services Research* 46, no. 4 (2011): 997.

84. K. E. Thorpe and D. H. Howard, "The Rise in Spending among Medicare Beneficiaries: The Role of Chronic Disease Prevalence and Changes in Treatment Intensity," *Health Affairs* 25, no. 5 (2006): 383.

85. R. Schneider, F. Staggers, C. N. Alexander, W. Sheppard, M. V. Rainforth, K. Kondwani, S. Smith, and C. Gaylord-King, "A Randomized Controlled Trial of Stress Reduction for Hypertension in Older African Americans," *Hypertension* 26, no. 5 (1995): 820.

86. R. Schneider, C. N Alexander, F. Staggers, D. W. Orme-Johnson, M. Rainforth, J. W. Salerno, W. Sheppard et al., "A Randomized Controlled Trial of Stress Reduction in African Americans Treated for Hypertension During One Year," *American Journal of Hypertension* 18 (2005): 88.

87. R. E. Herron, R. H. Schneider, J. V. Mandarino, C. N. Alexander, and K. G. Walton, "Cost-Effective Hypertension Management: Comparison of Drug Therapies with an Alternative Program," *American Journal of Managed Care* 2, no. 4 (1996): 427.

88. Eppley et al. (1989): 957; Alexander et al. (1991): 189.

89. Ibid.

90. Jayadevappa et al. (2007): 72.

91. S. Nidich, J. Z. Fields, M. Rainforth, R. Pomerantz, C. David, J. Kristeller, J. W. Salerno, and R. Schneider, "A Randomized Controlled Trial of the Effects of Transcendental Meditation on Quality of Life in Older Breast Cancer Patients," *Integrative Cancer Therapies* 8, no. 3 (2009): 228.

92. C. N. Alexander, E. J. Langer, R. I. Newman, H. M. Chandler, and J. L. Davies, "Transcendental Meditation, Mindfulness, and Longevity: An Experimental Study with the Elderly," *Journal of Personality and Social Psychology* 57, no. 6 (1989): 950.

93. R. H. Schneider, C. N. Alexander, F. Staggers, M. V. Rainforth, J. W. Salerno, A. Hartz, S. Arndt, V. A. Barnes, and S. I. Nidich, "Long-Term Effects of Stress Reduction on Mortality in Persons ≥ 55 Years of Age with Systemic Hypertension," *American Journal of Cardiology* 95 (2005): 1060.

94. Castillo-Richmond et al. (2000): 568; Kondwani et al. (2005): 181; Jayadevappa et al. (2007): 72; Schneider et al. (1995): 820; Schneider et al. (2005): 88; Schneider et al. (2012): 1.

95. M. Toomey, "The Effects of the Transcendental Meditation Program on Carotid Atherosclerosis and Cardiovascular Disease Risk Factors in Native Hawaiians," dissertation, Maharishi University of Management, 2007.

96. Eppley et al. (1989): 957; Alexander et al. (1991): 189; Alexander et al. (1994): 11.

97. Eppley et al. (1989): 957; Alexander et al. (1991): 189.

98. Alexander et al. (1994): 11.

99. Rainforth et al. (2007): 520.

100. Random assignment studies with TM: Pelletier (1974); Dillbeck (1977); Dillbeck (1982); Brooks and Scarano (1985); Alexander et al. (1989); Gaylord et al. (1989); Schneider et al. (1995); Maclean et al. (1997); Sheppard et al. (1997); Wenneberg et al. (1997); Castillo-Richmond et al. (2000); Barnes et al. (2003); Barnes and Davis et al. (2004); Barnes, Treiber et al. (2004); Kondwani et al. (2005); Schneider et al. (2005);

Paul-Labrador (2006); Jayadevappa et al. 2007); Nidich, Fields et al. (2009); Nidich and Rainforth et al. (2009); Tanner et al. (2009); Travis et al. (2009); Travis et al. (2010); Haaga et al. (2011); Barnes et al. (2012); Schneider et al. (2012); Elder et al. (2014).

101. TM Studies with blinded testing (i.e., testers were unaware of participants' treatment assignments: Schneider et al. (1995); Castillo-Richmond et al. (2000); Kondwani et al. (2005); Schneider et al. (2005); Paul-Labrador (2006); Jayadevappa et al. 2007); Toomey (2007); Nidich and Fields et al. (2009); Nidich and Rainforth et al. (2009); Tanner et al. (2009); Travis et al. (2009); Travis et al. (2010); Haaga et al. (2011); Schneider et al. (2012). Studies with structurally similar control groups (i.e., experimental and active control conditions were similar on time and attention received from trainers and expectations regarding home practice time): Alexander et al. (1989); Gaylord et al. (1989); Schneider et al. (1995); Castillo-Richmond et al. (2000); Kondwani et al. (2005); Schneider et al. (2005); Paul-Labrador (2006); Jayadevappa et al. 2007); Toomey (2007); Schneider et al. (2012).

102. Schneider et al. (2012): 1.

103. TM studies reporting correlations between intervention compliance and treatment outcomes: Orme-Johnson and John Kiehlbauch et al. (1977); Browne et al. (1990); Alexander et al. (1993); Schneider et al. (2012).

104. Schneider et al. (2012): 1.

105. Alexander et al. (1994): 11.

106. G. E. Browne, D. Fougére, A. Roxburgh, J. Bird, and H. D. Lovell-Smith, "Improved Mental and Physical Health and Decreased Use of Prescribed and Non-prescribed Drugs through the Transcendental Meditation Program," in *Scientific Research on Maharishi's Transcendental Meditation and TM-Sidhi Programme: Collected Papers*, vol. 3, edited by Roger Chalmers, Geoffrey Clements, Hartmut Schenkluhn, and Michael Weinless (Vlodrop, The Netherlands: Maharishi Vedic University Press, 1990), 1889.

107. R. K. Wallace, J. Silver, P. J. Mills, M. C. Dillbeck, and D. E. Wagoner, "Systolic Blood Pressure and Long-Term Practice of the Transcendental Meditation and TM-Sidhi Program: Effects of TM on Systolic Blood Pressure," *Psychosomatic Medicine* 45, no. 1 (1983): 41–46.

108. C. Patterson and L. W. Chambers, "Preventive Health Care," *Lancet* 345 (1995): 1611.

109. Blasdell (1990).

110. Orme-Johnson (1987): 493.

111. Ottoson (1977).

112. Rainforth et al. (2007): 520; Cooper and Aygen (1979): 24.

113. Alexander et al. (1994): 11.

114. Paul-Labrador et al. (2006): 1218.

115. Castillo-Richmond (2000): 568.

116. Brooks and Scarano (1985): 212.

117. Carter and Meyer (1990).

118. H. Schenkluhn and M. Geisler, "A Longitudinal Study of the Influence of the Transcendental Meditation Program on Drug Abuse," in *Scientific Research on the Transcendental Meditation Program: Collected Papers*, vol. 1, edited by David W. Orme-Johnson and John T. Farrow (Fairfield, IA: Maharishi International University Press, 1977), 544.

119. Schneider et al. (2012): 1.

120. Nidich et al. (2009): 228.

121. Jayadevappa et al. (2007): 72.

122. Eppley et al. (1989): 957.

123. Alexander et al. (1991): 189.

124. M. Dillbeck and D. W. Orme-Johnson, "Physiological Differences between Transcendental Meditation and Rest," *American Psychologist* 42 (1987): 879.

125. Nidich and Rainforth et al. (2009): 1326.

126. Throll (1990): 2112; Farinelli (1990): 1830; Monahan (1977): 729.

127. Sheppard et al. (1997): 341; Brooks and Scarano (1985): 212.

128. Schenkluhn and Geisler (1977): 544.

129. Orme-Johnson and Kiehlbauch et al. (1977): 556; Rainforth et al. (2003): 181.

130. Orme-Johnson and Kiehlbauch et al. (1977): 556.

131. J. H. Block and J. Block, "The Role of Ego-Control and Ego-Resiliency in the Organization of Behaviour," in *The Minnesota Symposia on Child Psychology*, edited by W. A. Collins, 39–101 (Hillsdale, NJ: Lawrence Erlbaum Associates, 1980).

132. B. Resnick, L. P. Gwyther, and K. A. Roberto, eds. *Resilience in Aging: Concepts, Research, and Outcomes* (New York: Springer, 2011).

133. Resnick, Gwyther, and Roberto (2011).

134. P. H. Finan, A. J. Zautra, and R. Wershba, "The Dynamics of Emotion in Adaptation to Stress," ch. 16 in *The Handbook of Stress Science*, edited by Richard Contrada and Andrew Baum (New York: Springer, 2011), 209.

135. Ibid.

136. K. L. Kumpfer, "Factors and Processes Contributing to Resilience," ch. 9 in *Resilience and Development: Positive Life Adaptations*, edited by Meyer D. Glantz and Jeannette Johnson (New York: Kluwer Academic Publishers, 1999), 179–224.

137. Resnick, Gwyther, and Roberto (2011).

138. Ibid.

139. Kumpfer (1999).

140. Resnick, Gwyther, and Roberto (2011).

141. H. Shecter, "The Transcendental Meditation Program in the Classroom: A Psychological Evaluation," in *Scientific Research on the Transcendental Meditation Program: Collected Papers*, vol. 1, edited by David W. Orme-Johnson and John T. Farrow (Fairfield, IA: Maharishi International University Press, 1977), 403.

142. F. Travis "Creative Thinking and the Transcendental Meditation Technique," *Journal of Creative Behavior* 13, no, 3 (1979): 169.

143. Alexander et al. (1989): 950.

144. Alexander et al. (1991): 189.

145. Nidich and Rainforth et al. (2009): 1326.

146. S. Sawhney "Effects of the TM Technique on Anxiety, Emotional Intelligence, and Trust: Implications for Supply Chain Management," doctoral dissertation, Maharishi University of Management, 2012.

147. Alexander and Swanson et al. (1993): 245.

148. D. W. Orme-Johnson, "Autonomic Stability and Transcendental Meditation," *Psychosomatic Medicine* 35 (1973): 341–49.

149. Orme-Johnson and Kiehlbauch et al. (1977): 556.

150. F. Travis, D. A. Haaga, J. S. Hagelin, M. Tanner, S. Nidich, and C. Gaylord-King, "Effects of Transcendental Meditation Practice on Brain Functioning and Stress Reactivity in College Students," *International Journal of Psychophysiology* 71, no. 2 (2009): 170–76.

151. Alexander and Swanson et al. (1993): 245.

152. P. Fry and C. Keys, eds., *New Frontiers in Resilient Aging: Well-Being in Late Life* (Cambridge: Cambridge University Press, 2010).

153. E. Norlyk Herriott and D. P. Heaton, "Spiritual Dimensions of Entrepreneurship in Transcendental Meditation and TM-Sidhi Program Practitioners," *Journal of Management, Spirituality, and Religion* 6, no. 3 (2009): 195–208.

154. Ibid.

155. H. Chandler, C. N. Alexander, and D. P. Heaton, "Transcendental Meditation and Post-Conventional Self-Development: A 10-Year Longitudinal Study," *Journal of Social Behavior and Personality* 17 (2005): 93.

156. S. R. Cook-Greuter, "Mature Ego Development: A Gateway to Ego Transcendence?" *Journal of Adult Development* 7, no. 4 (2000): 227–40.

157. Chandler et al. (2005): 93.

158. C. N. Alexander, J. L. Davies, C. A. Dixon, M. C. Dillbeck, S. M. Druker, R. M. Detzel, J. M. Muehlman, and D. W. Orme-Johnson, "Growth of Higher Stages of Consciousness: Maharishi's Vedic Psychology of Human Development," in *Higher Stages of Human Development: Perspectives on Adult Growth*, edited by Charles N. Alexander and Ellen J. Langer (New York: Oxford University Press, 1990), 310–11.

159. Travis (1979): 169; Alexander et al. (1991): 228; Chandler et al. (2005): 93.

160. Travis and Haaga et al. (2009): 170.

161. F. Travis, "Beyond Waking, Dreaming and Sleeping: Perspectives from Research on Meditation Experiences," in *States of Consciousness: Experimental Insights into Meditation, Waking, Sleep and Dreams States of Consciousness*, edited by Dean Cvetkovic and Irena Cosic (New York: Springer, 2011), 223–34.

162. Ibid.

163. Ibid.

BIBLIOGRAPHY

Alexander, C. N., Langer, E. J., Newman, R. I. Chandler, H. M. and Davies, J. L. "Transcendental Meditation, Mindfulness, and Longevity: An Experimental Study with the Elderly." *Journal of Personality and Social Psychology* 57, no. 6 (1989): 950–64.

Alexander, C. N., Rainforth, M., and Gelderloos, P. "Transcendental Meditation, Self-Actualization, and Psychological Health: A Conceptual Overview and Statistical Meta-Analysis." *Journal of Social Behavior and Personality* 6, no. 5 (1991): 189–247.

Alexander, C. N., Robinson, P., and Rainforth, M. V. "Treating and Preventing Alcohol, Nicotine and Drug Abuse through Transcendental Meditation: A Review and Statistical Meta-analysis." *Alcoholism Treatment Quarterly* 11, no. 1 (1994): 11–84.

Alexander, C. N., Davies, J. L., C. A. Dixon, M. C. Dillbeck, Steven M. Druker, R. M. Retzel, J. M. Muehlman, and D. W. Orme-Johnson. "Growth of Higher Stages of Consciousness: Maharishi's Vedic Psychology of Human Development." In *Higher Stages of Human Development: Perspectives on Adult Growth*, edited by Charles N. Alexander and Ellen J. Langer, 286–340. New York: Oxford University Press, 1990.

Alexander, C. N., Gerald Swanson, Maxwell Rainforth, Thomas Carlisle, Christopher Todd, and Robert Oates. "Effects of the Transcendental Meditation Program on Stress Reduction, Health, and Employee Development: A Prospective Study in Two Occupational Settings." *Anxiety, Stress, and Coping* 6 (1993): 245–62.

Anderson, D. R., William Whitmer, Ron Z. Goetzel, Ronald J. Ozminkowski, Jeffrey Wasserman, Seth Serxner, and the Health Enhancement Research Organization. "The Relationship between Modifiable Health Risks and Group-Level Health Care Expenditures." *American Journal of Health Promotion* 15, no. 1 (2000): 45–52.

Aron, A., and Elaine N. Aron. "Rehabilitation of Juvenile Offenders through the Transcendental Meditation Program: A Controlled Study." In *Scientific Research on Maharishi's Transcendental Meditation and TM-Sidhi Programme: Collected Papers*, vol. 3, edited by Roger Chalmers, Geoffrey Clements, Hartmut Schenkluhn, and Michael Weinless, 2163–66. Vlodrop, The Netherlands: Maharishi Vedic University Press, 1990.

Barnes, V. A., Lynnette B. Bauza, and Frank A. Treiber. "Impact of Stress Reduction on Negative School Behavior in Adolescents." *Health and Quality of Life Outcomes* 1, no. 10 (2003).

Barnes, V. A., Frank A. Treiber, and Maribeth. H. Johnson. "Impact of Transcendental Meditation on Ambulatory Blood Pressure in African American Adolescents." *American Journal of Hypertension* 17, no. 4 (2004): 366–69.

Barnes, V. A., Harry C. Davis, James B. Murzynowski, and Frank A. Treiber. "Impact of Meditation on Resting and Ambulatory Blood Pressure and Heart Rate in Youth." *Psychosomatic Medicine* 66, no. 6 (2004): 909–14.

Barnes, V. A., Gaston K. Kapuku, and Frank A. Treiber. "Impact of Transcendental Meditation on Left Ventricular Mass in African American Adolescents." *Evidence-Based Complementary and Alternative Medicine* (2012).

Bekkouche, N. S., Sari Holmes, Kerry S. Whittaker, and David S. Krantz. "Stress and the Heart: Psychosocial Stress and Coronary Heart Disease." In *The Handbook of Stress Science*, edited by Richard Contrada and Andrew Baum, 385–98. New York: Springer, 2011.

Blair, C., Douglas Granger, and Rachel Peters Razza. "Cortisol Reactivity Is Positively Related to Executive Function in Preschool Children Attending Head Start Child Development." *Child Development* 76 (2005): 554–67.

Blasdell, K. S. "Acute Immunoreactivity, Transcendental Meditation, and Type A/B Behavior." Abstract of Doctoral Dissertation, Department of Physiological and Biological Sciences." *Dissertation Abstracts International* 50, no. 10 (1990): 4806B.

Block, J. H., and Jeanne Block. "The Role of Ego-Control and Ego-Resiliency in the Organization of Behaviour." In *The Minnesota Symposia on Child Psychology*, edited by W. A. Collins, 39–101. Hillsdale, NJ: Lawrence Erlbaum Associates, 1980.

Brook, R. D., Lawrence J. Appel, Melvyn Rubenfire, Gbenga Ogedegbe, John D. Bisognano, William J. Elliott, and Flavio D. Fuchs et al. "Beyond Medications and

Diet: Alternative Approaches to Lowering Blood Pressure: A Scientific Statement from the American Heart Association." *Hypertension* 61, no. 6 (2013): 1360–83.

Brooks, J. S. and Thomas Scarano. "Transcendental Meditation in the Treatment of Post-Vietnam Adjustment." *Journal of Counseling and Development* 64 (1985): 212–14.

Browne, G. E., David Fougére, Alistair Roxburgh, John Bird, and H. David Lovell-Smith. "Improved Mental and Physical Health and Decreased Use of Prescribed and Non-Prescribed Drugs through the Transcendental Meditation Program." In *Scientific Research on Maharishi's Transcendental Meditation Program: Collected Papers*, edited by Roger Chalmers, Geoffrey Clements, Hartmut Schenkluhn, and Michael Weinless, 1884–99. Fairfield, IA: Maharishi International University Press, 1990.

Carter, R. and Jo E. Meyer. "The Use of the Transcendental Meditation Technique with Severely Disturbed Psychiatric Inpatients." In *Scientific Research on Maharishi's Transcendental Meditation and TM-Sidhi Programme: Collected Papers*, vol. 3, edited by Roger Chalmers, Geoffrey Clements, Hartmut Schenkluhn, and Michael Weinless, 2112–14. Vlodrop, The Netherlands: Maharishi Vedic University Press, 1990.

Castillo-Richmond, A., Robert H. Schneider, Charles N. Alexander, Robert Cook, Hector Myers, Sanford Nidich, Chinelo Haney, Maxwell V. Rainforth, and John W. Salerno. "Effects of Stress Reduction on Carotid Atherosclerosis in Hypertensive African Americans." *Stroke* 31 (2000): 568–73.

Chalmers, R., Geoffrey Clements, Hartmut Schenkluhn, and Michael Weinless, eds. *Scientific Research on Maharishi's Transcendental Meditation and TM-Sidhi Programme: Collected Papers*, vols. 2–4. Vlodrop, The Netherlands: Maharishi Vedic University Press, 1990.

Chandler, H., Charles N. Alexander, and Dennis P. Heaton. "Transcendental Meditation and Post-Conventional Self-Development: A 10-Year Longitudinal Study." *Journal of Social Behavior and Personality* 17 (2005): 93–121.

Cohen, S., Denise Janicki-Deverts, William J. Doyle, Gregory E. Miller, Ellen Frank, Bruce S. Rabin, and Ronald B. Turner. "Chronic Stress, Glucocorticoid Receptor Resistance, Inflammation, and Disease Risk." *Proceedings of the National Academy of Sciences USA* 109, no. 16 (2012): 5995–99.

Cohen, S. B. and Frederick Rohde. "The Concentration in Health Expenditures over a Two-Year Time Interval, Estimates for the U.S. Population, 2005–2006." In *Medical Expenditure Panel Survey: Statistical Briefs*. Rockville, MD: U.S. Agency for Healthcare Research and Quality, 2009.

Colten, H. R. and Bruce M. Altevogt, eds. *Sleep Disorders and Sleep Deprivation: An Unmet Public Health Problem*. Washington, DC: National Academies Press, 2006.

Contrada, R. and Andrew Baum, eds. *The Handbook of Stress Science*. New York: Springer, 2011.

Cook-Greuter, S. R. "Mature Ego Development: A Gateway to Ego Transcendence?" *Journal of Adult Development* 7, no. 4 (2000): 227–40.

Cooper, M. J. and Maurice M. Aygen. "Transcendental Meditation in the Management of Hypercholesterolemia." *Journal of Human Stress* 5, no. 4 (1979): 24–27.

Dillbeck, M. C. "The effect of Transcendental Meditation on Anxiety Level." *Journal of Clinical Psychology* 33 (1977): 1076–78.

Dillbeck, M. C. "Meditation and Flexibility of Visual Perception and Verbal Problem Solving." *Memory and Cognition* 10, no. 3 (1982): 207–15.

Dillbeck, M. C., ed. *Scientific Research on Maharishi's Transcendental Meditation and TM-Sidhi Programme: Collected Papers.* Volume 6. Fairfield, IA: Maharishi International University Press, 2011.

Dillbeck, M. C., Vernon A. Barnes, Robert Schneider, Fred Travis, and Kenneth G. Walton, eds. *Scientific Research on Maharishi's Transcendental Meditation and TM-Sidhi Programme: Collected Papers.* Volume 7. Fairfield, IA: Maharishi International University Press, 2013.

Dillbeck, M. and David W. Orme-Johnson. "Physiological Differences between Transcendental Meditation and Rest." *American Psychologist* 42 (1987): 879–81.

Elder, C., Sanford Nidich, Francis Moriarty, and Randi Nidich. "Effect of Transcendental Meditation on Employee Stress, Depression, and Burnout: A Randomized Controlled Study." *Permanente Journal* 18, no. 1 (2014): 19–23.

Eppley, K. R., Allan I. Abrams, and Jonathon Shear. "Differential Effects of Relaxation Techniques on Trait Anxiety: A Meta-analysis." *Journal of Clinical Psychology* 45, no. 6 (1989): 957–74.

Farinelli, L. "Possibilita di applicationi della technologia della conscienza in aspetti di medicina preventiva: Una ricerca pilota." In *Scientific Research on Maharishi's Transcendental Meditation and TM-Sidhi Programme: Collected Papers.* Volume 3. Edited by Roger Chalmers, Geoffrey Clements, Hartmut Schenkluhn, and Michael Weinless, 1830–45. Vlodrop, The Netherlands: Maharishi Vedic University Press, 1990.

Finan, P. H., Alex J. Zautra, and Rebecca Wershba. "The Dynamics of Emotion in Adaptation to Stress." In *The Handbook of Stress Science*, edited by Richard Contrada and Andrew Baum, 209–20. New York: Springer, 2011.

Fries, J. F., C. Everett Koop, Carson E. Beadle, Paul P. Cooper, Mary Jane England, Roger F. Greaves, Jacque J. Sokolov, Daniel Wright, and the Health Project Consortium. "Reducing Health Care Costs by Reducing the Need and Demand for Medical Services." *New England Journal of Medicine* 329 (1993): 321–25.

Fry, P. and Corey Keys, eds. *New Frontiers in Resilient Aging: Well-Being in Late Life.* Cambridge: Cambridge University Press, 2010.

Gaylord, C., David W. Orme-Johnson, and Fred Travis. "The Effects of the Transcendental Meditation Technique and Progressive Muscle Relaxation on EEG Coherence, Stress Reactivity, and Mental Health in Black Adults." *International Journal of Neuroscience* 46 (1989): 77–86.

Grosswald, S. J., William R. Stixrud, Fred Travis, and Mark A. Bateh. "Use of the Transcendental Meditation Technique to Reduce Symptoms of Attention Deficit Hyperactivity Disorder (ADHD) by Reducing Stress and Anxiety: An Exploratory Study." *Current Issues in Education* 10, no. 2 (2008).

Gutman, D. A. and Charles B. Nemeroff. "Stress and Depression." In *The Handbook of Stress Science*, edited by Richard Contrada and Andrew Baum, 345–58. New York: Springer, 2011.

Haaga D. A., Sarina Grosswald, Carolyn Gaylord-King, Maxwell Rainforth, Melissa Tanner, Fred Travis, Sanford Nidich, and Robert H. Schneider. "Effects of the Transcendental Meditation Program on Substance Use among University Students." *Cardiology Research and Practice* (2011). DOI: 10.4061/2011/537101.

Haynes, C. T., J. Russell Hebert, William Reber, and David W. Orme-Johnson. "The Psychophysiology of Advanced Participants in the Transcendental Meditation Program: Correlations of EEG Coherence, Creativity, H-Reflex Recovery, and Experience of Transcendental Consciousness. " In *Scientific Research on the Transcendental Meditation Program: Collected* Papers. Volume 1. Edited by D. W. Orme-Johnson and John T. Farrow, 208–12. Fairfield, IA: Maharishi International University Press, 1977.

Herron, R. E. "Changes in Physician Costs among High-Cost Transcendental Meditation Practitioners Compared with High-Cost Nonpractitioners over 5 Years." *American Journal of Health Promotion* 26, no. 1 (2011): 56–60.

Herron, Robert E. and Kenneth Cavanaugh. "Can the Transcendental Meditation Program Reduce the Medical Expenditures of Older People? A Longitudinal Cost-Reduction Study in Canada." *Journal of Social Behavior and Personality* 17 (2005): 415–42.

Herron, R. E. and Stephen L. Hillis. "The Impact of the Transcendental Meditation Program on Government Payments to Physicians in Quebec: An Update." *American Journal of Health Promotion* 14, no. 5 (2000): 284–91.

Herron, R. E., Stephen L. Hillis, Joseph V. Mandarino, David W. Orme-Johnson, and Kenneth G. Walton. "The Impact of the Transcendental Meditation Program on Government Payments to Physicians in Quebec." *American Journal of Health Promotion* 10, no. 3 (1996): 208–16.

Herron, R. E., Robert H. Schneider, Joseph V. Mandarino, Charles N. Alexander, and Kenneth G. Walton. "Cost-Effective Hypertension Management: Comparison of Drug Therapies with an Alternative Program." *American Journal of Managed Care* 2, no. 4 (1996): 427–37.

Jauch, D. A. and William T. Carpenter Jr. "Reactive Psychosis: I. Does the Pre-DSM-III Concept Define a Third Psychosis?" *Journal of Nervous and Mental Disease* 176, no. 2 (1988): 72–81.

Jayadevappa, R., Jerry C. Johnson, Bernard S. Bloom, Sanford Nidich, Shashank Desai, Sumedha Chhatre, Donna B. Raziano, and Robert Schneider. "Effectiveness of Transcendental Meditation on Functional Capacity and Quality of Life of African Americans with Congestive Heart Failure: A Randomized Control Study." *Ethnicity and Disease* 17, no. 1 (2007): 72–77.

Klemons, I. M. "Changes in Inflammation in Persons Practicing the Transcendental Meditation Technique." In *Scientific Research on the Transcendental Meditation Program: Collected Papers*. Volume 1. Edited by D. W. Orme-Johnson and John T. Farrow, 287–91. Fairfield, IA: Maharishi International University Press, 1977.

Komisar, H. "The Effects of Rising Health Care Costs on Middle-Class Economic Security." In *Insight on the Issues*. Washington, DC: AARP Public Policy Institute, 2013. www.aarp.org/content/dam/aarp/research/public_policy_institute/security/2013/impact-of-rising-healthcare-costs-AARP-ppi-sec.pdf.

Kondwani, K., Robert Schneider, Charles N. Alexander, Carlos Sledge, Frank Staggers, B. Mawiyah Clayborne, and William Sheppard et al. "Left Ventricular Mass Regression with the Transcendental Meditation Technique and a Health Education Program in Hypertensive African Americans." *Journal of Social Behavior and Personality* 17 (2005): 181–200.

Kumpfer, K. L. "Factors and Processes Contributing to Resilience." In *Resilience and Development: Positive Life Adaptations.* Edited by Meyer D. Glantz and Jeannette Johnson, 179–224. New York: Kluwer Academic Publishers, 1999.

Liegey D., Angela. and Jeffrey N. Swanson. "Physical Heath Outcomes of Trauma." In *The Handbook of Stress Science.* Edited by Richard Contrada and Andrew Baum, 373–84. New York: Springer, 2011.

Lovell-Smith, H. D. "Transcendental Meditation and Three Cases of Migraine." *New Zealand Medical Journal* 98 (1985): 443–45.

MacLean C. R., Kenneth G. Walton, Stig R. Wenneberg, Debra K. Levitsky, Joseph P. Mandarino, R. Waziri R, Steven L. Hillis, and Robert H. Schneider. "Effects of the Transcendental Meditation Program on Adaptive Mechanisms: Changes in Hormone Levels and Responses to Stress after 4 Months of Practice." *Psychoneuroendocrinology* 22 (1997): 277–95.

Miller, G., Charles Roehrig, Paul Hughes-Cromwick, and Craig Lake. "Quantifying National Spending on Wellness and Prevention." *Advances in Health Economics and Health Services Research* 19 (2008): 1–24.

Mills, W. W. and John T. Farrow. "The Transcendental Meditation Technique and Acute Experimental Pain." *Psychosomatic Medicine* 43 (1981): 157–64.

Miskiman, D. E. "Long-Term Effects of the Transcendental Meditation Program in the Treatment of Insomnia." In *Scientific Research on the Transcendental Meditation Program: Collected Papers.* Volume 1. Edited by D. W. Orme-Johnson and John T. Farrow, 299–300. Fairfield, IA: Maharishi International University Press, 1977.

Monahan, R. J. "Secondary Prevention of Drug Dependence through the Transcendental Meditation Program in Metropolitan Philadelphia." *International Journal of the Addictions* 12, no. 6 (1977): 729–54.

Nidich, S., Jeremy Z. Fields, Maxwell Rainforth, Rhoda Pomerantz, Cella David, Jean Kristeller, John W. Salerno, and Robert Schneider. "A Randomized Controlled Trial of the Effects of Transcendental Meditation on Quality of Life in Older Breast Cancer Patients." *Integrative Cancer Therapies* 8, no. 3 (2009): 228–34.

Nidich, S. I., Maxwell V. Rainforth, David A. Haaga, John S. Hagelin, John W. Salerno, Fred Travis, and Melissa Tanner et al. "A Randomized Controlled Trial on Effects of the Transcendental Meditation Program on Blood Pressure, Psychological Distress, and Coping in Young Adults." *American Journal of Hypertension* 22, no. 12 (2009): 1326–31.

Norlyk Herriott, Eva and Dennis P. Heaton. "Spiritual Dimensions of Entrepreneurship in Transcendental Meditation and TM-Sidhi Program Practitioners." *Journal of Management, Spirituality, and Religion* 6, no. 3 (2009): 195–208.

Orme-Johnson, D. W. "Autonomic Stability and Transcendental Meditation." *Psychosomatic Medicine* 35 (1973): 341–49.

Orme-Johnson, D. W. "Medical Care Utilization and the Transcendental Meditation Program." *Psychosomatic Medicine* 49 (1987): 493–507.

Orme-Johnson, D. W. and John T. Farrow, eds. *Scientific Research on the Transcendental Meditation Program: Collected Papers.* Volume 1. Fairfield, IA: Maharishi International University Press, 1977.

Orme-Johnson, D. W. and Robert E. Herron. "An Innovative Approach to Reducing Medical Care Utilization and Expenditures." *American Journal of Managed Care* 3, no. 1 (1997): 135–44.

Orme-Johnson, D. W., John Kiehlbauch, Richard Moore, and John Bristol. "Personality and Autonomic Changes in Prisoners Practicing the Transcendental Meditation Technique." In *Scientific Research on the Transcendental Meditation Program: Collected Papers*. Volume 1. Edited by D. W. Orme-Johnson and John T. Farrow, 556–61. Fairfield, IA: Maharishi International University Press, 1977.

Orme-Johnson, D. W., Robert H. Schneider, Young D. Son, Sanford Nidich, and Zang-Hee Cho. "Neuroimaging of Meditation's Effect on Brain Reactivity to Pain." *NeuroReport* 17, no. 12 (2006): 1359–63.

Ottoson, J. "Transcendental Meditation." Stockholm, Sweden: Socialstrytelsen, 1977.

Patterson, C. and Larry W. Chambers. "Preventive Health Care." *Lancet* 345 (1995): 1611–15.

Paul-Labrador, M., Donna Polk, James H. Dwyer, Ivan Velasquez, Sanford Nidich, Maxwell Rainforth, Robert Schneider, and Noel Bairey Merz. "Effects of Randomized Controlled Trial of Transcendental Meditation on Components of the Metabolic Syndrome in Subjects with Coronary Heart Disease." *Archives of Internal Medicine* 166 (2006): 1218–24.

Pelletier, K. R. "Influence of Transcendental Meditation upon Autokinetic Perception." *Perceptual and Motor Skills* 39 (1974): 1031–34

Pelletier, K. R. and Robert Lutz. "Healthy People—Healthy Business: A Critical Review of Stress Management Programs in the Workplace." *American Journal of Health Promotion* 2, no. 3 (1988): 5–12.

Rainforth, M., Charles N. Alexander, and Kenneth L. Cavanaugh. "The Transcendental Meditation Program and Criminal Recidivism in Folsom State Prisoners: A 15-Year Follow-up Study." *Journal of Offender Rehabilitation* 36 (2003): 181–204.

Rainforth, M. V., Robert H. Schneider, Sanford I. Nidich, Carolyn Gaylord-King, John W. Salerno, and James W. Anderson. "Stress Reduction Programs in Patients with Elevated Blood Pressure: A Systematic Review and Meta-analysis." *Current Hypertension Reports* 9, no. 6 (2007): 520–28.

Reschovsky, J. D., Jack Hadley, Cynthia B. Saiontz-Martinez, and Ellyn R. Boukus. "Following the Money: Factors Associated with the Cost of Treating High-Cost Medicare Beneficiaries." *Health Services Research* 46, no. 4 (2011): 997–1021.

Resnick, B., Lisa P. Gwyther, and Karen A. Roberto, eds. *Resilience in Aging: Concepts, Research, and Outcomes*. New York: Springer, 2011.

Sawhney, S. "Effects of the TM Technique on Anxiety, Emotional Intelligence, and Trust: Implications for Supply Chain Management." Maharishi University of Management, 2012.

Schenkluhn, H. and Matthias Geisler. "A Longitudinal Study of the Influence of the Transcendental Meditation Program on Drug Abuse." In *Scientific Research on the Transcendental Meditation Program: Collected Papers*. Volume 1. Edited by D. W. Orme-Johnson and John T. Farrow, 544–55. Fairfield, IA: Maharishi International University Press, 1977.

Schneider, R., Charles N Alexander, Frank Staggers, David W. Orme-Johnson, Maxwell Rainforth, John W. Salerno, and William Sheppard et al. "A Randomized Controlled Trial of Stress Reduction in African Americans Treated for Hypertension During One Year." *American Journal of Hypertension* 18 (2005): 88–98.

Schneider, R. H., Charles N. Alexander, Frank Staggers, Maxwell V. Rainforth, John W. Salerno, Arthur Hartz, Stephen Arndt, Vernon A. Barnes, and Sanford I. Nidich. "Long-Term Effects of Stress Reduction on Mortality in Persons ≥ 55 Years of Age with Systemic Hypertension." *American Journal of Cardiology* 95 (2005): 1060–64.

Schneider, R. H., Clarence E. Grim, Maxwell V. Rainforth, Theodore Kotchen, Sanford I. Nidich, Carolyn Gaylord-King, John W. Salerno, Jane Morley Kotchen, and Charles N. Alexander. "Stress Reduction in the Secondary Prevention of Cardiovascular Disease: Randomized Controlled Trial of Transcendental Meditation and Health Education in Blacks." *Circulation: Cardiovascular Quality and Outcomes* 2, no. 5 (2012): 1–9.

Schneider, R., Frank Staggers, Charles N. Alexander, William Sheppard, Maxwell V. Rainforth, Kofi Kondwani, Sandra Smith, and Carolyn Gaylord-King. "A Randomized Controlled Trial of Stress Reduction for Hypertension in Older African Americans." *Hypertension* 26, no. 5 (1995): 820–27.

Shecter, H. "The Transcendental Meditation Program in the Classroom: A Psychological Evaluation." In *Scientific Research on the Transcendental Meditation Program: Collected Papers*. Volume 1. Edited by D. W. Orme-Johnson and John T. Farrow, 403–9. Fairfield, IA: Maharishi International University Press, 1977.

Sheppard, W., Frank Staggers, and Lucille John. "The Effects of a Stress Management Program in a High Security Government Agency." *Anxiety, Stress, and Coping* 10 (1997): 341–50.

Starfield, B. "Is U.S. Health Really the Best in the World?" *JAMA* 284, no. 4 (2000): 483–85.

Tanner, M. A., Fred Travis, Carolyn Gaylord-King, David A. Haaga, Sarina Grosswald, and Robert H. Schneider. "The Effects of the Transcendental Meditation Program on Mindfulness." *Journal of Clinical Psychology* 65 (2009): 574–89.

Thorpe, K. E. and David H. Howard. "The Rise in Spending among Medicare Beneficiaries: The Role of Chronic Disease Prevalence and Changes in Treatment Intensity." *Health Affairs* 25, no. 5 (2006): 378–88.

Throll, D. A. "The Effects of the Transcendental Meditation Technique upon Adolescent Personality." In *Scientific Research on Maharishi's Transcendental Meditation and TM-Sidhi Programme: Collected Papers*. Volume 2. Edited by Roger Chalmers, Geoffrey Clements, Hartmut Schenkluhn, and Michael Weinless, 1087–95. Vlodrop, The Netherlands: Maharishi Vedic University Press, 1990.

Tjoa, A. "Meditation, Neuroticism and Intelligence: A Follow-up." *Gedrag: Tijdschrift voor Psychologie* 3, no. 3 (1975): 167–82.

Toomey, M. "The Effects of the Transcendental Meditation Program on Carotid Atherosclerosis and Cardiovascular Disease Risk Factors in Native Hawaiians." Dissertation, Maharishi University of Management, 2007.

Travis, F. "Creative Thinking and the Transcendental Meditation Technique." *Journal of Creative Behavior* 13, no. 3 (1979): 169–180.

Travis, F. "Beyond Waking, Dreaming and Sleeping: Perspectives from Research on Meditation Experiences." In *States of Consciousness: Experimental Insights into Meditation, Waking, Sleep and Dreams States of Consciousness*. Edited by Dean Cvetkovic and Irena Cosic, 223–34. New York: Springer, 2011.

Travis, F., David A. Haaga, John S. Hagelin, Melissa Tanner, Sanford Nidich, and Gaylord-King Carolyn. "Effects of Transcendental Meditation Practice on Brain Functioning and Stress Reactivity in College Students." *International Journal of Psychophysiology* 71, no. 2 (2009): 170–76.

Travis, F., David A. Haaga, John S. Hagelin, Melissa Tanner, Alarik Arenander, Sanford Nidich, Carolyn Gaylord-King, Sarina Grosswald, Maxwell Rainforth, and Robert H. Schneider. "A Self-Referential Default Brain State: Patterns of Coherence, Power, and Eloreta Sources during Eyes-Closed Rest and Transcendental Meditation Practice." *Cognitive Processing* 11, no. 1 (2010): 21–30.

U.S. Centers for Disease Control. "Heart Disease and Stroke Prevention: Addressing the Nation's Leading Killers." 2011.

U.S. Department of Labor, Bureau of Labor Statistics. "Economic Report of the President. Table B–60: Consumer Price Indexes for Major Expenditure Classes, 1969–2012." U.S. Government Printing Office, www.gpo.gov/fdsys/pkg/ERP -2013/pdf/ERP-2013-table60.pdf.

U.S. National Institute of Aging. "Global Health and Aging." Bethesda, MD: National Institutes of Health, 2011. www.nia.nih.gov/research/publication/ global-health-and-aging/humanitys-aging.

Van den Berg, W. P. and Bert Mulder. "Psychological Research on the Effects of the Transcendental Meditation Technique on a Number of Personality Variables." *Gedrag: Tijdschrift voor Psychologie* 4 (1976): 206–18.

Wallace, R. K., D. W. Orme-Johnson, and Michael C. Dillbeck, eds. *Scientific Research on Maharishi's Transcendental Meditation and TM-Sidhi Programme: Collected Papers.* Volume 5. Fairfield, IA: Maharishi International University Press, 1991.

Wallace, R. K., Joel Silver, Paul J. Mills, Michael C. Dillbeck, and Dale E. Wagoner. "Systolic Blood Pressure and Long-Term Practice of the Transcendental Meditation and TM-Sidhi Program: Effects of TM on Systolic Blood Pressure." *Psychosomatic Medicine* 45, no. 1 (1983): 41–46.

Wenneberg, S. R., Robert H. Schneider, Kenneth G. Walton, Christopher R. Maclean, Debra K. Levitsky, John W. Salerno, R. Keith Wallace, Joseph V. Mandarino, Maxwell V. Rainforth, and R. Waziri. "A Controlled Study of the Effects of the Transcendental Meditation Program on Cardiovascular Reactivity and Ambulatory Blood Pressure." *International Journal of Neuroscience* 89 (1997): 15–28.

Williams, P. G., Timothy W. Smith, Heather E. Gunn, and Bert N. Uchino. "Personality and Stress: Individual Differences in Exposure, Reactivity, Recovery, and Restoration." In *The Handbook of Stress Science.* Edited by Richard Contrada and Andrew Baum, 231–46. New York: Springer, 2011.

Wilson, A. F., Ronald W. Honsberger, John T. Chiu, and Harold S. Novey. "Transcendental Meditation and Asthma." *Respiration* 32 (1975): 74–80.

Zamarra, J. W., Robert H. Schneider, Italo Besseghini, Donald K. Robinson, and John W. Salerno. "Usefulness of the Transcendental Meditation Program in the Treatment of Patients with Coronary Artery Disease." *American Journal of Cardiology* 77, no. 10 (1996): 867–70.

ELEVEN

Addressing Societal Problems through Transcendental Meditation: Aging, Prison Rehabilitation, and Collective Health

David W. Orme-Johnson, Ph.D., and
David F. O'Connell, Ph.D., M.S., CFC, DABPS

In this chapter, the scope of the research expands beyond individual health concerns. We consider the wider impact of Transcendental Meditation (TM®) practice on the health of society. With the increasing number of seniors requiring medical and supportive care, the effects of TM on the aging process are presented. Another area of great concern, the ever-expanding problem of crime and criminal recidivism, is then examined from the perspective of TM's effects in the prison environment. The chapter concludes with a presentation on the effects of the practice of TM as mentioned by a large groups of researchers and practitioners on the collective consciousness and health of a society—a phenomenon known as the Maharishi Effect, which has immense potential to raise the quality of life worldwide.

TM RESEARCH ON AGING AND THE ELDERLY

The American Academy of Anti-Aging Medicine has indicated that 90 percent of adult illnesses are due to the degenerative process of aging. Research on the impact of TM on aging has been conducted over the past four decades. In the following section, we address the issue of why TM might be expected to improve the aging process, and how it might improve well-being among the elderly.

Mechanics of How TM Works

Basic research indicates that TM works in two complementary ways: (1) by reducing stress, and (2) by increasing orderliness of brain functioning.

MECHANISM 1: STRESS REDUCTION

In 1929, physiologist Walter Bradford Cannon described the fight or flight response, a pattern of physiological reactions that occur when an organism is faced with a life-challenging situation.[1] The fight or flight response is a hyperarousal state which includes rapid increases in heart rate, cardiac output, respiratory rate, blood pressure, skin conductance, and plasma lactate and cortisol, among other changes. This response helps the individual survive a dangerous emergency by rapidly mobilizing the body's energy reserves and deploying them to the brain and muscles for flight or fight, whichever seems more appropriate for the given situation. The fight or flight response is a highly adaptive mechanism that has been fine-tuned over millions of years of evolution. However, problems arise with chronic stressors, such as the psychosocial stress of being a minority person in a racist society.[2] Repeated elicitation of the fight or flight response over a long period of time by chronic stressors depletes the body's resources, wearing down its tissues and systems. Chronic stressors may cause long-lasting elevations of the major stress hormone cortisol, which weakens the body's ability to muster a robust cortisol response when emergency challenges do arise.[3] Chronically elevated cortisol levels may cause neuronal death, may damage the brain,[4] may cause hypertension,[5] may contribute to drug use and addictions,[6] and may age the body.[3,7]

In 1970, R. K. Wallace, in his doctoral dissertation at the University of California, Los Angeles, discovered that the physiological effects of TM are just the opposite of the fight or flight response, a pattern he called a "wakeful hypometabolic physiologic state."[8-11] A subsequent meta-analysis of thirty-two physiological studies found that starting from a resting baseline, TM decreases respiratory rates and plasma lactate and elevates basal skin resistance more than ordinary rest in non-meditating controls.[12] This meta-analysis also found that stress indicators (spontaneous skin resistance responses, heart rate, respiratory rate, and plasma lactate) were lower when people who practice TM were not meditating than in non-meditating control subjects. Evidence also suggests that cortisol levels decrease during TM and remain lower throughout the day and night.[5] This suggests that regular reduction of stress markers during meditation results in lowering their levels throughout the day. Thus TM reduces physiological stress parameters during the practice and lowers them throughout the day (see table 11.1).

Thus the first mechanism by which TM could be understood to benefit health is that TM reduces the effects of both acute and chronic stress, and chronic stress is a risk factor for many, if not all, diseases. When such a potent stress-reducing practice is added to one's daily routine, it could be expected to neutralize elevated levels of cortisol and other stress-related imbalances caused by frustration, fear, and anger and prevent their ac-

Table 11.1.   Comparison of the Effects of the Fight or Flight Response and TM

Fight or Flight: Hyperarousal Stress Response	*TM: Wakeful Hypometabolic State*
Increased metabolic rate	Decreased metabolic rate
Faster breathing	Slower Breathing
Faster heart rate	Slower heart rate
Increased cardiac output	Decreased cardiac output
Increased blood pressure	Decreased blood pressure
Increased muscle tension	Decreased muscle tension
Sweaty palms	Dry palms
Increased cortisol	Decreased cortisol

cumulation to deleterious levels that damage the body, thus healing the body and preventing disease.[2,5,6,13]

MECHANISM 2: INCREASED ORDERLINESS OF BRAIN FUNCTIONING

The "wakeful" part of Wallace's "wakeful hypometabolic physiologic state" refers to his observation that TM increases alpha1 EEG (8 to 10 Hz) readings in the frontal executive areas of the cerebral cortex, which then spread throughout the brain.[9–11] Subsequent research has found that this EEG signature is highly coherent,[14,15] indicating that the various areas of the brain are working together in concert in a holistic way. High coherence is seen especially during the deepest period of meditation, a period of pure consciousness and respiratory suspension.[16–20] In time, regular experience of the high coherence state during TM habituates the system to maintain higher EEG coherence outside the practice and during other activities, such as during a computer task.[21,22] A major review of the effects of different meditation techniques found over a dozen studies consistently reporting that TM increases alpha EEG coherence with no evidence that mindfulness or other techniques do.[23]

The functional significance of increased alpha EEG coherence is that its rhythm orchestrates the separate activities of different areas of the cerebral cortex to work together in concert, much as the rhythm of the conductor's baton sets the timing that coordinates the diverse instruments in an orchestra to bring forth harmony and music from chaos.[24–28] Research has shown that EEG alpha coherence during TM is correlated with creativity,[29] concept learning,[30] moral reasoning,[21,31] and self-esteem[21] and is inversely correlated with anxiety and neuroticism.[21]

Such increases in the orderliness of brain functioning during and outside TM could be expected to benefit health by making a person more aware of advances in preventative medicine, more compliant with healthful recommendations of diet, exercise, and non-smoking, and more likely to comply with prescriptions and otherwise take responsibility for their health. It is also likely that increased orderliness of brain function-ing would facilitate the healing process by increasing the communication among bodily systems during the extra deep rest provided by TM.

Evidence That TM Improves the Aging Process

Aging is the "footprint of the elephant," that is, an elephant's foot-print is so big that all the other animals' footprints can fit into it,[32-36] and in the same way, aging is the holistic outcome of life that subsumes all other outcomes. It is essentially the bottom line. Successful aging is the ultimate gauge that one has effectively managed stress over one's lifes-pan. All of the more than six hundred studies on TM provide evidence that TM improves the aging process. We will consider two categories of research on TM and aging: the effects of TM on markers of biologi-cal age, and direct evidence that it reduces mortality and improves the quality of life in old age.

BIOLOGICAL AGE

Early studies focused on biological markers for aging, such as near-point vision, blood pressure, and vital capacity.[37] This research demon-strated that TM practitioners, with a mean age of 50, who had practiced TM for 5 years, had biological ages 12 years younger than non-meditating controls. Subsequent research indicates that TM reduces a whole host of age-related variables.

BLOOD PRESSURE

Blood pressure (BP) tends to rise with age and is a risk factor for cardio-vascular disease. Forty-five percent of coronary heart disease deaths and 51 percent of stroke deaths are attributable to high systolic blood pressure (SBP).[38] TM has been shown to lower BP levels and reduce cardiovascular risk in adults and adolescents.[13] Randomized clinical trials have found that TM lowers BP in both normotensive[39] and hypertensive patients,[40,41] and it may reduce use of BP medication.[40]

A risk-subgroup analysis of older hypertensive African Americans (55 years and older, mean age 66.6 ± 7.3 years) found that TM reduced SBP and diastolic blood pressure (DBP) for both sexes and for subjects high or low on several measures of hypertension risk—psychosocial stress, obesity, alcohol use, physical inactivity, and dietary sodium/potassium ratio—indicating that the practice was effective for all subgroups.[42]

A meta-analysis of nine randomized controlled trials found that TM lowered SBP/DBP on average by 4.7/3.2 mmHg compared with control groups.[43] Subjects in the meta-analysis ranged in age from adolescents (15–18 years) to seniors (mean age 81.3 ±9.8 years), and TM was effective for all age groups. Subjects included normotensive, pre-hypertensive, and hypertensive individuals. Subgroup analyses of four hypertensive groups and three high-quality studies showed similar reductions.

Another meta-analysis of the effects of stress-reduction programs on hypertension patients evaluated high-quality studies that used active controls, adequate baseline measurement, and blinded BP assessment.[44] Meta-analysis was used to calculate BP changes. The results for BP decreases associated with biofeedback, relaxation-assisted biofeedback, progressive muscle relaxation, and stress-management training were not statistically significant. However, TM significantly lowered BP by 5.0/2.8 mmHg. BP reductions of this magnitude are suggested to result in significant decreases in cardiovascular disease risk.[45]

In 2013, the American Heart Association issued a scientific statement, based on their review of the evidence, which concluded that TM and *only* TM could be recommended to doctors as a meditative means to reduce BP.

> TM may be considered in clinical practice to lower BP. Because of many negative studies or mixed results and a paucity of available trials, all other meditation techniques (including MBSR [mindfulness-based stress reduction]) received a "Class III, no benefit, Level of Evidence C" recommendation. Thus, other meditation techniques are not recommended in clinical practice to lower BP at this time.[46]

METABOLIC SYNDROME AND INSULIN RESISTANCE

Metabolic syndrome in the elderly is a proposed risk factor for cardiovascular morbidity and mortality, especially stroke and coronary heart disease, as well as for diabetes mellitus type.[47] A randomized clinical trial studied the effects of sixteen weeks of TM practice on metabolic syndrome in 103 subjects, approximately 66 years old, and with stable coronary heart disease.[48] At sixteen weeks post-test, TM subjects showed decreased insulin resistance as measured by the homeostasis model assessment, an index of glucose regulation calculated from fasting plasma glucose and insulin levels. SBP and mean arterial pressure were lower and heart rate variability increased in the TM group, indicating an improvement in cardiac autonomic nervous system tone.

MYOCARDIAL ISCHEMIA

The effects of TM on the cardiac response to a standard exercise tolerance protocol were studied in 55-year-old men with documented coronary artery disease and symptoms of angina. After a mean of 7.6 months of TM practice, the TM group showed a significant reduction in rate pressure product (the product of heart rate and BP) compared with wait-list control subjects. TM subjects also increased in the maximum workload they could tolerate before angina symptoms occurred and showed a delayed appearance of electrocardiographic abnormalities during exercise (delayed onset of ST segment depression).[49]

CAROTID ATHEROSCLEROSIS

TM also may reverse arterial blockage in older people. A randomized controlled trial of 60 African American subjects, mean age 55 years, compared the effects of TM with a heart disease education-control group on carotid intima-media thickness, a validated surrogate measure for coronary and cerebral atherosclerosis.[50] The results indicated a statistically significant decrease in carotid intima-media thickness in the TM group by 0.098 mm (95 percent confidence interval [CI] [-0.198, 0.003 mm]) compared with an increase of 0.054 mm (95 percent CI [-0.05, 0.158 mm]) in the control group (p = .038 for difference between groups), suggesting that TM may reduce carotid atherosclerosis in hypertensive African Americans. The literature indicates that changes of this magnitude predict a reduction in heart attacks by 11 percent[51] and stroke by 7.7 percent to 15 percent.[52]

HEART FAILURE

A six-month randomized pilot trial of older African American patients (55 years or older) recently hospitalized for chronic heart failure found that the TM group significantly improved in functional capacity on a six-minute walk test compared with control subjects who received only health education. TM subjects also had reduced depression and only half the hospitalizations as health-education controls.[53]

DEHYDROEPIANDROSTERONE SULFATE

The practice of TM has also been found to lead to elevated levels of serum dehydroepiandrosterone sulfate (DHEAS), a hormone that tends to decrease with age and has been implicated in maintaining immune system integrity and keeping the body strong and vital.[54]

P300

P300 latency is an endogenous potential, which reflects processes involved in stimulus evaluation and categorization. It can be used as a measure of the effectiveness of treatments to enhance cognitive functioning and treat cognitive impairment. A study found less age-related decline in P300 latency in elderly TM practitioners relative to controls.[55]

REVERSAL OF AGING FOR OTHER AGE-RELATED PARAMETERS

The above results show that TM helps suppress the detrimental effects of aging. This has been found for a wide range of other measures as well. Reflex latency, susceptibility to stress, and insomnia, which all increase with age, are decreased by TM. Cardiovascular efficiency, vital capacity, cerebral blood flow, EEG alpha power, neuromuscular coordination, and periodontal health, which all decrease with age, are increased by TM. TM slows age-related cognitive declines as well; it improves fluid intelligence (the capacity to think logically and solve problems in novel situations), creativity, learning ability, memory, cognitive flexibility, self-evaluation of health, and well-being, which all decline with age.[56]

MEDICAL CARE UTILIZATION

Several studies have also illustrated the global effects of TM on health in that it reduces hospitalization rates in all disease categories (figure 11.1).[57,58] These studies also found that TM reduced both hospitalization and outpatient doctor visits across all age categories. Significantly, the greatest proportional reductions were for people over forty (figure 11.2). This evidence from large field studies supports the view that the cumulative effects of daily stress reduction through TM prevents the

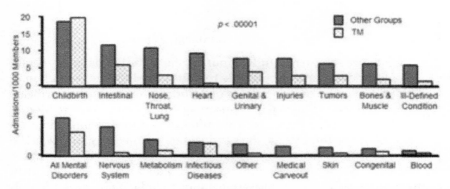

Figure 11.1.   A five-year study of health insurance statistics of approximately 2,000 TM practitioners showing hospitalization rates in all disease categories

Note: This five-year study found that the TM group had lower hospitalization rates in all disease categories compared to normative data on other groups. Only rates of normal childbirth were comparable for TM and other groups. This illustrates the holistic effects of regular stress-reduction through TM practice on health and implies that TM may slow the aging process.

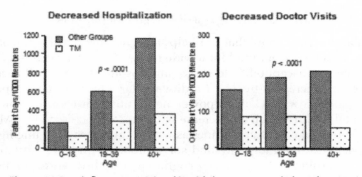

Figure 11.2.   A five-year study of health insurance statistics of approximately 2,000 TM practitioners showing hospitalization rates in all age categories

Note: The same study as shown in Figure 11.1 also found that TM practice reduced hospitalization and doctor visits across all age categories, with the largest reductions for meditators over 40. Hospitalization increased with age in both groups, but it increased much more slowly in the TM group, 69% less for people over 40. Similarly, doctor visits also increased with age for other groups but declined slightly for the TM group. For subjects over 40, the rate of doctor visits was 74% less for TM subjects compared to other groups. These results suggest that TM practice slows the aging process.

accumulation of imbalances caused by stress, thus reducing sickness rates and slowing the aging process.

The following studies directly show that TM decreases mortality and improves the quality of life.

DECREASED MORTALITY IN INSTITUTIONALIZED ELDERLY

A randomized long-term study of nursing home residents by psychologist Charles Alexander highlights the benefits of TM for the institutionalized elderly.[39] A total of 73 residents of 8 nursing homes in the northeast region of the United States with a mean age of 81 years were randomly assigned to one of three groups: TM, mindfulness meditation, and a relaxation group. At three years, the survival rate for the TM group was 100 percent versus 87 percent for the mindfulness group and 75 percent for the relaxation group. Overall, the TM group did significantly better than controls on measures of cognitive flexibility, systolic blood pressure, ratings of behavioral flexibility, and treatment efficacy. No one necessarily wants to live longer if they are going to be sick and unhappy during life extension. The study found that in addition to the objective measures, TM made the elders "feel less old."

DECREASED MORTALITY IN OLDER HYPERTENSION PATIENTS

More recent randomized controlled trials confirm the finding of Alexander et al.[39] that TM lowers mortality rates for older meditators.[40] This study reported that the stress-reducing effects of TM resulted in lowered mortality rates for individuals over 55 years of age suffering from systemic hypertension. Reductions in all-cause mortality in the elderly have been shown to be sustained in two long-term studies of 8 and 15 years respectively.[59,60]

DECREASED MORTALITY IN OLDER HEART DISEASE PATIENTS

A controlled 10-year trial of 201 black men and women (mean age approximately 59 years) with coronary heart disease who were randomized to TM or a health education program found that TM produced a 48 percent risk reduction in a composite of all-cause mortality, heart attacks, or stroke. The TM group also showed a 24 percent risk reduction in the secondary end-point composite composed of cardiovascular mortality, revascularizations, and cardiovascular hospitalizations, BP, psychosocial stress factors, and lifestyle behaviors.[61] The health education group controlled for the amount of attention patients received, their expectation of benefits, and their program structure, which, like that of many of the other studies, controlled for placebo effects.

Summary of the Effects of TM on Aging

We have seen that the physiological effects of TM are in the opposite direction of the effects of stress, that the practice cultivates lower levels of stress throughout the day, and that it has immediate and long-term effects on increasing alpha1 EEG coherence, which coordinates the diverse activities of the brain for higher levels of perception, cognition, and motor behavior. We have also seen that its effects help suppress a large number of age-related parameters, such as high BP, various categories of cardiovascular disease, and feeling old. And finally, we have observed direct evidence from well-controlled studies that TM actually decreases mortality rates. These results provide strong, cross-validating evidence that TM is beneficial for slowing the aging process and actually lengthening the lifespan with a higher quality of life.

With the baby boomers' health burden upon us, the medical management of this concern looms large and demands proactive measures. The inclusion of TM in the prevention and treatment of problems associated with aging appears to be a vital approach to addressing these health problems, and further research on TM and aging appears quite promising and worthwhile.

RESEARCH ON TM WITH PRISON INMATES, CORRECTIONS, AND CRIMINAL RECIDIVISM

The rate of crimes committed and the way a society deals with criminal behavior are important indicators of the overall health of a society. Research indicates that prison populations are soaring, with 1 out of 100 Americans behind bars, and, unfortunately, the effectiveness of rehabilitation programs for prison inmates and parolees is low. As of 2008, 1 in every 31 Americans has been involved in the criminal justice system. Criminal recidivism remains high despite increases in funds to combat it and an expansion in prison treatment programs.[62]

Reversing the Neuroendocrine Abnormalities Associated with Crime and Aggression

Just as TM reverses physiological and neuroendocrine factors associated with aging, it also reverses imbalances associated with crime. The reason is that the abnormalities caused by chronic stress that accelerate aging are the same or highly similar to the ones that predispose the individual to crime. Walton and Levitsky found that TM resulted in significant normalization of abnormal neuroendocrine functioning associated with aggression and crime. For example, whereas crime is associated with lower levels of serotonin and high levels of cortisol, the evidence indicates that TM increases serotonin and lowers cortisol.[63] Normalization of stress-related physiological abnormalities associated with crime is the basis of the psychological and behavioral improvements in criminal behavior produced by TM practice, as documented below.

Psychological Improvements

Over thirty studies have been conducted on the impact of TM on psychological and behavioral changes in prison inmates.[64,65] A narrative and quantitative review of 1,500 inmates in eight correctional institutions showed that TM produced marked improvements in health, psychological development, and behavior.[65]

One of the best studies was by Charles Alexander on maximum-security inmates, reported in his doctoral dissertation at Harvard.[64–66] These cross-sectional and longitudinal studies revealed that TM practitioners improved significantly on several measures of mental health and psychological development compared to groups in other rehabilitation programs. Alexander predicted that the Loevinger test of ego development[67] "may provide outer behavioral 'signs' of internal shifts in self-organization that may result from association of the awareness of the knower (the ego) with progressively deeper levels of the mind. Ego development typically freezes by around 18–20 years of age or by the end of formal education."[68] Using Loevinger's test, Alexander found that the TM inmates grew more in cognitive complexity, character, and social development in one year than college students over a four-year period. By contrast, there was no significant improvement in subjects participating in four other prison programs (drug rehabilitation, counseling, a Muslim group, a Christian group). The TM subjects progressed from the "conformist" stage (corresponding to a dominance of concrete thinking) to the "self-aware" stage (corresponding to a dominance of the onset of reflective functioning of the intellect). In a second one-year longitudinal study, inmates who were already meditating and who were initially at the "self-aware" stage moved to the "conscientious" stage, corresponding to a dominance of mature form of abstract reflection, the highest level typically obtained in adult samples.[69] Ego development is a holistic measure of overall personality structure, and it indicated that TM develops the person away from a dependent, exploitive psychological orientation commonly found with criminals to one of a more responsible, self-monitoring, self-respecting orientation, such as is found in law-abiding citizens.[69,70] Other significant changes in the TM group compared to controls included decreases in aggression, anxiety, depression, and schizophrenic symptoms.

Other studies with inmates practicing TM showed decreased resentment, neuroticism, negativism, suspicion, verbal hostility, anger, and paranoid anxiety.[71–73] In addition, TM has been shown to have equally positive effects on the psychological functioning and behavior of juvenile offenders.

Behavioral Improvements

Rehabilitation research has also documented objective behavioral changes in inmates practicing the TM technique. These include fewer sleep disturbances, reduced substance abuse, and perhaps most importantly, decreased rule infractions and physical violence in the prison.[71–73]

Decreased Recidivism: Fewer Returns to Prison

The bottom line on whether a prison rehabilitation program works or not is recidivism, or the rate at which inmates commit new crimes and are re-incarcerated after they have been released into society. A 52-month follow-up of the Alexander Harvard study found that the group of those who learned TM while in prison had 33 percent fewer repeat offenders than the control groups.[66]

Rainforth and colleagues conducted a 15-year follow-up study of inmates who learned TM while in prison. They found the impact of TM on criminal recidivism was long lasting, a reduction of 43 percent in the TM group compared to matched controls over the 15-year period.[74]

TM in a National Prison System

Perhaps the most dramatic demonstration of the impact of TM on a criminal justice system was reported by Anklesaria and King.[75] These researchers found that TM essentially changed the entire penitentiary system in the African country of Senegal. TM was widely adopted as a rehabilitation program in 31 of the 34 prisons in the country, with 11,000 prisoners learning TM (only three remotely located prisons were not included in the project). Overall, reports on inmates included reductions in insomnia, negativity, escape attempts, aggression, fights, and murders. On the positive side, there was a marked increase in general positive affect, self-confidence, and pro-social behavior. Objective measures showed an 81 percent reduction in rule infractions and a 43 percent reduction in medical utilization at three months. Benefits for prison staff and guards included reduced absenteeism, less paranoid anxiety, fewer disciplinary infractions, and increased self-confidence, self-control, conscientiousness, health, esprit de corps, and respect for superior officers.

Senegal occasionally grants a presidential amnesty during which all prisoners in the country are released. Usually 90 percent of the inmates return to prison within one month after the amnesty. However, for the prisoners who learned TM, the number of those who returned to prison after an amnesty was less than 10 percent after six months.

Judges Sentencing Offenders to TM

In a pioneering, community-based corrections program in St. Louis, Missouri, eight judges sentenced over one hundred probationers (with offenses ranging from drunk driving to manslaughter) to a TM program with remarkable success, including lower recidivism rates and increased pro-social behaviors.[76]

Judge David Mason, who spearheaded the project, explains TM this way:

It's a simple technique that involves two 20-minute periods a day wherein a person gains a very deep level of rest. During this process of deep rest, the physiology becomes normalized, thinking becomes clearer, self-esteem grows, enlightenment of self and others grows, so that by the time people have gone through the process, their ability to deal with the world around them, to deal with the stresses of the world around them, to find some personal peace within, and to express peace without, is greatly enhanced.

In discussion of the project, it's noted that in the project's early stages,

some community groups raised questions as to its validity. They were concerned that the project might be imposing a religious practice (other than theirs) upon probationers. However, after investigating the situation, Mason concluded that their concerns arose from a lack of knowledge about the nature and mechanics of the TM technique. His investigation confirmed what the teachers of the technique had said, namely, that the practice was a purely mechanical one, based on the natural tendency of the mind to seek a state of greatest happiness. Mason could see that no specific belief system or lifestyle was required.[76]

The participants were mostly poor, illiterate substance abusers who lived in impoverished areas of St. Louis. They learned the standard TM technique (two hours a day over four consecutive days) and then were given a 13-week follow-up program during which they attended one-and-a-half hour classes twice a week in which they received knowledge about the nature of TM, a simple breathing technique, and stretching exercises (yoga asanas). The result was unprecedented participation in the program. Participants commonly reported on the ease and calmness they derived from the program. A typical comment was "I've had excellent experiences right from the start. I was amazed by the effortlessness of the practice. After my very first meditation, I kept saying, 'I didn't do anything,'—and yet I had experienced all the symptoms of correct meditation: deep physical and mental relaxation and greater calmness after meditation. It seemed as though my body was just weightless."[76]

Probationers consistently reported improvements in diverse areas of their lives, including work, home, and relationships with other people, as well as decreased substance abuse. The project has gained the support of judges at all levels of the state judiciary, as well as corrections officials, counsel appearing before the court, legislators, the project participants, and their families.

An Enlightened View

In reflecting on his experience with TM for criminal rehabilitation and its importance as an effective approach to change criminal behavior, Arthur John Anderson, former director of the Criminal Justice Division in Little Rock, Arkansas, commented,

The thrust of our criminal justice system has been obvious: to impose orderliness from the outside inward through the codification and enforcement of laws and the restructuring of the environment . . . But orderliness does not begin from the outside. The secret of orderliness is that it is already there, within each individual . . . to secure orderly thinking, we must go to the source of thought, which is consciousness. Depending on its quality, consciousness is the ultimate source of crime or of suffering or of harmony and happiness. The practice of TM leads to contact with this source from which all change, criminal or otherwise, emanates.[77]

The robust body of research on the positive impact of TM on criminal behavior shows that TM has been one of the most effective, and grossly underutilized, rehabilitation programs to date for inmates and parolees. Despite this widely published finding and the large body of research documenting its effectiveness, TM has never been adopted in the U.S. prison system or criminal justice system.

INCREASED COHERENCE IN COLLECTIVE CONSCIOUSNESS: THE MAHARISHI EFFECT

A Field-Theoretic Perspective of Society

This theory proposes that individuals in society directly interact at a distance via a common underlying field of collective consciousness, in addition to their usual interactions on the levels of the senses and extensions of the senses through phones, radio, TV, the Internet, etc. This idea has appeared in many forms throughout history as the perennial philosophy—a set of ideas found in virtually all traditions throughout history. It holds that there is a transcendental field of consciousness common to everyone and everything at the basis of natural law, that humans can directly experience this universal consciousness in the transcendental level of their own minds, and that this experience is the means to create a more ideal individual and society.[78-80] In some traditions, the transcendental field is considered in religious terms. In other traditions, both in the East and the West, it is conceptualized without a God concept, as the Being, the Self, the Tao, or the Atman.

In twentieth-century social science, the idea was perceived under Jung's "collective unconscious," a collective memory shared by all the individuals of a species that organizes individual personal experiences in a similar way according to archetypal patterns.[81,82] E. Durkheim, one of the founders of the discipline of sociology, wrote of a "collective consciousness," the mind of society that is created when the consciousness of individuals is grouped and combined instead of remaining isolated.[83] G. Fechner, best known for developing methods of measuring sensory thresholds, conceived of a "general consciousness" which is a transcendental continuum of consciousness that connects all individual minds at their basis.[84] However, the idea has not entered into mainstream science because there has not been a way to test it. Without a means to operationally define basic concepts that can be measured and experimentally manipulated, the theories stall in the doldrums of philosophical speculation.

The most recent elaboration of the theory is by Maharishi Mahesh Yogi, who provided practical technologies for increasing coherence in collective consciousness and predicted, measurable effects on objective social indicators like rates of sickness, crime, violent deaths, and terrorism. For the first time in history, the availability of a technology to influence collective consciousness has brought the field-theoretic perceptive of society into mainstream science, allowing sociological experiments on the unprecedented scales of cities, states, nations, and the whole world. Collectively, these studies have demonstrated an unparalleled means of improving the quality of life in society and creating world peace.[85,86]

The Structure of Collective Consciousness

In Maharishi's view, every level of collective life has a corresponding level of collective consciousness, which exists in a nested hierarchy of family consciousness, community consciousness, city consciousness, state consciousness, national consciousness, world consciousness and, ultimately, a transcendental field of pure consciousness at the basis of natural law. Each individual reciprocally interacts with all levels of the collective. Our thoughts and feelings to some extent influence everyone else in the world through the various strata of collective consciousness. If we are feeling grumpy or happy, those influences will be added to the mix that permeates all levels of society, and everyone else in the world will be influenced by it to some degree. In Maharishi's view, the collective effects will be stronger closer to home, to the family and community, and in those who we are most genetically similar, identical twins more than fraternal twins, and so on. This is because similar nervous systems will give rise to similar consciousness, which will be more tuned to each other.

Reciprocally, all the various layers of collective consciousness influence our feelings, thoughts, and behaviors. A war in the Middle East, whether or not we watch the news, affects us. Collective consciousness, then, can be seen as the sum total of all contributions by all the individuals in the population. If the individuals in society are predominantly stressed, then anyone entering into its collective consciousness will notice a feeling of stress impinging on them. We notice the differences in collective consciousness when we cross a national border, or travel from one city to another, such as between New York and San Francisco.

How Do You Change Society?

In Maharishi's view, those who are in charge of the different levels of the collective—the mayors, governors, and presidents—will most

acutely feel the effects of the respective levels of collective consciousness they rule, and they will be most controlled by them. They will be
the least able to make innovative changes. This is because collective
consciousness is the intelligence that guides the decisions and actions of
government, not the individual politicians. Just as the individual's mind
is the intelligence that guides the hand as it writes or does anything,
the "government is the innocent mirror of collective consciousness."[87]
Moreover, the type and quality of a national government is the emergent property of the national consciousness. If the individuals in society
are highly adversarial and dominated by an ethos of "every man for
himself," that influence in collective consciousness will give rise to a
totalitarian government. Without a strong system of law and order, such
a population will be completely chaotic and dangerous, and society as
an organized social structure will not exist. A measure of the degree of
intrinsic disorderliness of society is the number of laws on the books
and the proportion of the population that makes up lawyers, police, and
other members of the criminal justice system. On the other hand, if the
individuals in the population are self-ruling, cooperative, and helpful to
each other, then the population will need a minimal government. Cooperation has a powerful adaptive advantage over selfish interests, and it
is the hallmark of successful civilizations.

This is not to say that government can be changed by educating the
population in a new philosophy. In Maharishi's model, the *individual is the
unit of collective consciousness*, and only by increasing the integration of the
individual on the fundamental level of more coherent physiological functioning will they have the broad comprehension and ability to focus from
which cooperative and harmonious behavior is spontaneously the natural
consequence. It can't be contrived by mood making. In this approach,
unless the individuals are changed at the root level of their physiologies,
collective consciousness will not be changed, and a new government will
always turn out to be qualitatively the same as the old. Preaching to the
population will not change society in any significant way. Changing the
government will not change the quality of life in society in any fundamental way. The men and women in power do not rule, fundamentally.
Collective consciousness does, and if collective consciousness does not
change, then the new rulers and their methods will be quite similar to the
old ones, and they have the same limitations. Old despots will only be re-
placed by new ones. Thus Maharishi's theme of social change is radically
different from the usual methodology of changing government to change
society, whether peacefully through elections, or violently through revo-
lution. Electing new government officials or adopting a particular type of
government will not fundamentally change society. On the other hand, in
Maharishi's view, any form of government—totalitarian, military, demo-

cratic, socialist, communist, monarchic—will benefit by increasing the co-herence level in the population. This is because the rulers, operating in the focal point of collective consciousness, will now be supported by society's coherence, and they will be able to create and implement programs that will truly be to everyone's advantage. Otherwise, the hands of leadership are tied. Even a leader who may be fully enlightened personally will not be able to do much as a ruler unless the quality of collective consciousness is substantially improved. Parents want to give all good things to their children, but if the children misbehave, parents can't. Interestingly, pri-vate individuals who are more removed from the focal point of collective consciousness have more degrees of freedom for independent, innovative action than members of government. We are now seeing this with a new generation of philanthropists who are implementing significant world-wide health and training programs.

In Maharishi's view, the answer to *how to change society* lies in hav-ing recourse to the most fundamental level of collective consciousness, the transcendental field of universal pure consciousness, because that is the source of order in the universe. Only from that level of intelligence can we integrate all the diverse desires and tendencies in society into a harmonious whole. This idea may still be several steps away from the current formulations of a unified field theory in physics; however, logically, whatever is the most fundamental level of natural law, whatever was there before the Big Bang, whatever will be there after the universe completely dissipates, as inflationary cosmology predicts, that infinite compactification of order must be inherent within the universe at its fun-damental levels, in some potential form or another. Laws of nature are structures of order and intelligence that are conserved under all condi-tions. Intelligence must be conserved. Even when matter and energy were not there, before the Big Bang, there must have been a primordial form of intelligence or order that guided the evolution of an exquisitely ordered universe. How can order evolve from disorder? We know that in ther-modynamic systems, lowering temperature can reduce entropy. Random agitations of water molecules in steam and water can be transformed into fine, crystalline structures of ice by just lowering the temperature. Where did the order come from? In this case, reducing the thermal agitation of the molecules by lowering the temperature allowed the subtler electro-static forces intrinsic in the geometry of the molecules to come into play to arrange themselves into crystal lattices. The order was already there within the system, one just had to lower the agitation to let it manifest. Analogously, in Maharishi's theory, the source of order in all individuals is transcendental consciousness, the transcendental basis of their minds, beyond the mind's activity. All that is needed to access it is a method of reducing the agitation in the mind, the stresses, and thoughts.

Natural selection no doubt is a powerful mechanism of the evolution of structure and function. Whatever continues to exist, that is what we find existing around us. It is a tautology, actually. That which exists, exists. But what is it about fundamental force and matter fields that they self-organize into subatomic particles, atoms, molecules, and when conditions are right, they further self-organize into organic molecules, tissues, and life forms? Mainstream science has not yet understood how consciousness connects with the standard model of the Lagrangian of the universe, a mathematical theory that sorts out all the relationships between the force and matter fields that create, sustain, and dissipate the universe. The Lagrangian was created in the minds of scientists, and the fact that it fits (almost) with physical reality is in itself a demonstration of the intrinsic parity of the human mind and natural law. Logical processes, intuition, and systematic feedback from sensory observation have molded the human mind in the image of the unified field. The fact that the human mind can know the fundamental laws of nature is because it is that, in essence.

Hagelin advanced this discussion by demonstrating that the structure and function of consciousness described in Vedic literature is parallel to the structure and function of the standard model of physics.[88,89] Similarly, Nader showed how the fundamental structure and function of consciousness described in Vedic literature are parallel to the structure and function of neurophysiology.[90] These are important steps in showing that the universe and the human physiology are ultimately structured out of consciousness.

Physicists on Universal Consciousness

Even though consciousness is not yet formally recognized as part of the scientific description of natural law, many of our greatest scientists have intuited that consciousness is fundamental. Einstein put it this way: "Everyone who is seriously involved in the pursuit of science becomes convinced that a spirit is manifest in the laws of the Universe—a spirit vastly superior to that of man, and one in the face of which we with our modest powers must feel humble."[91] In another example, Sir James Jeans, the eminent British physicist and mathematician who was the first to propose that matter is continuously created throughout the universe, said,

> Thirty years ago, we thought, or assumed that we were heading towards an ultimate reality of a mechanical kind . . . Into this wholly mechanical world . . . life had stumbled by accident . . . Today there is a wide measure of agreement, which on the physical side of science approaches almost unanimously, that the stream of knowledge is heading towards a non-mechanical reality; the universe begins to look more like a great thought than a great machine. Mind no longer appears as an accidental intruder into the realm

of matter; we are beginning to suspect that we ought rather to hail it as the creator and governor of the realm of matter—not of course our individual minds, but the mind in which the atoms of which our individual minds have grown exist as thoughts.[92]

Jeans further wrote,

When we view ourselves in space and time, our consciousnesses are obviously the separate individuals of a particle-picture, but when we pass beyond space and time, they may perhaps form ingredients of a single continuous stream of life. As it is with light and electricity, so may it be with life; the phenomena may be individuals carrying on separate existences in space and time, while in the deeper reality beyond space and time we may all be members of one body.[93]

Eugene Wigner, Nobel laureate and pioneer of measurement theory, explains this change in science's perspective on consciousness: "When the province of physical theory was extended to encompass microscopic phenomena, through the creation of quantum mechanics, the concept of consciousness came to the fore again: it was not possible to formulate the laws of quantum mechanics in a fully consistent way without reference to consciousness."[94]

Max Planck, the first physicist to discern the quantized nature of the apparently physical world, was led by the implications of his studies to state, "I regard consciousness as fundamental. I regard matter as derivative from consciousness."[95] More recently, H. P. Stapp, a physicist at the Lawrence Berkeley Laboratory, long acknowledged for his contributions to the S matrix approach to quantum mechanics, concluded his book *Mind, Matter and Quantum Mechanics* by saying that quantum "particles" and their interactions are "idea-like" rather than "matter-like."[96]

This view has been similarly expressed by the formulations of other eminent physical scientists, for example, Sir Arthur Eddington's "mind stuff" and Wolfgang Pauli's "unity of all being."[93] In an article on quantum mechanics appearing in *Scientific American*, French physicist Bernard D'Espagnat summarized the field by stating, "The doctrine that the world is made up of objects whose existence is independent of human consciousness turns out to be in conflict with quantum mechanics and with the facts established by experiment."[97]

In the context of collective consciousness, Maharishi put it this way: "This transcendental level of nature's functioning is the level of infinite correlation. When the group awareness is brought in attunement with that level, then a very intensified influence of coherence radiates and a great richness is created. Infinite correlation is a quality of the transcendental level of nature's functioning from where orderliness governs the universe."[98]

Measuring Collective Consciousness

To be considered a science, the terms of a theory have to be operational so that they can be measured, and the theory has to make falsifiable predictions. Measurement has two aspects: sensory perception of something, such as a dial on an instrument, with an observer reporting what was seen, and the ability for others to also look at the dial to verify what was seen. In principle, the unified field, as the totality of everything, cannot be measured by anything outside of itself. The part cannot apprehend the whole. An element of a set cannot do justice to the totality of the whole set. Here the objective methodology of modern science fails. You can't measure the unified field by instruments of science because they are themselves subsets of the field. However, the unified field, as a field of consciousness, has the potential for self-awareness. It can directly "measure" itself in its self-referral state. The usual tripartite division of the mind is into an observer (say, the scientist), the process of observing (the instruments of science), and the observed (the object under observation). The Vedic tradition of India holds that the transcendental Self is the knower at the inner end of any sensory experience. Who is the knower who looks out onto the world? It is the Self. The Self is not seen because it is that by which everything is seen, and it is in a sense mixed with sensory experiences. The sensory experience "hides" it, much as the projected movie hides the movie screen. One sees the action, not the ground on which the action in playing. However, if the movie is made progressively dimmer, there will be a point where the movie is lost to awareness and the screen becomes predominant. The way to experience pure transcendental consciousness is to follow any of the channels of the senses back to their origin. For example, Patanjali, one of the great Maharishis (seers) in the Vedic tradition begins his *Yoga Sutras* with "Now is the teaching on Yoga." Yoga means the integration of the individual mind with the cosmic mind, so he is about to teach how to get there. The second sutra provides the formula: "Yoga is the complete settling of the activity of the mind."[99] This is operationalized by TM, in which the meditators follow a mantra (a thought of a sound without meaning known from tradition and scientific research to have a completely positive effect) back to its origin until, transcending the finest level of the mantra, the experiencer experiences pure consciousness. This fulfills the first requirement of measurement, a systematic way anyone can experience something. Although it is not experienced through the senses, and is not open to direct observation through the senses and their scientific extensions, it is experienced by following any sense back to its origin, the Self. In principle, anyone can experience pure consciousness just by following the systematic procedure.

TM fulfills the second requirement of measurement that others can use it to verify the experience of pure consciousness for themselves. The supporting evidence is the highly similar reports of pure consciousness by people from all over the world practicing TM in association with their common physiological signature of transcending, as well as similar reports by people from many traditions throughout history.[100] A caveat is that a healthy, fully functional nervous system is needed for the experience. But this is not unique to transcending. In any area of measurement, highly tuned instruments are needed for the measurements to be valid. The brain is the instrument for measuring pure consciousness. Tuning it occurs during the process because the process provides a deep coherent rest that sets the optimal conditions for the body's myriad self-repair mechanisms to function, as we have seen earlier in this chapter in the sections on aging and prison rehabilitation. Successful aging and rehabilitation are two areas of measurement that verify—through multiple, cross-validating measurements—that experiencing transcending is a powerful means to create order in the individual.

To summarize, we have argued that pure consciousness cannot be directly measured by anything outside itself (i.e., not by the instruments of objective referral science), but it can be "measured" in the self-referral state of scientists' own consciousness via the instrumentality of highly refined nervous systems, and practicing transcending refines the nervous system, creating order in the individual, the basic unit of collective consciousness. The next step in the measurement problem is how to measure these individuals' influence on the larger society.

There are precedents for attempting to measure collective consciousness in the history of the social science. Gustav Fechner (1801–1887), the founder of psychophysics, is best known for developing methods of measuring sensory thresholds, which are the smallest amounts of energy that the senses can detect. What motivated his studies of thresholds was his experience of a single, transcendental continuum of "general consciousness" underlying the discontinuities of numerous, localized, individual minds associated with different people, as mentioned earlier. Like many others throughout history, Fechner somehow managed to slip into an experience of unbounded transcendental consciousness. Puzzled by why we don't always experience this level of reality, he reasoned that it must lie just beyond ordinary sensory experience, and that if we could only lower our sensory threshold sufficiently, then we would experience general consciousness.

Fechner illustrated his idea with a model in which individual minds were likened to separate islands in the water, apparently separated and isolated from each other when seen from the perspective of the surface of the water. But if the level of the water were lowered sufficiently, the "islands" would appear as mountains that were *connected at their base* by the ground of general consciousness. Fechner reasoned that if one's sensory threshold were insensitive, as is usually the case, then each individual mind and person would experience itself as isolated from the other. But if the sensory thresholds were sufficiently refined, the individual would experience the continuity of consciousness connecting all minds at their base.[84]

The problem is that objective measurement of sensory thresholds does not refine the senses to the level where they can transcend to experience general consciousness. Measurements of sensory thresholds are only objective measures of the abilities of the sensory apparatuses, not a means for lowering sensory thresholds. In the end, Fechner's approach did not achieve his intended goal. However, it did create the highly useful field of psychophysics, while the field of psychology continues to evolve its object-referral methods, all but forgetting about general consciousness. (For further discussion of this concept, see "Some Conceptual Precedents for a Field Theoretic View of Consciousness from *The Perennial Philosophy*, Social Sciences, and Quantum Physics."[79])

How Many Meditators Are Needed?

In Maharishi's theory, not everyone in society needs to meditate to create coherence in collective consciousness. This is because coherence is more powerful than incoherence. As early as 1960, Maharishi maintained that even 1 percent of the population practicing TM would be sufficient to create a measureable influence on social indicators because the influence of coherent members of a system is greater than the influence of disorderly members.[98] This takes advantage of a general principle in science that the influence of the coherent elements in a system is proportional to their number squared, whereas the influence of the incoherent elements is only proportional to their number. Ten men pulling on a rope together can overcome ninety-nine men pulling at odds with each other at the other end of the rope. In our International Peace Project in the Middle East, discussed in the *Journal of Conflict Resolution*, we addressed the question of how many meditators would be needed to influence the larger society in the following way.

> With the introduction of the more advanced TM-Sidhi program in 1976, Maharishi anticipated an even more marked influence of coherence in collective consciousness. He predicted that when the TM-Sidhi program was practiced in a group by as few as the square root of one percent the TM-Sidhi program was practiced in a measurable effect on standard indices of quality of life. This prediction is based on a field theoretic model describing

the coherent superposition of amplitudes, in which the intensity of the effect generated is proportional to the square of the number of participants.[88] For example, in coherent systems such as lasers, the coherent elements in the system have an influence that is proportional to their number squared, whereas incoherent elements generally have an influence that is proportional only to their number. Thus the predicted population size influenced by a given number of TM and TM-Sidhi program participants would be tentatively modeled by the polynomial:

$$ME = aN_1 + bN_2^2 \ (1)$$

where ME (Maharishi Effect) is defined as the size of the population that is positively influenced by the number of independent meditators distributed throughout the population (N_1), and the number of individuals practicing the more advanced TM-Sidhi program collectively in one place (N_2). The quadratic term reflects the proposed coherent influence resulting from constructive interference of the group of N_2 subjects. Coefficients a and b are empirically defined constants, with data suggesting that both have an estimated value of approximately 10^2 (for values of N over 100). The absence of a constant term follows from the assumption that the effect vanishes (and does not diverge) as N tends to zero (cubic and higher-order terms are neglected because they have no clear theoretical motivation). The apparent necessity for having a single group meet at one time and place to produce this $\sqrt{ }$ 1 percent effect may again be understood with reference to coherent physical systems such as lasers. In these systems, close proximity of elements is required to ensure that they have sufficient opportunity to stimulate coherent behavior in other members of the group.[101]

What Is Predicted to Happen in Society?

Given a formula for what size population will be influenced by a given number of meditators and TM-Sidhi participants, what does the theory predict will happen in society? The theory broadly holds that life in society will become completely evolutionary and "supported by natural law."[98] This means that people will grow in self-actualizing values of infinite correlation inherent in the unified field rather than in conflict. However, many, if not most, scientists think of natural law as value neutral. Why then would infusing an influence of the unified field result in only positive effects on society? We have suggested the following explanation.

Through its long evolutionary history and the process of natural selection, the brain and physiology have become "hardwired" with intrinsic pleasure/pain circuits and homeostatic feedback mechanisms, which have the obvious adaptive advantage of directing life away from physical damage and towards life-promoting influences. Maslow (1968) and others have extended this line of reasoning to say that the positive qualities of self-actualization are as fundamental to our biological makeup as the motivations for self-preservation and reproduction. Consider the potential adaptive advantages of the qualities of self-actualization: being "present" oriented rather than being distracted by non-useful thoughts and feelings; having broad comprehension and increased ability to focus sharply; increased ability to integrate dichotomies into greater wholes; heightened perception; spontaneous skilled behavior; increased empathy and ability to function cooperatively with others (Maslow, 1968).

All of these qualities have obvious adaptive advantages, for modern human life as well as for hunting mastodons. An implication of Darwin and Maslow's work is that such self-actualizing qualities are inherent in the human genome, arising as the species evolved through its interaction with various environments. A further implication is that self-actualizing qualities are inherent in the very structure of natural law itself and are not arbitrary human conceptions. A fundamental tenet of science is that all the actors and the entire field of action are entirely comprised of the same elementary particles, forces, etc. and are governed by the same laws of nature. Furthermore, if the unified field is the basis of existence, then all that exists must in some way be inherent in it, even in seed form.

Maslow speculated that self-actualizing qualities inherent in every individual become expressed through experiences that he called "peak experiences" and "Being cognition," which are experiences pertaining to pure consciousness (Alexander et al., 1990, 1991). A meta-analysis of 42 treatment outcomes found that regular practice of the TM technique produced a three-fold greater increase in self-actualizing qualities than other meditation and relaxation techniques (Alexander et al., 1991).[102] This result supports the hypothesis that systematic transcending is the key factor contributing to the development of self-actualization. [103]

Social Indicators

If a sufficient number of individuals in society did agree with the total potential of natural law inherent in the unified field and begin to spontaneously express its more highly adaptive qualities of greater cooperation and harmony and infinite correlation of individual desires with the needs of society, how would that be measured in the larger society? What we have been able to do is use social indicators, such as crime rate, hospitalization, financial markets, war casualties, terrorism, international cooperation, etc., as indices of social trends. Even without measuring any intermediate steps (such as the meditators becoming more coherent, other people within their sphere of influence becoming more self-actualized and synergetic, etc.), we find that equation 1 makes specific, verifiable (and falsifiable) predictions that a given number of meditators and TM-Sidhi participants in a population will have positive effects on social indicators. Which social indicators?

Social indicators have many challenges to validity, such as the under-reporting of crime data, ongoing trends, and cycles in time-series data that may obscure and confound exogenous effects, the influence of political and military events, aberrant weather patterns, and the difficulty in interpreting most financial data, etc. Even an objective measure such as war casualties (assuming that they have been accurately reported and are not being manipulated for political purposes), cannot be interpreted as a positive trend in society (the way we got around that one was by using the numbers reported by actors on both sides of the war[86]). There could be circumstances where increased war casualties are an index of good triumphing over evil. Is the war clearing the way for a more just and equitable society? One would have to be omniscient to say for sure if a change in any social indicator was truly positive in a universal sense of evolutionary change that was in the best interest of all. Short of that, we were limited to examining variables that appeared to have a face validity of being positive, such as crime, terrorism, violent deaths, etc.

Some Studies on the Maharishi Effect

Over the past four decades, the Maharishi theory was vigorously studied in 51 research projects in over 15 countries, and results have been published in 38 peer-reviewed scientific journals and other research periodicals, papers, books, and doctoral dissertations.[104,105] The discovery of the effects of TM on collective consciousness was named the *Maharishi Effect*, following the tradition in science of naming a scientific discovery or breakthrough after its founder (e.g., the Meisner effect, the Doppler effect, the Planck scale, Schrodinger equations, etc.). The first studies pertain to the first part of equation 1, the prediction that 1 percent or more of the members of a population individually practicing TM will be sufficient to create positive trends in their cities, specifically on crime rates.

ONE PERCENT STUDIES

The initial study, which demonstrated the existence of the Maharishi Effect, assessed crime rates based on FBI and local police department data in eleven cities that had 1 percent of their population practicing TM.[106] The results indicated a significant 16 percent decrease in crime in the 1 percent cities compared to controls with matched demographics in the year following which 1 percent of the population becoming meditators. Later, when twenty-four U.S. cities with 1 percent of their population practicing TM were identified and included in the study, these results were replicated. This research indicated that the crime rate decreased significantly over the six years, subsequent to the attainment of 1 percent meditating, when controlling for several demographic variables.[107] This initial research was expanded in a study that applied causal analyses of crime trends over a period of seven years in 160 U.S. cities and 50 standard statistical metropolitan areas (which represented 50 percent of the U.S. population). The study revealed that U.S. cities and metropolitan areas which had a higher percentage of TM practitioners in their population showed a six-year period of decreased crime rate trends while statistically controlling for demographic variables known to influence crime.[108] The causal analysis showed that a rise in meditators in a metropolitan area predicted decreased crime in subsequent years, but not the other way around. Change in crime trends did not predict subsequent change in the proportion of meditators, supporting a causal interpretation that TM caused the crime to decrease.

$\sqrt{1}$ PERCENT STUDIES

A later, more striking research result involving significant improvements on a quality of life index was discovered while studying groups practicing the advanced TM-Sidhi program. Whereas with TM the minimum requirement was 1 percent of the population practicing it, with the TM-Sidhi program the requirement was as little as the square root of 1 percent of the population practicing it. For example, five studies in diverse populations found improvement in quality of life indices, including crime, deaths, pollution, cigarette and alcohol consumption, unemployment, motor vehicle fatalities, and accidents.[109]

A study published in *Social Indicators Research* revealed that an established, ongoing group of more than one thousand TM-Sidhi practitioners in Fairfield, Iowa, had an impact on U.S. violent deaths (homicides, suicides, traffic fatalities), reducing them by over one hundred deaths per week from 1979 to 1985. This and most of the other studies on the Extended Maharishi Effect used time-series analysis to demonstrate that beneficial changes were a function of the size of the meditating group. As the group of meditators increased, the violent deaths decreased proportionately, controlling for cyclical patterns, long-term trends, and stochastic drift in data on violent deaths. This was seen as indicating a coherent group producing an increased level of coherence in the collective consciousness in the United States. A similar time-series analysis found a decrease in violent deaths in Canada as well when the Fairfield group reached the square root of 1 percent of the population of North America.[85]

A major experimental test of the application of the Maharishi Effect to resolve international conflicts was carried out in 1983 in Israel during the war with Lebanon. Using daily time-series data, the results indicated major reductions in war casualties and war intensity in Lebanon, in addition to many other improved social indicators in Israel (reduced crime, decreased auto accidents, fewer fires, improved national mood, and rises in the stock market), where the group was located. The magnitude of war casualties and war intensity varied with size of the meditating group: as the number of meditators rose, there was a corresponding reduction in war deaths and war intensity, controlling for trends and cycles (such as weekend effects) in the data.[101,110]

Causality was supported by the finding that the effects on social indicators were simultaneous with (same day) or lag 1 (the next day) as the change in the size of the creating group. The theory that the TM and TM-Sidhi group created a holistic, unified influence on society was supported by the finding that the results were stronger for a composite index of all the variables taken together than for any of the single variables. Apparently, as in signal averaging, adding the variables all together canceled out the idiosyncratic variances specific to the individual variables and added the common component of the effect of the coherence creating group, increasing the signal-to-noise ratio. Subsequent reanalysis of the data also showed that the results held up controlling for the major political and military events of the time.[103] This result on the war in Lebanon has been replicated seven times.[86]

Subsequent studies of the Maharishi Effect on global conflicts were carried out with large groups of meditators, many as large as seven thousand, which was the square root of 1 percent of the world's population at that time. These studies found that as the number of group meditators approached seven thousand, there was a 30 percent reduction in world conflicts as measured by content analysis of the *New York Times* and the *London Times*, and a 70 percent reduction in terrorism as indicated by a database compiled by the Rand Corporation.[111]

These data seriously challenge the basic assumption of current social sciences that individuals in society only interact directly through sensory/behavioral channels. These data also support the view that we all influence each other at a distance with no apparent physical connections between us. Critics of the theory and research have not been able to explain away the phenomenon. For those interested, these scholarly exchanges of criticisms and rebuttals, which were published in peer-reviewed journals, have been summarized in detail elsewhere, along with references to the original papers.[112]

Applying the Maharishi Effect

Large groups of TM practitioners can and already do exist. The formation of large groups of meditators in institutions such as homes for the elderly, prisons, schools, the military, hospitals, and the government could result in increasing the quality of life and reducing problems and suffering for members of the institution as well as for society as a whole. This is already happening in some Latin American countries with funding from and the efforts of the David Lynch Foundation, a nonprofit organization with the goal of making TM available to all people.[113,114]

CONCLUSION

The ultimate aspiration of the healthcare system could be defined as achieving lasting mental and physical health for all people. But seriously contemplating this idea, much less having a vision of its fulfillment and a viable approach to its realization, appears absurdly idealistic. With the advent of the psychophysiological technologies of the TM and TM-Sidhi programs, however, and the evidence that they can and do improve aging, criminal rehabilitation, and world health, as presented here, this ancient concept shifts from the realm of philosophical speculation into a practical, evidence-based solution to many of the recalcitrant problems of contemporary civilization. When this finding is considered along with all the research on TM and its contributions to lowered morbidity and mortality rates due to the effects of TM on specific disease conditions, there is an overwhelming case for considering TM a standard program of care, a *best practice* for a broad range of mental and physical disorders and maladaptive social behaviors.

NOTES

1. B. W. Cannon. *Bodily Changes in Pain, Hunger, Fear, and Rage* (New York: Appleton-Century-Crofts, 1929).

2. R. H. Schneider, Egan, B., and Johnson, E. et al. "Anger and Anxiety in Borderline Hypertension." *Psychosomatic Medicine* 48 (1986): 242–48.

3. R. Sapolsky, Krey, L., and McEwens, B. "The Neuroendocrinology of Stress and Aging: The Glucocorticoid Cascade Hypothesis." *Endocrine Review* 7, no. 3 (1986): 284–301.

4. R. M. Sapolsky. *Stress, the Aging Brain, and the Mechanisms of Neuron Death* (Cambridge, MA: MIT Press, 1992).

5. K. G. Walton, Pugh, N., Gelderloos, P., and Macrae, P. "Stress Reduction and Preventing Hypertension: Preliminary Support for a Psychoneuroendocrine Mechanism." *Journal of Alternative and Complementary Medicine* 1, no. 3 (1995): 263–83.

6. K. G. Walton and Levitsky, D. "A Neuroendocrine Mechanism for the Reduction of Drug Use and Addictions by Transcendental Meditation." In Self-

Recovery—Treating Addictions Using Transcendental Meditation and Maharishi Ayur-Veda. Edited by O'Connell, D. F. and Alexander, C. N., 89–118 (Binghamton, NY: Harrington Park Press, 1994).

7. K. G. Walton, Fields, J. Z., and Harris, D. A. et al. "Stress and Aging: Reduced Cortisol Response to Glucose in Postmenopausal Women Practicing the Transcendental Meditation Program." *Society for Neuroscience Abstracts* 24 (1998): 1764.

8. R. K. Wallace. "Physiological Effects of Transcendental Meditation." *Science* 167 (1970): 1751–54.

9. R. K. Wallace. "The Physiological Effects of Transcendental Meditation: A Proposed Fourth Major State of Consciousness." In *Scientific Research on the Transcendental Meditation Program: Collected Papers,* edited by Orme-Johnson, D. W. and Farrow, J. T., 43–78 (Livingston Manor, NY: MIU Press, 1970).

10. R. K. Wallace. "The Physiology of Meditation." *Scientific American* 226 (1972): 84–90.

11. R. K. Wallace, Benson, H., and Wilson, A. F. "A Wakeful Hypometabolic Physiologic State." *American Journal of Physiology* 221 (1971): 795–99.

12. M. C. Dillbeck and Orme-Johnson, D. W. "Physiological Differences between Transcendental Meditation and Rest." *American Psychologist* 42 (1987): 879–81.

13. V. A. Barnes and Orme-Johnson, D. W. "Prevention and Treatment of Cardiovascular Disease in Adolescents and Adults through the Transcendental Meditation Program: A Research Review Update." *Current Hypertension Reviews* 8, no. 3 (2012): 227–42.

14. P. H. Levine. "The Coherence Spectral Array (Cospar) and Its Application to the Spatial Ordering of the EEG." *Proceedings of the San Diego Biomedical Symposium* 15 (1976): 237–47.

15. P. H. Levine, Hebert, R., Haynes, C. T., and Strobel, U. "EEG Coherence During the Transcendental Meditation Technique." In *Scientific Research on the Transcendental Meditation Program: Collected Papers,* edited by Orme-Johnson, D. W. and Farrow, J., 187–207 (Livingston Manor, NY: Maharishi European Research University Press, 1977).

16. K. Badawi, Wallace, R. K., Orme-Johnson, D., and Rouzere, A. M. "Electrophysiologic Characteristics of Respiratory Suspension Periods Occurring During the Practice of the Transcendental Meditation Program." *Psychosomatic Medicine* 46, no. 3 (1984): 267–76.

17. J. T. Farrow and Hebert, J. R. "Breath Suspension During the Transcendental Meditation Technique." *Psychosomatic Medicine* 44, no. 2 (1982): 133–53.

18. F. T. Travis and Pearson, C. "Pure Consciousness: Distinct Phenomenological and Physiological Correlates of 'Consciousness Itself.'" *International Journal of Neuroscience* 100, nos. 1–4 (1999): 77–89.

19. F. T. Travis and Wallace, R. K. "Autonomic Patterns During Respiration Suspensions: Possible Markers of Transcendental Consciousness." *Psychophysiology* 34 (1997): 39–46.

20. F. T. Travis and Wallace, R. K. "Autonomic and EEG Patterns During Eyes-Closed Rest and Transcendental Meditation (TM) Practice: The Basis for a Neural Model of TM Practice." *Consciousness and Cognition* 8, no. 3 (1999): 302–18.

21. F. T. Travis and Arenander, A. "Cross-Sectional and Longitudinal Study of Effects of Transcendental Meditation Practice on Interhemispheric Frontal Asymmetry and Frontal Coherence." *International Journal of Neuroscience* 116, no. 12 (2006): 1519–38.

22. F. T. Travis, Haaga, D., and Hagelin, J. S. et al. "Effects of Transcendental Meditation Practice on Brain Functioning and Stress Reactivity in College Students." *International Journal of Psychophysiology* 71, no. 2 (2009): 170–76.

23. B. R. Cahn and Polich, J. "Meditation States and Traits: EEG, ERP, and Neuroimaging Studies." *Psychological Bulletin* 132, no. 2 (2006): 180–211.

24. F. C. Hummel and Gerloff, C. G. "Interregional Long-Range and Short-Range Synchrony: A Basis for Complex Sensorimotor Processing." *Progress in Brain Research* 159 (2006): 223–36.

25. S. Palva and Palva, J. M. "New Vistas for α-frequency Band Oscillations." *Trends in Neurosciences* 30, no. 4 (2007): 150–58.

26. P. Sauseng and Klimesch, W. "What Does Phase Information of Oscillatory Brain Activity Tell Us About Cognitive Processes?" *Neuroscience and Biobehavioral Reviews* 32, no. 5 (2008): 1001–13.

27. R. W. Thatcher. "Coherence, Phase Differences, Phase Shift, and Phase Lock in EEG/ERP Analyses." *Developmental Neuropsychology* 37, no. 6 (2012): 476–96.

28. R. W. Thatcher, Biver, C. J., and North, D. "Spatial-Temporal Current Source Correlations and Cortical Connectivity." *Clinical EEG and Neuroscience* 38, no. 1 (2007): 35–48.

29. D. W. Orme-Johnson and Haynes, C. T. "EEG Phase Coherence, Pure Consciousness, Creativity and TM-Sidhi Experiences." *International Journal of Neuroscience* 13 (1981): 211–17.

30. M. C. Dillbeck, Orme-Johnson, D. W., and Wallace, R. K. "Frontal EEG Coherence, H-reflex Recovery, Concept Learning, and the TM-Sidhi Program." *International Journal of Neuroscience* 15, no. 3 (1981): 151–57.

31. S. I. Nidich, Ryncarz, R. A., and Abrams, A. I. et al. "Kohlbergian Moral Perspective Responses, EEG coherence, and the Transcendental Meditation and TM-Sidhi Program." *Journal of Moral Education* 12, no. 3 (1983): 166–73.

32. R. Chalmers, Clements, G., Schenkluhn., H., and Weinless, M., eds. *Scientific Research on Maharishi's Transcendental Meditation and TM-Sidhi Program: Collected Papers*, Volumes 2–4 (Vlodrop, The Netherlands: Maharishi Vedic University Press, 1989).

33. M. C. Dillbeck, ed. *Scientific Research on Maharishi's Transcendental Meditation and TM-Sidhi Program: Collected Papers*. Volume 6 (Vlodrop, The Netherlands: Maharishi Vedic University Press, 2011).

34. D. W. Orme-Johnson and Farrow, J. T., eds. *Scientific Research on Maharishi's Transcendental Meditation and TM-Sidhi Program: Collected Papers*. Volume 1 (Livingston Manor, NY: Maharishi International University Press, 1977).

35. R. K. Wallace, Orme-Johnson, D. W., and Dillbeck, M. C., eds. *Scientific Research on Maharishi's Transcendental Meditation and TM-Sidhi Program: Collected Papers*. Volume 5 (Fairfield, IA: Maharishi International University Press, 1990).

36. M. C. Dillbeck, Barnes, V. A., and Schneider, R. H. et al., eds. *Scientific Research on the Transcendental Meditation and TM-Sidhi Program: Collected Papers*. Volume 7 (Vlodrop, The Netherlands: Maharishi Vedic University Press, 2013).

37. R. K. Wallace, Dillbeck, M., Jacobe, E., and Harrington, B. "The Effects of the Transcendental Meditation and TM-Sidhi Program on the Aging Process." *International Journal of Neuroscience* 16 (1982): 53–58.

38. G. Stevens, Mascarenhas, M., and Mathers, C. "Global Health Risks: Progress and Challenges." *Bulletin of the World Health Organization* 87, no. 646 (2009).

39. C. N. Alexander, Langer, E. J., and Newman, R. I. et al. "Transcendental Meditation, Mindfulness, and Longevity: An Experimental Study with the Elderly." *Journal of Personality and Social Psychology* 57, no. 6 (1989): 950–64.

40. R. H. Schneider, Alexander, C. N., and Staggers, F. et al. "Long-Term Effects of Stress Reduction on Mortality in Persons ≥ 55 Years of Age with Systemic Hypertension." *American Journal of Cardiology* 95, no. 9 (2005): 1060–64.

41. R. H. Schneider, Staggers, F., and Alexander, C. N. et al. "A Randomized Controlled Trial of Stress Reduction for Hypertension in Older African Americans." *Hypertension* 26 (1995): 820–27.

42. C. N. Alexander, Schneider, R. H., and Barnes, V. A. et al. "Effects of Transcendental Meditation on Psychological Risk Factors, Cardiovascular and All-Cause Mortality: A Review of Meta-analyses and Controlled Clinical Trials." Paper presented at the Tenth Conference of the European Health Psychology Society, Dublin, Ireland, 1996.

43. J. W. Anderson, Liu, C. H., and Kryscio, R. J. "Blood Pressure Response to Transcendental Meditation: A Meta-analysis." *American Journal of Hypertension* 21, no. 3 (2008): 310–16.

44. M. V. Rainforth, Schneider, R. H., and Nidich, S. I. et al. "Stress Reduction Programs in Patients with Elevated Blood Pressure: A Systematic Review and Meta-analysis." *Current Hypertension Reports* 9, no. 6 (2007): 520–28.

45. J. A. Staessen, Thijisq, L., and Fagard, R. et al. "Systolic Hypertension in Europe (Syst-Eur) Trial Investigators (2004). Effects of Immediate Versus Delayed Antihypertensive Therapy on Outcome in the Systolic Hypertension in Europe Trial." *Journal of Hypertension* 22 (2004): 847–57.

46. R. D. Brook, Appel, L. J., and Rubenfire, M. et al. "Beyond Medications and Diet: Alternative Approaches to Lowering Blood Pressure, A Scientific Statement from the American Heart Association." *Hypertension*, no. 61 (2013).

47. K. Denys, Cankurtaran M., Janssens W., and Petrovic, M. "Metabolic Syndrome in the Elderly: An Overview of the Evidence." *Acta Clinica Belgica* 64 (2009): 23–34.

48. M. Paul-Labrador, Polk, D., and Dwyer, J. H. et al. "Effects of a Randomized Controlled Trial of Transcendental Meditation on Components of the Metabolic Syndrome in Subjects with Coronary Heart Disease." *Archives of Internal Medicine* 166 (2006): 1218–24.

49. J. W. Zamarra, Schneider, R. H., and Besseghini, I. et al. "Usefulness of the Transcendental Meditation Program in the Treatment of Patients with Coronary Artery Disease." *American Journal of Cardiology* 78 (1996): 77–80.

50. A. Castillo-Richmond, Schneider, R. H., and Alexander, C. N. et al. "Effects of Stress Reduction on Carotid Atherosclerosis in Hypertensive African Americans." *Stroke* 31 (2000): 568–73.

51. J. T. Salonen and Salonen, R. "Ultrasound B-mode Imaging in Observational Studies of Atherosclerotic Progression." *Circulation* 87, suppl. 3 (1993): II56–II65.

52. D. H. O'Leary, Polak, J. F., and Kronmal, R. A. et al. "Carotid-Artery Intima and Media Thickness as a Risk Factor for Myocardial Infarction and Stroke in Older Adults: Cardiovascular Health Study Collaborative Research Group." *New England Journal of Medicine* 340, no. 1 (1999): 14–22.

53. R. Jayadevappa, Johnson, J. C., and Bloom, B. S. et al. "Effectiveness of Transcendental Meditation on Functional Capacity and Quality of Life of African Americans with Congestive Heart Failure: A Randomized Control Study." *Ethnicity and Disease* 17 (2007): 72–77.

54. J. L. Glaser, Brind, J. L., and Vogelman, J. H. et al. "Elevated Serum Dehydroepiandrosterone Sulfate Levels in Practitioners of Transcendental Meditation (TM) and TM-Sidhi Programs." *Journal of Behavioral Medicine* 15, no. 4 (1992): 327–41.

55. P. H. Goddard. "Reduced Age Related Declines of P300 Latency in Elderly Practicing Transcendental Meditation." *Psychophysiology* 26 (1989): 529.

56. R. Chalmers. "Effects of the Transcendental Meditation Program Opposite to Detrimental Effects of the Aging Process." www.truthabouttm.org/truth/TM Research/TMResearchSummary/SummaryContinued/index.cfm#Ageing.

57. D. W. Orme-Johnson. "Medical Care Utilization and the Transcendental Meditation Program." *Psychosomatic Medicine* 49 (1987): 493–507.

58. D. W. Orme-Johnson and Herron, R. E. "An Innovative Approach to Reducing Medical Care Utilization and Expenditures." *American Journal of Managed Care* 3, no. 1 (1997): 135–44.

59. C. N. Alexander, Barnes, V. A., and Schneider, R. H. et al. "A Randomized Controlled Trial of Stress Reduction on Cardiovascular and All-Cause Mortality in the Elderly: Results of 8- and 15-Year Follow-ups." *Circulation* 93, no. 3 (1996): P19.

60. V. Barnes, Schneider, R., and Alexander, C. et al. "Impact of Transcendental Meditation on Mortality in Older African Americans with Hypertension—Eight Year Follow-up." *Journal of Social Behavior and Personality* 17, no. 1 (2005): 201–16.

61. R. H. Schneider, Grim, C. E., and Rainforth, M. A. et al. "Stress Reduction in the Secondary Prevention of Cardiovascular Disease: Randomized Controlled Trial of Transcendental Meditation and Health Education in Blacks." *Circulation: Cardiovascular Quality and Outcomes* 2, no. 5 (2012): 1–9.

62. Pew Center on the States. *State of Recidivism: The Revolving Door of America's Prisons* (Washington, DC: Pew Charitable Trusts, 2011).

63. K. G. Walton and Levitsky D. K. "Stress-Induced Neuroendocrine Abnormalities in Aggression and Crime—Apparent Reversal by the Transcendental Meditation Program." *Journal of Offender Rehabilitation* 36 (2003): 67–87.

64. M. A. Hawkins, Orme-Johnson, D. W., and Durchholz, C. F. "Fulfilling the Rehabilitative Ideal through the Transcendental Meditation and TM-Sidhi Programs: Primary, Secondary, and Tertiary Prevention." *Journal of Social Behavior and Personality* 17, no. 1 (2005): 443–88.

65. M. C. Dillbeck and Abrams, A. I. "The Application of the Transcendental Meditation Program to Corrections: Meta-analysis." *International Journal of Comparative and Applied Criminal Justice* 11, and no. 1 (1987): 111–32.

66. C. N. Alexander, Rainforth, M. V., and Frank, P. R. et al. "Walpole Study of the Transcendental Meditation Program in Maximum Security Prisoners III: Reduced Recidivism." *Journal of Offender Rehabilitation* 36, no. 3 (2003): 161–80.

67. J. Loevinger. *Ego Development: Conceptions and Theories* (San Francisco: Jossey-Bass, 1976).

68. C. N. Alexander, Davies, J. L., and Dixon, C. A. et al. "Growth of Higher Stages of Consciousness: Maharishi's Vedic Psychology of Human Development." Edited by Alexander, C. N., and Langer, E. L., *Higher Stages of Human Development: Perspectives on Adult Growth* (New York: Oxford University Press, 1990), 331.

69. C. N. Alexander and Orme-Johnson, D. W. "Walpole Study of the TM Program in Maximum Security Prisoners II: Longitudinal Study of Development and Psychopathology." *Journal of Offender Rehabilitation* 36, nos. 1–4 (2003): 127–60.

70. C. N. Alexander, Walton, K. G., and Goodman, R. S. "Walpole Study of the TM Program in Maximum Security Prisoners I: Cross-Sectional Differences in Development and Psychopathology." *Journal of Offender Rehabilitation* 36, no. 1 (2003): 97–125.

71. A. Abrams and Siegel, L. "The Transcendental Meditation Program and Rehabilitation at Folsom State Prison: A Cross-Validation Study." *Criminal Justice and Behavior* 5 (1978): 3–20.

72. A. I. Abrams. "Transcendental Meditation and Rehabilitation at Folsom Prison: Response to a Critique." *Criminal Justice and Behavior* 6, no. 1 (1979): 13–21.

73. S. W. Gore, Abrams, A. I., and Ellis, G. "The Effects of Statewide Implementation of the Maharishi Technology of the Unified Field in the Vermon Department of Corrections." In *Scientific Research on Maharishi's Transcendental Meditation and TM-Sidhi Programme*. Edited by Chalmers, R., Clements, G., Schenkluhn, H., and Weinless, M., 2453–64 (Vlodrop: The Netherlands: Maharishi Vedic University Press, 1984).

74. M. V. Rainforth, Bleick, C., Alexander, C. N., and Cavanaugh, K. L. "The Transcendental Meditation Program and Criminal Recidivism in Folsom State Prisoners: A 15-Year Follow-up Study." *Journal of Offender Rehabilitation* 36 (2003): 181–204.

75. F. K. Anklesaria and King, M. S. "The Transcendental Meditation Program in the Senegalese Penitentiary System." *Journal of Offender Rehabilitation* 36, nos. 1–4 (2003): 303–18.

76. F. Anklesaria and King, M. S. "The Enlightened Sentencing Project: A Judicial Innovation." *Journal of Offender Rehabilitation* 36, nos. 1–4 (2003): 39.

77. A. J. Anderson. "Law, Justice, and Rehabilitation." In A *Symphony of Silence: An Enlightened Vision*. Edited by Eliss, G. A., 283–90 (North Charleston, SC: CreateSpace, 2012).

78. A. Huxley. *The Perennial Philosophy* (New York: Harper Collins Publishers, 2009).

79. D. W. Orme-Johnson. "Some Conceptual Precedents for a Field Theoretic View of Consciousness from *The Perennial Philosophy*, Social Sciences, and Quantum Physics.

80. www.truthabouttm.org/truth/SocietalEffects/Rationale-Research/index.cfm.

81. M. M. Yogi. *Creating an Ideal Society* (West Germany: Maharishi European Research University Press, 1977).

82. J. Campbell. *Hero with a Thousand Faces* (New York: Pantheon Books, 1949).

83. C. G. Jung. *The Archetypes and the Collective Unconscious* (New York: Bollingen Foundation, 1959).

84. E. Durkheim. "Society and Individual Consciousness. In *Theories of* Society. Edited by Parsons, T., Shils, E., Naegele, K. D., and Pitts, J. R., 720–24 (Glencoe, IL: Free Press, 1961).

85. W. James. "Human Immortality: Two Supposed Objections to the Doctrine" (New York, 1898).

86. P. Assimakis and Dillbeck, M. C. "Time Series Analysis of Improved Quality of Life in Canada: Social Change, Collective Consciousness, and the TM-Sidhi Program." *Psychological Report* 76 (1995): 1171–93.

87. J. L. Davies and Alexander, C. N. "Alleviating Political Violence through Reducing Collective Tension: Impact Assessment Analysis of the Lebanon War." *Journal of Social Behavior and Personality* 17, no. 1 (2005): 285–338.

88. M. M. Yogi. *Maharishi's Absolute Theory of Government: Automation in Administration* (India: Maharishi Prakashan, Age of Enlightenment Publications, 1995).

89. J. S. Hagelin. "Is Consciousness the Unified Field? A Field Theorist's Perspective." *Modern Science and Vedic Science* 1, no. 1 (1987): 29–88.

90. J. S. Hagelin. "Restructuring Physics from Its Foundation in Light of Maharishi's Vedic Science." *Modern Science and Vedic Science* 3, no. 1 (1989): 3–72.

91. T. Nader. *Human Physiology—Expression of Veda and the Vedic Literature* (Vlodrop, The Netherlands: Maharishi University Press, 1995).

92. A. Einstein. "Albert Einstein Quotes on Spirituality." Judaism Online, www.simpletoremember.com/articles/a/einstein/.

93. J. Jeans. *The Mysterious Universe* (New York: Macmillan, 1932).

94. L. Dossey. *Recovering the Soul* (New York: Bantam Books, 1989).

95. E. Wigner. *Symmetries and Reflections* (Woodbridge, CT: Ox Bow Press, 1967).

96. D. B. Klein. *The Concept of Consciousness: A Survey* (Lincoln: University of Nebraska Press, 1984).

97. H. Stapp. *Mind, Matter and Quantum Mechanics* (New York: Springer-Verlag, 1993).

98. B. D'Espagnat. "The Quantum Theory and Reality." *Scientific American* 241, no. 5 (1979): 158–181.

99. M. M. Yogi. *Life Supported by Natural Law* (Washington, DC: Age of Enlightenment Press, 1986).

100. T. Egenes. *Maharishi Patanjali Yoga Sutra*. Translated by Thomas Egenes (Fairfield, IA: 1st World Publishing, 2010).

101. C. Pearson. *Supreme Awakening: Experiences of Higher States of Consciousness Across Time and Across the World* (Fairfield, IA: Maharishi University of Management Press, 2012).

102. D. W. Orme-Johnson, Alexander, C. N., and Davies, J. L. et al. "International Peace Project: The Effects of the Maharishi Technology of the Unified Field." *Journal of Conflict Resolution* 32, no. 4 (1988): 776–812.

103. C. N. Alexander, Rainforth, M. V., and Gelderloos, P. "Transcendental Meditation, Self-Actualization and Psychological Health: A Conceptual Overview and Statistical Meta-analysis." *Journal of Social Behavior and Personality* 6, no. 5 (1991): 189–247.

104. D. W. Orme-Johnson and Oates, R. M. "A Field-Theoretic View of Consciousness: Reply to Critics." *Journal of Scientific Exploration* 32, no. 2 (2009): 139–66.

105. D. W. Orme-Johnson. "Preventing Crime through the Maharishi Effect." *Journal of Offender Rehabilitation* 36, nos. 1–4 (2003): 257–82.

106. D. W. Orme-Johnson. "Theory and Research on Conflict Resolution through the Maharishi Effect." *Modern Science and Vedic Science* 5, nos. 1–2 (1991): 76–98.

107. C. L. Borland and Landrith, G. S. III. "Improved Quality of Life through the Transcendental Meditation Program: Decreased Crime Rate." In *Scientific Research on the Transcendental Meditation Program: Collected Papers*. Edited by Orme-Johnson, D. W., 651–58 (Livingston Manor, NY: Maharishi European Research University Press, 1977).

108. M. C. Dillbeck, Landrith, G. S. III, and Orme-Johnson, D. W. "The Transcendental Meditation Program and Crime Rate Changes in a Sample of Forty-Eight Cities." *Journal of Crime and Justice* 4 (1981): 25–45.

109. M. C. Dillbeck, Banus, C. B., Polanzi, C., and Landrith, G. S. III. "Test of a Field Model of Consciousness and Social Change: Transcendental Meditation and TM-Sidhi Program and Decreased Urban Crime." *Journal of Mind and Behavior* 9, no. 4 (1988): 457–86

110. M. C. Dillbeck, Cavanaugh, K. L., and Glenn, T. et al. "Consciousness as a Field: The Transcendental Meditation and TM-Sidhi Program and Changes in Social Indicators." *Journal of Mind and Behavior* 8, no. 1 (1987): 67–104.

111. D. W. Orme-Johnson, Alexander, C. N., and Davies, J. L. "The Effects of the Maharishi Technology of the Unified Field: Reply to a Methodological Critique." *Journal of Conflict Resolution* 34 (1990): 756–68.

112. D. W. Orme-Johnson, Dillbeck, M. C., and Alexander, C. N. "Preventing Terrorism and International Conflict: Effects of Large Assemblies of Participants in the Transcendental Meditation and TM-Sidhi Programs." *Journal of Offender Rehabilitation* 36 (2003): 283–302.

113. D. W. Orme-Johnson. "Scholarly Exchanges on the Maharishi Effect: Critics and Rebuttals." www.truthabouttm.org/truth/SocietalEffects/Critics-Rebuttals/index.cfm#IPPME.

114. D. Lynch. "David Lynch Foundation Schools." www.davidlynchfoundation.org/schools.html.

BIBLIOGRAPHY

Abrams, A. and Siegel, L. "The Transcendental Program and Rehabilitation at Folsom Prison: A Cross-validation Study." *Criminal Justice and Behavior* 5 (1978): 3–20.

Abrams, A. "Transcendental Meditation and Rehabilitation at Folsom Prison: Response to a Critique. *Criminal Justice and Behavior* 6 (1979): 13–21.

Alexander, C. N., Langer, E. J., and Newman, R. I. et al. "Transcendental Meditation, Mindfulness and Longevity: An Experimental Study with the Elderly." *Journal of Personality and Social Psychology and Personality* 57, no. 6 (1989): 950–64.

Alexander, C. N. Davies, J. L., and Dixon, C. A. et al. *Growth of Higher Stages of Consciousness: Maharishi's Vedic Psychology of Human Development*. Edited by

Alexander, C. N. and Langer, E. L. *Higher Stages of Human Development: Perspectives on Adult Growth.* New York: Oxford University Press, 1990.

Alexander, C. N., Rainforth, M. V., and Gelderloos, P. "Transcendental Meditation, Self -Actualization and Psychological Health: A Conceptual Overview and Statistical Meta-analysis." *Journal of Social Behavior and Personality* 6, no. 5 (1991): 189–247.

Alexander, C. N., Barnes, V. A., and Schneider, R. H. et al. "A Randomized Controlled Trial of Stress Reduction on Cardiovascular and All-Cause Mortality in the Elderly: Results of 8- and 15-Year Follow-ups." *Circulation* 93, no. 3 (1996): 19.

Alexander, C. N., Schneider, R. H., and Barnes, V. A. et al. "Effects of Transcendental Meditation on Psychological Risk Factors, Cardiovascular and All-Cause Mortality: A Review of Meta-analyses and Controlled Clinical Trials." Paper Presented at the Tenth Conference of the European Health Psychology Society, Dublin, Ireland, 1996.

Alexander, C. N. and Orme-Johnson, D. W. "Walpole Study of the TM Program in Maximum Security Prisoners II: Longitudinal Study of Development and Psychopathology." *Journal of Offender Rehabilitation* 36, nos. 1–4 (2003): 127–160.

Alexander, C. N., Rainforth, M. V., and Frank, P. R. et al " Walpole Study of the Transcendental Meditation Program in Maximum Security Prisoners III: Reduced Recidivism." *Journal of Offender Rehabilitation* 36, no. 3 (2003): 161–80.

Alexander, C. N. Walton, K. G., and Goodman, R. S. "Walpole Study of the TM Program in Maximum Security Prisoners I: Cross Sectional Differences in Development and Psychopathology." *Journal of Offender Rehabilitation* 36, no. 1 (2003): 97–125.

Anderson, J. W., Liu, C. H., Kryscio, R. J. "Blood Pressure Response to Transcendental Meditation: A Meta-analysis." *American Journal of Hypertension* 21, no. 3 (2008): 310–16.

Anderson, A. J. "Law, Justice and Rehabilitation." In *A Symphony of Silence: An Enlightened Vision.* Edited by Eliss, G. A., 283–90. North Charleston, SC: CreateSpace, 2012.

Anklesaria, F. K. and King, M. S. "The Transcendental Meditation Program in the Senegalese Penitentiary System." *Journal of Offender Rehabilitation* 36, no. 1–4 (2003): 303–18.

Anklesaria, F. K. and King, M. S. "The Enlightened Sentencing Project: A Judicial Innovation." *Journal of Offender Rehabilitation* 36, nos. 1–4 (2003): 35–46.

Assimakis, P. and Dillbeck, M. C. "Time Series Analysis of Improved Quality of Life in Canada: Social Change, Collective Consciousness, and the TM-Sidhi Program." *Psychological Reports* 76 (1995): 1171–93.

Badawi, K., Wallace, R. K., Orme-Johnson, D. W., and Rouzere, A. M. "Electrophysiologic Characteristics of Respiratory Suspension Periods Occurring During the Practice of the Transcendental Meditation Program." *Psychosomatic Medicine* 46, no. 3 (1984): 267–76.

Barnes, V., Schneider, R., and Alexander, C. et al. "Impact of Transcendental Meditation on Mortality in Older African Americans with Hypertension—Eight Year Follow-up." *Journal of Social Behavior and Personality* 17, no. 1 (2005): 201–16.

Barnes, V. A. and Orme-Johnson, D. W. "Prevention and Treatment of Cardiovascular Disease in Adolescents and Adults through the Transcendental Meditation Program: A Research Review Update." *Current Hypertension Reviews* 8, no. 3 (2012): 227–42.

Borland, C. L. "Improved Quality of Life through the Transcendental Meditation Program: Decreased Crime Rate." In *Scientific Research on the Transcendental Meditation Program: Collected Papers.* Edited by Orme-Johnson, D. W. and Farrow, J. T., 651–58. Livingston Manor, NY: Maharishi European Research University Press, 1977.

Brook, R. D., Appel, L. J., and Rubenfire, M. et al. "Beyond Medications and Diet: Alternative Approaches to Lowering Blood Pressure; A Scientific Statement from the American Heart Association." *Journal of the American Heart Association* 61 (2013).

Cahn, B. R. and Polich, J. "Meditation States and Traits: EEG, ERP and Neuroimaging Studies." *Psychological Bulletin* 132, no. 2 (2006): 180–211.

Campbell, J. *Hero with a Thousand Faces.* New York: Pantheon Books, 1949.

Cannon, B. W. *Bodily Changes in Pain, Hunger, Fear and Rage.* New York: Appleton-Century-Crofts, 1929.

Castillo-Richmond, A., Schneider, R. H., and Alexander, C. N. et al. "Effects of Stress Reduction on Carotid Atherosclerosis in Hypertensive African Americans." *Stroke* 31 (2000): 568–73.

Chalmers, R., Clements, G., Schenkluhn, H., and Weinless, M., eds. *Scientific Research on Maharishi's Transcendental Meditation and TM-Sidhi Program: Collected Papers.* Volumes 2–4. Vlodrop, The Netherlands: Maharishi Vedic University Press, 1989.

Chalmers, R. "Effects of the Transcendental Meditation Program Opposite to Detrimental Effects of the Aging Process." www.truthabouttm.org/truth/TM ResearchSummary/SummaryContinued/index.cfm#Ageing.

Davies, J. L. and Alexander, C. N. "Alleviating Political Violence through Reducing Collective Tension: Impact Assessment Analysis of the Lebanon War." *Journal of Social Behavior and Personality* 17, no. 1 (2005): 285–338.

Denys, K., Cankurtaran, M., Janssens, W., and Petrovic, M. "Metabolic Syndrome in the Elderly: An Overview of the Evidence." *Acta Clinica Belgica* 64 (2009): 23–34.

D'Espagnat. "The Quantum Theory and Reality." *Scientific American* 241, no. 5 (1979): 158–81.

Dillbeck, M. C., Orme-Johnson, D. W., and Wallace, R. K. "Frontal EEG Coherence, H-Reflex, Concept Learning and the TM-Sidhi Program." *International Journal of Neuroscience* 15, no. 3 (1981): 151–57.

Dillbeck, M. C., Landrith, G. III, and Orme-Johnson, D. W. "The Transcendental Meditation Program and Crime Rate Changes in a Sample of Forty-Eight Cities." *Journal of Crime and Justice* 4 (1981): 25–45.

Dillbeck, M. C. and Orme-Johnson, D. W. "Physiological Differences between Transcendental Meditation and Rest." *American Psychologist* 42 (1987): 879–81.

Dillbeck, M. C. and Abrams, A. I. "The Application of the Transcendental Meditation Program to Corrections: Meta-analysis. *International Journal of Comparative and Applied Criminal Justice* 11, no. 1 (1987): 111–32.

Dillbeck, M. C., Cananaugh, K. L., and Glen, T. et al. "Consciousness as a Field: The Transcendental Meditation and TM-Sidhi Program and Changes in Social Indicators." *Journal of Mind and Behavior* 8, no. 1 (1987): 67–104.

Dillbeck, M. C., Banus, C. B., Polanzi, C., and Landrith, G. S. III "Test of a Field Model of Consciousness and Social Change: Transcendental Meditation and TM-Sidhi Program and Decreased Urban Crime." *Journal of Mind and Behavior* 9, no. 4 (1988): 457–86.

Dillbeck, M. C., ed. *Scientific Research on Maharishi's Transcendental Meditation and TM-Sidhi Program: Collected Papers.* Volume 6. Vlodrop, The Netherlands: Maharishi Vedic University Press, 2011.

Dillbeck, M. C., Barnes, V. A., and Schneider, R. H. et al., eds. *Scientific Research on the Transcendental Meditation Program: Collected Papers.* Volume 7. Vlodrop, The Netherlands: Maharishi Vedic University Press, 2013.

Dossey, L. *Recovering the Soul.* New York: Bantam Books, 1989.

Durkheim, E. "Society and Individual Consciousness." In *Theories of Society.* Edited by Parsons, T., Shils, E., Naegele, K. D., and Pitts, J. R., 720–24. Glencoe, IL: Free Press, 1961.

Egenes, T. *Maharishi Patanjali Yoga Sutra.* Translated by Thomas Egenes. Fairfield, IA: 1st World Publishing, 2010.

Einstein, A. "Albert Einstein Quotes on Spirituality." www.simpletoremember.com/articles/a/einstein/.

Farrow, J. T. and Hebert, J. R. "Breath Suspension During the Transcendental Meditation Technique." *Psychosomatic Medicine* 44, no. 2 (1982): 133–53.

Glaser, J. L., Brind, J. L., and Vogelman, J. H. et al. "Elevated Serum Dehydroepiandrosterone Sulfate Levels in Practitioners of Transcendental Meditation and TM-Sidhi Programs." *Journal of Behavioral Medicine* 15, no. 4 (1992): 327–41.

Goddhard, P. H. "Reduced Age Related Declines of P300 Latency in Elderly Practicing Transcendental Meditation." *Psychophysiology* 26 (1989): 529.

Hagelin, J. S. "Is Consciousness the Unified Field? A Field Theorist's Perspective." *Modern Science and Vedic Science* 1, no. 1 (1987): 29–88.

Hagelin, J. S. "Restructuring Physics from Its Foundation in Light of Maharishi's Vedic Science." *Modern Science and Vedic Science* 3, no. 1 (1989): 3–72.

Hawkins, M. A., Orme-Johnson, D. W., and Durchholz, C. F. "Fulfilling the Rehabilitative Ideal through the Transcendental Meditation and TM-Sidhi Programs: Primary, Secondary and Tertiary Prevention." *Journal of Social Behavior and Personality* 17, no. 1 (2005): 443–88.

Hummel, F. C. and Gerloff, C. G. "Interregional Long-Range and Short-Range Synchrony: A Basis for Complex Sensorimotor Functioning." *Progress in Brain Research* 159 (2006): 223–36.

Huxley, A. *The Perennial Philosophy: Harper Perennial Modern Classics.* New York: Harper Collins Publishers, 2009.

James, W. "Human Immortality: Two Supposed Objections to the Doctrine." New York, 1898.

Jayadevappa, R., Johnson, J. C., and Bloom, B. S. et al. "Effectiveness of Transcendental Meditation on Functional Capacity and Quality of Life of African Americans with Congestive Heart Failure: A Randomized Controlled Study." *Ethnicity and Disease* 17 (2007): 72–77.

Jeans, J. *The Mysterious Universe.* New York: Macmillan,1932.

Jung, C. G. *The Archetypes and the Collective Unconscious.* New York: Bollingen Foundation, 1959.

Klein, D. B. *The Concept of Consciousness: A Survey.* Lincoln: University of Nebraska Press, 1984.

Levine, P. H. "The Coherence Spectral Array (Cospar) and Its Application to the Spatial Ordering of the EEG." *Proceedings of the San Diego Biomedical Symposium* 15 (1976): 237–47.

Levine, P. H., Hebert, R., Haynes, C. T., and Strobel, U. "EEG Coherence During the Transcendental Meditation Technique." In *Scientific Research on the Transcendental Meditation Program: Collected Papers.* Edited by Orme-Johnson, D. W. and Farrow, J., 187–207. Livingston Manor, NY: Maharishi European Research University, 1977.

Loevinger, J. *Ego Development: Conceptions and Theories.* San Francisco: Jossey-Bass, 1976.

Lynch, D. www.davidlynchfoundation.org/schools.html.

Maharishi, M. Y. *Creating an Ideal Society.* West Germany: Maharishi European Research University Press, 1977.

Maharishi, M. Y. *Life Supported by Natural law.* Washington, DC: Age of Enlightenment Press, 1986.

Maharishi, M. Y. *Maharishi's Absolute Theory of Government: Automation in Administration.* India: Maharishi Prakashan, Age of Enlightenment Publications, 1995.

Nader, T. *Human Physiology-Expression of Veda and the Vedic Literature.* Vlodrop, Holland: Maharishi University Press, 1995.

Nidich, S. I., Ryncarz, R. A., and Abrams, A. I. et al. "Kohlbergian Moral Perspective Responses, EEG Coherence and the Transcendental Meditation and TM-Sidhi Program." *Journal of Moral Education* 12, no. 3 (19830: 166–73.

O'Leary, D. H., Polak, J. F., and Kronmal, R. A. et al. "Carotid-Artery Intima and Media Thickness as a Risk Factor for Myocardial Infarction and Stroke in Older Adults. Cardiovascular Health Study Collaborative Research Group. *New England Journal of Medicine* 340, no. 1 (1999): 14–22.

Orme-Johnson, D. W. and Farrow, J. T., eds. *Scientific Research on Maharishi's Transcendental Meditation and TM-Sidhi Program: Collected Papers.* Livingston Manor, NY: Maharishi International University Press, 1977.

Orme-Johnson, D. W. and Haynes, C. T. "EEG Phase Coherence, Pure Consciousness, Creativity and TM-Sidhi Experiences." *International Journal of Neuroscience* 13 (1981): 211–17.

Orme-Johnson, D. W. "Medical Care Utilization and the Transcendental Meditation Program." *Psychosomatic Medicine* 49 (1987): 493–507.

Orme-Johnson, D. W., Alexander, C. N., and Davies, J. L. et al. "International Peace Project: The Effects of the Maharishi Technology of the Unified Field." *Journal of Conflict Resolution* 32, no. 4 (1988): 776–812.

Orme-Johnson, D. W., Alexander, C. N., and Davies, J. L. "The Effects of the Maharishi Technology of the Unified Field: Reply to a Methodological Critique." *Journal of Conflict Resolution* 34 (1990): 756–68.

Orme-Johnson, D. W. "Theory and Research on Conflict Resolution through the Maharishi Effect." *Modern Science and Vedic Science* 5, nos. 1–2 (1991): 76–98.

Orme-Johnson, D. W. and Herron, R. E. "An Innovative Approach to Reducing Medical Care Utilization and Expenditures." *American Journal of Managed Care* 3, no. 1 (1997): 135–44.

Orme-Johnson, D. W. "Preventing Crime through the Maharishi Effect." *Journal of Offender Rehabilitation* 36, nos. 1–4 (2003): 257–82.

Orme-Johnson, D. W., Dillbeck, M. C., and Alexander, C. N. "Preventing Terrorism and International Conflict: Effects of Large Assemblies of Participants in the Transcendental Meditation and TM-Sidhi Programs." *Journal of Offender Rehabilitation* 36 (2003): 283–302.

Orme-Johnson, D. W. and Oates, R. M." A Field-Theoretic View of Consciousness: Reply to Critics." *Journal of Scientific Exploration* 32, no. 2 (2009): 139–66.

Orme-Johnson, D. W. "Scholarly Exchanges on the Maharishi Effect: Critics and Rebuttals." www.truthabouttm.org / truth / SocietalEffects / Critics-Rebuttals / index.cfm#IPPME.

Orme-Johnson, D. W. "Some Conceptual Precedents for a Field Theoretic View of Consciousness from *The Perennial Philosophy*, Social Sciences and Quantum Physics." www.truthabouttm.org / truth / SocietalEffects / Rationale-Research / index.cfm.

Palva, S. and Palva, J. M. "New Vistas for Alpha Frequency Band Oscillations." *Trends in Neurosciences* 30, no. 4 (2007): 150–58.

Paul-Labrador, M., Polk, D., and Dwyer, J. H. et al. "Effects of a Randomized Controlled Trial of Transcendental Meditation on Components of the Metabolic Syndrome in Subjects with Coronary Artery Disease." *Archives of Internal Medicine* 166 (2006): 1218–24.

Pearson, C. *Supreme Awakening: Experiences of Higher States of Consciousness across Time and across the World.* Fairfield, IA: Maharishi University of Management Press, 2012.

Pew Center on the States. *State of Recidivism: The Revolving Door of America's Prisons.* Washington, DC: Pew Charitable Trusts, 2011

Rainforth, M. V., Bleick, C., Alexander, C. N., and Cavanaugh, K. L. "The Transcendental Meditation Program and Criminal Recidivism in Folsom State Prisoners: A 15-Year Follow-up Study." *Journal of Offender Rehabilitation* 36 (2003): 181–204.

Salonen, J. T. and Salonen, R. "Ultrasound B-mode Imaging in Observational Studies of Athersclerotic Progression." *Circulation* 87, suppl. 3 (1993): II56–II65.

Sapolsky, R., Krey, L., and McEwens, B. "The Neuroendocrinology of Stress and Aging: The Glucocorticoid Cascade Hypothesis. *Endocrine Review* 7, no. 3 (1986): 284–301.

Sapolsky, R. M. *Stress, the Aging Brain, and the Mechanisms of Neuron Death.* Cambridge, MA: MIT Press, 1992

Sauseng, P. and Klimesch, W. "What Does Phase Information of Oscillatory Brain Activity Tell Us About Cognitive Processes?" *Neuroscience and Biobehavioral Reviews* 32, no. 5 (2008): 1001–13.

Schneider, R. H., Egan, B., and Johnson, E. et al. "Anger and Anxiety in Borderline Hypertension." *Psychosomatic Medicine* 48 (1986): 242–48.

Schneider, R. H., Staggers, F., and Alexander, C. N. et al. "A Randomized Controlled Trial of Stress Reduction for Hypertension in Older African Americans." *Hypertension* 26 (1995): 820–27.

Schneider, R. H., Alexander, C. N., and Staggers, F. et al. "Long-Term Effects of Stress Reduction on Mortality in Persons ≥ 55 Years of Age with Systemic Hypertension." *American Journal of Cardiology* 95, no. 9 (2005): 1060–64.

Schneider, R. H., Grim, C. E., and Rainforth, M. A. et al. "Stress Reduction in the Secondary Prevention of Cardiovascular Disease: Randomized Controlled Trial of Transcendental Meditation and Health Education in Blacks." *Circulation: Cardiovascular Quality and Outcomes* 5, no. 6 (2012): 750–58.

Staessen, J. A., Thijisq, L., and Fagard, R. et al. "Systolic Hypertension in Europe (Syst-Eur) Trial Investigators: Effects of Immediate versus Delayed Antihypertensive Therapy on Outcome in the Systolic Hypertension in Europe Trial." *Journal of Hypertension* 22 (2004): 847–57.

Stapp, H. *Mind, Matter and Quantum Mechanics*. New York: Springer-Verlag, 1993

Stevens, G., Mascarenhas, M., and Mathers, C. "Global Health Risks: Progress and Challenges." *Journal of Personality and Social Psychology* 57, no. 6 (1989): 950–64.

Thatcher, R. W., Biver, C. J., and North, D. "Spatial-Temporal Current Source Correlations and Cortical Connectivity." *Clinical EEG and Neuroscience* 38, no. 1 (2007): 35–48.

Thatcher, R. W. "Coherence, Phase Differences, Phase Shift, and Phase Lock in EEG/ERP Analyses." *Developmental Neuropsychology* 37, no. 6 (2012): 476–96.

Travis, F. T. and Wallace, R. K. "Autonomic Patterns During Respiration Suspensions: Possible Markers of Transcendental Consciousness." *Psychophysiology* 34 (1997): 39–46.

Travis, F. T. and Pearson, C. "Pure Consciousness: Distinct Phenomenological and Physiological Correlates of 'Consciousness Itself.'" *International Journal of Neuroscience* 100, nos. 1–4 (1999): 77–89.

Travis, F. T. and Wallace, K. "Autonomic and EEG Patterns During Eyes-Closed Rest and Transcendental Meditation (TM) Practice." *Consciousness and Cognition* 8, no. 3 (1999): 302–18.

Travis, F. T. and Arenander, A. "Cross-Sectional and Longitudinal Study of Effects of Transcendental Meditation Practice on Interhemispheric Frontal Asymmetry and Frontal Coherence." *International Journal of Neuroscience* 116, no. 12 (2006): 1519–38.

Travis, F. T., Haaga, D., and Hagelin, J. S. et al. "Effects of Transcendental Meditation Practice on Brain Functioning and Stress Reactivity in College Students." *International Journal of Psychophysiology* 71, no. 2 (2009): 170–76.

Wallace, R. K. "Physiological Effects of Transcendental Meditation." *Science* 167 (1970): 1751–54.

Wallace, R. K. "The Physiological Effects of Transcendental Meditation: A Proposed Fourth Major State of Consciousness." In *Scientific Research on the Transcendental Meditation Program: Collected Papers*. Edited by Orme-Johnson, D. W. and Farrow, J. T., 43–78. Livingston Manor, NY: MIU Press, 1970).

Wallace, R. K., Benson, H., and Wilson, A. F. "A Wakeful Hypometabolic Physiologic State." *American Journal of Physiology* 221 (1971): 795–99.

Wallace, R. K. "The Physiology of Meditation." *Scientific American* 226 (1972): 84–90.

Wallace, R. K., Dillbeck, M. C., Jacobe, E., and Harrington, B. "The Effects of the Transcendental Meditation and TM-Sidhi Program on the Aging Process." *International Journal of Neuroscience* 16 (1982): 53–58.

Wallace, R. K., Orme-Johnson, D. W., and Dillbeck, M. C., eds. *Scientific Research on Maharishi's Transcendental meditation and TM_Sidhi Program: Collected Papers.* Volume 5. Fairfield, IA: Maharishi International University Press, 1990.

Walton, K. G. and Levitsky, D. "A Neuroendocrine Mechanism for the Reduction of Drug Use and Addictions by Transcendental Meditation." In *Self-Recovery— Treating Addictions Using Transcendental Meditation and Maharishi Ayurveda.* Edited by O'Connell, D. F. and Alexander, C. N., 89–118. Binghampton, NY: Harrington Park Press,1994.

Walton, K. G., Pugh, N., Gelderloos, P., and Macrae, P. "Stress Reduction and Preventing Hypertension: Preliminary Support for a Psychoendocrine Mechanism." *Journal of Alternative and Complementary Medicine* 1, no. 3 (1995): 263–83.

Walton, K. G., Fields, J. Z., and Harris, D. et al. "Stress and Aging: Reduced Cortisol Response to Glucose in Postmenopausal Women Practicing the Transcendental Meditation Program." *Society for Neuroscience Abstracts* 24 (1998): 1764.

Walton, K. G. and Levitsky, D. K. " Stress-Induced Neuroendocrine Abnormalities in Aggression and Crime-Apparent Reversal by the Transcendental Meditation Program." *Journal of Offender Rehabilitation* 36 (2003): 67–87.

Wigner, E. *Symmetries and Reflections.* Woodbridge, CT: Ox Bow Press, 1967.

Zamarra, J. W., Schneider, R. H., and Besseghini, I. et al. "Usefulness of the Transcendental Meditation Program in the Treatment of Patients with Coronary Artery Disease." *American Journal of Cardiology* 78 (1996): 77–80.

Index

AA. *See* Alcoholics Anonymous
ACE. *See* Adverse Childhood Experience Study
ACTH. *See* adrenocorticotropic hormone
adaptation, 91, 222–23; from natural selection, 265–66; to stress, 47
addictions: AA for, 158–60, 162, 165; adjunct treatment in, 159; anxiety and, 163; brain-wave coherence in, 164–65; comorbidity in, 160; environment in, 166; meditation comparisons and, 158–59; meta-analyses in, 158–59; neurophysiology in, 158; personality disorders and, 162–63; physiology and, 163–64, 167; psychological effects and, 161–62; recommendations in, 166–67; social relationships in, 165–66; spirituality in, 165; for students, 160
ADHD. *See* attention-deficit hyperactivity disorder
adjunct treatment, 151–52, 159
adjustment reaction, 142
adolescent mental health: anxiety research in, 57–58, 182–83; ASDs in, 185–86; mood disorders in, 183–85;

prevention in, 187; self-injury in, 187; substance abuse and, 186–87
adolescents, 160, 177, 185–87; ADHD and, 183, 188–90, 194; African Americans, 181, 184, 190; BP in, 76–77, 181, 190; brain-wave coherence and, 181–82; case studies of, 193–95; cortisol in, 181; depression in, 137, 179, 183–84; learning in, 188–92; morals of, 178; parents and, 193–94; peer support for, 192; presentations to, 192–93; Quiet Time program for, 190–92, 194–95; restful alertness for, 180; stress in, 181
adrenalin, 89, 91
adrenocorticotropic hormone (ACTH), 52
Adverse Childhood Experience Study (ACE), 51
Afghanistan veterans, 126, 128–29
African Americans, 215; adolescents, 181, 184, 190; alcohol abuse by, 159–60; BP in, 73, 76–77, 246–47; CVD and, 55, 75–76, 251; depression in, 139; hypertension for, 73; obesity in, 100–101
Age of Enlightenment, 13

Age of Reason, 13
aggression, 252
aging: adaptability in, 222–23; biological age in, 246; BP in, 246–47; Canada's healthcare costs related to, 213; carotid atherosclerosis in, 248; DHEAS in, 248; healthcare resource use in, 211–13, *249*, 249–50, *250*; mechanics of, 243–46, *245*; metabolic syndrome and insulin resistance in, 247; mortality in, 215, 250–51; myocardial ischemia in, 247–48; orderliness of brain functioning in, 245–46; P300 in, 248–49; stress-reduction in, 244–45, *245*
AIDS, 106
alcohol abuse, 74, 157; by African Americans, 159–60
Alcoholics Anonymous (AA), 158–60, 162, 165
aldosterone, 71–72
Alexander, Charles, 73, 163, 187, 250–53
alienation. *See* loneliness
allergies, *207*
alpha EEG coherence, 245
alternative explanations, 216
ambulatory BP, 77
American Academy of Anti-Aging Medicine, 243
American Heart Association, 29, 56, 205
American Indians. *See* Native Americans
American Psychological Association, 48–49
Anderson, A. J., 74, 255–56
anger, 184; for depression, 141; in girls, 190
angina pectoris, 75
Anklesaria, F. K., 254
ANS. *See* autonomic nervous system
antidepressant medications, 138, 142–44, 149
anxiety, 182; addictions and, 163; causes of, 121; description of, 89; symptoms of, 121–22; in type-2 diabetes, 92–93; type-2 diabetes from, *90*, 91. *See also* post-traumatic stress disorder
anxiety research, 131–32, 185–86; in adolescent mental health, 57–58, 182–83; case studies on, 127–29; GABA in, 164; meta-analyses on, 92, 123–24, *124*, 183; on psychiatric patients, 122; race and ethnicity in, 57–58, 122–23, 182–83; on students, 122–23, 127–28, 182–83; trait anxiety in, 92, 122–24, *124*, 182–83
apneustic breathing, 33
Aristotle, 27
Arnsten, A. F. T., 188–89
asanas (gentle exercise routines), 17
ASDs. *See* autism spectrum disorders
asthma, *207*, 209
atherosclerosis, *207*, 209
atherosclerotic vascular disease, 100
athletes, 37
attention, 188–92; direction of, 5; focused attention meditation, 28, 30–31; on negativity, 8–9
attention deficit hyperactivity disorder (ADHD), 183, 188–90, 194, 209
autism spectrum disorders (ASDs), 185–86
automatic self-transcending meditation, 28–29, 31. *See also* Transcendental Meditation
automotive employees, 222
autonomic nervous system (ANS), 53
autonomic stability, 221
autonomy, 106
Ayurveda. *See* Maharishi Ayurveda
Ayurvedic physician (*vaidya*), 144–45

Badawi, K., 33
Barnes, V. A., *124*, 181, 184, 187, 190
behavior, *124*, *207*, 220, 253
behavioral *rasayanas* (daily and seasonal routines), 17
behavior disorders, 188–92
Being. *See* transcendental consciousness

belief: Maharishi Vedic Science and Technology and, 8, 12, 18; TM related to, 107, 255
Benn, R., 190
Bhagavad Chetana (refined cosmic consciousness), x–xi, 11, 36
biofeedback, 74, 159–60
biological age, 246
biology, 141
bipolar disorder, 151–52
Black, David, 185–86
blind testing, 217
blood glucose: daily routine and, 96–97; loneliness from, 89, *90*, 91; pandemic of, 87; stress and, 89, 91; type-2 diabetes and, 87–88, 91–92
blood pressure (BP), 70; in adolescents, 76–77, 181, 190; in African Americans, 73, 76–77, 246–47; in aging, 246–47; AHA and, 29, 56; breathing and, 56; reactivity, 76; SBP, 72–75; in youth, 76–77. *See also* hypertension
Blue Cross/Blue Shield, 210–12, *211*
the blues, 138
body purification therapies (*panchakarma*), 17
BP. *See* blood pressure
Brahma Chetana (unity consciousness), x–xi, 11, 36
Brahman, x–xi
Brahmananda Saraswati, 11
brain, 224, 246; conscious experience of, 15; cortical idling of, 34; depression and, 26; development of, 179; frontal executive system in, 26, 189, 245; glucocorticoids and, 51; habits and, 27; IBS and, 51; mind-body interactions and, 51–52; stress and, 49–52, 58; of youth, 179. *See also* neuroplasticity
Brain Integration Scale, 36–37, 224
brain-wave coherence, 6, 131, 146; in addictions, 164–65; with ADHD, 189–90; adolescents and, 181–82; cosmic consciousness and, 36; definition of, 164; markers in,

28–29; orderliness of, 245–46; psychological integration and, 224; transcendental consciousness and, 33–34
breast cancer, 215
breathing, 56; apneustic, 33
breathing exercises (*pranayama*), 17
breath rate, 33
Brooks, James, 29, *30*, 92
Bruch, Hilda, 94
Buddhist traditions, 34

California Healthy Kids Survey, 191
California Standards Test, 191
Canada, 268
Canada's healthcare costs, 212; aging related to, 213; high-cost patients in, 213, *214*; prescription medications in, 213–14
Canadian Consumer Price Index, 213
cancer mortality, 75, 215
Cannon, Walter Bradford, 91, 244
cardiovascular disease (CVD), 73–74, 78, *207*; in African Americans, 55, 75–76, 251; controlled studies on, 55–56, 209–10, *210*; mortality from, 75–76, 224–25, 251; physiological mechanisms related to, 71–72; risk factors of, 69; stress and, 55–56, 70–72
carotid atherosclerosis, 75; in aging, 248
CASA. *See* National Center on Addiction and Substance Abuse
case studies: of adolescents, 193–95; on anxiety research, 127–29; on depression, 148–50; on Quiet Time program, 194–95
CDC. *See* Centers for Disease Control and Prevention
cellular health, 56–57
Center for Epidemiologic Studies Depression Scale (CES-D), 139
Center for Wellness and Achievement in Education (CWAE), 190–92
Centers for Disease Control and Prevention (CDC), 137, 185

CES-D. *See* Center for Epidemiologic Studies Depression Scale
character issues, 162–63
Charaka Samhita, 145
CHD. *See* coronary heart disease
checking procedure, for TM, 4, 8
Chen, K. W., 124
childbirth, 211, 249, *249*
children: ADHD in, 209; depression in, 137; IBS in, 101; PTSD in, 125. *See also* adolescents
children and stress, 51; ethnicity in, 57–58; income related to, 179; pregnancy related to, 26
chronic stress, 47–52, 70–71, 129; in addictions, 163; on CVD, 55, 76; on development, 179; fight or flight response and, 244; inflammation from, 53–54
Ciampolini, Mario, 95, 101
cognitive effects, *220*
coherence, 258–59, 264–65. *See also* brain-wave coherence
Colbert, R. D., 192
collective consciousness: coherence in, 258–59, 264–65; individuals in, 257–58; leaders in, 257–58; Maharishi on, 257–59, 261; measurement of, 262–64; order in, 259–60; pure consciousness for, 259–60; rulers in, 258–59; social science on, 256–57; structure of, 257; unified field theory and, 259. *See also* Maharishi Effect
college students, 178; brain functioning of, 224; hypertension in, 73
comorbidity, 138, 160
compassion meditation, 28
completely holistic approach: fragmented approach compared to, 16–17; individual as cosmic in, 15–16; as natural vs. artificial, 16–17; parts in, 16; without reductive physicalism, 15–16; without side-effects, 16; unified field theory and, 17

composite index of variables, 269
concentration, 5–6
Congolese refugees, 126–27
consciousness: as core issue, 13; development of, x–xi; ego development and, 223–24; Lagrangian and, 260; mainstream view of, 13; physics and, 13–14, 260–61; stabilization of, 15; as unified field, 14–15; Vedic literature related to, 260. *See also* higher states of consciousness; *specific states of consciousness*
consciousness-based education, 3, 13
contemplation, 5–6
coronary heart disease (CHD), 215; African Americans and, 55, 75–76; mortality from, 75–76, 209–10, *210*, 224–25, 251
corrections. *See* prison inmates
cortical idling, 34
corticotrophin releasing hormone (CRP), 52
cortisol, 1, 52, 71, 252; in adolescents, 181; ASDs and, 185; for eating, 97; inflammation and, 53–54; stress and, 53–54, 163–64, 244–45, *245*; in type-2 diabetes, 91–92
cosmic consciousness (*nitya-samadhi*; *Turyatit Chetana*), 11; brain-wave coherence and, 36; Maharishi on, 35; physiological patterns in activity and, 36; sleep in, 35–36
costs. *See* healthcare costs; healthcare resource use
C-reactive protein (CRP), *102*, 102–3
creativity, 106
crime: in one percent cities, 267–68; probationers and, 254–55; serotonin related to, 252. *See also* prison inmates
Crohn's disease, *102*, 102–3
CRP. *See* corticotrophin releasing hormone; C-reactive protein
CVD. *See* cardiovascular disease
CWAE. *See* Center for Wellness and Achievement in Education

DA. *See* dopamine
daily and seasonal routines
 (behavioral *rasayanas*), 17
daily routine (*dinacharya*): blood
 glucose and, 96–97; reflux
 esophagitis and, 98–99; in type-2
 diabetes and Maharishi Ayurveda,
 96–100
David Lynch Foundation, ix, 129,
 192–93, 270
Davis, J., 34
dehydroepiandrosterone sulfate
 (DHEAS), 72, 248
depression, *90, 91*; adjunct treatment
 in, 151–52; in adolescents, 137, 179,
 183–84; in African Americans, 139;
 anger for, 141; biology for, 141;
 bipolar disorder with, 152; brain
 and, 26; case study on, 148–50;
 causes of, 141; in children, 137;
 comorbidity with, 138; description
 of, 89; in girls, 183; happiness
 related to, 147–50; Maharishi
 Ayurveda and, 139–40, 144–45;
 measurement of, 150; medications
 for, 138, 142–44, 149; minor,
 144; neurovegetative signs of,
 137–38; object referral and, 147–50;
 prevalence of, 137–38; Self and,
 146–47; self referral in, 150–51;
 stress for, 141, 184; suicides in,
 148–49, 153; symptoms of, 140–41;
 treatment drawbacks for, 143–44,
 149; treatment of, 139, 142–45, 148–
 49; types of, 142–44; unawareness
 of, 137–38; Western perspective on,
 140–44
D'Espagnat, Bernard, 261
DHEAS. *See* dehydroepiandrosterone
 sulfate
diabetes, 108, 209. *See also* type-1
 diabetes; type-2 diabetes
*Diagnostic and Statistical Manual of
 Psychiatry–V*, 122, 142
Dierke, James, 191
Dillbeck, Michael, 92
dinacharya. See daily routine

directedness, 106
disease care, 205
District of Columbia Veterans Home
 (Occoquan, Virginia), 159–60
dopamine (DA), 54, 163–64
Dornelas, E. M., 124
dose-response relationship, 217
dreaming state of consciousness
 (*Swapn Chetana*), 11
Durkheim, E., 256
dysthymic disorder, 142

E. *See* epinephrine
ECT. *See* electro-convulsive therapy
Eddington, Arthur, 14, 261
education, 190–92; consciousness-
 based, 3, 13; health education
 control groups, 209–10, *210*, 213–14,
 217; TM instruction, 4–5
EEG, 6, 36
EEG gamma synchrony, 6
effect sizes, 29
effortlessness, 5–6, 13, 16, 255
ego development: consciousness and,
 223–24; Loevinger test of, 252–53
EH. *See* essential hypertension
EHS. *See* empty hollow sensation
Einstein, Albert, 260
Elder, C., 92–93
electro-convulsive therapy (ECT)
 (shock treatment), 143
Emeran, M., 51
EMG biofeedback, 159–60
emotional eating, 92
emotional effects, *220*
emotional instability, *207*
emotional stress, 55
emotions, negative, 92–93, *124*
empty hollow sensation (EHS), 94–95,
 101
enlightenment, 13; in Buddhist
 tradition, 34; development of, x–xi,
 7, 9; in Vedic tradition, 34–35. *See
 also* higher states of consciousness
entrepreneurs, 223
environment, 166; Maharishi
 Sthapatya-Veda, 17; Self and, 10–11

environmental stress, 71–72
epinephrine (E), 54, 72
Eppley, K., 92
essential hypertension (EH), 69, 78;
     rise in, 76; stress reactivity and,
     70–71; stress-reduction for, 71
ethnicity, 57–58. *See also* race and
     ethnicity
evidence strength, 216–17
experience, 27; conscious, of brain, 15;
     of transcendental consciousness,
     262–63; of unified field, 14–15, 262,
     265–66
Extended Maharishi Effect, 268

Farrow, J. T., 33
Fechner, Gustav, 256, 263–64
fight or flight response, 52, 54,
     129; chronic stress and, 244;
     noradrenergic system and, 189; TM
     compared to, 244–45, *245*
Finkelstein, Evan, 165
5-HIAA. *See* 5-hydroxyindoleacetic
     acid
focused attention meditation, 28, 30–31
food: EHS and, 94–95, 101; hunger
     recognition, 94–95, 98, *99*, 101–2;
     overeating, 92; sugar, 93; for type-2
     diabetes and Maharishi Ayurveda,
     93–94
frontal executive system, 26, 189, 245
Fry, Prem, 222–23
functional capacity, 75

GABA. *See* gamma-aminobutyric acid
GAD. *See* general adaptation
     syndrome
gamma-aminobutyric acid (GABA),
     164
Gelderloos, P., 187
general adaptation syndrome (GAD),
     91
gentle exercise routines (*asanas*), 17
Gen Xers, 49
GH. *See* growth hormone
girls: anger in, 190; depression in, 183
glucocorticoids, 51

Grave's disease, 103–4, *104*
Grosswald, Sarina, 190
growth hormone (GH), 96–97

habits, 27. *See also* neuroplasticity
Hagelin, John, 260
Hamilton Depression Rating Scale
     (HAM-D), 150
happiness, 147–50
hatha yoga, 10
Hawaiians, Native, 139, 215
headaches, *207*, 209; migraine, 105–6
healing, 38. *See also* natural healing
health, 37–38
healthcare costs: in Canada, 212–14,
     214; in U.S., 212
healthcare professionals, 27;
     spirituality and, 107; stress and, 48
healthcare resource use, 206; in aging,
     211–13, *249*, 249–50, *250*; Blue
     Cross/Blue Shield in, 210–11,
     211; childbirth in, 211, 249, *249*;
     hospital admissions in, *211*, 211–12;
     outpatient visits in, 211–12
health education control groups, 209–
     10, *210*, 213–14, 217
heart failure. *See* aging; cardiovascular
     disease; coronary heart disease
Hebert, J. Russell, 33
Herron, Robert, 212–14, *214*, 216
higher states of consciousness, 7,
     10–11; Brain Integration Scale
     and, 36–37; health related to,
     37–38; Maharishi on, 34–35; for
     mental health, 153. *See also* cosmic
     consciousness; refined cosmic
     consciousness; unity consciousness
Hispanics, 57–58
holistic approach. *See* completely
     holistic approach
HOMA. *See* homeostasis model
     assessment
homeostasis, 52–53
homeostasis model assessment
     (HOMA), 88
hormones, 71–72, 146; research on, 54;
     in sleep, 96

hospitalization. *See* healthcare resource use

HPA. *See* hypothalamic-pituitary-adrenal (HPA) axis

hunger recognition, 101–2; in type-2 diabetes and Maharishi Ayurveda, 94–95, 98, *99*

5-hydroxyindoleacetic acid (5-HIAA), 54

hypertension: for African Americans, 73; in college students, 73; drug therapy for, 72; EH, 69–71, 76, 78; meditation comparisons for, 29; stress and, 70

hypervigilance, 129

hypothalamic-pituitary-adrenal (HPA) axis, 52–53, 71, 188

IBS. *See* irritable bowel syndrome

illicit drug use, 157, 159; marijuana, 193

illness, 51–57

immunity. *See* resilience

income, 179

individuals: in collective consciousness, 257–58; as cosmic, 15–16

Infante, J. R., 54

inflammation: cortisol and, 53–54; subclinical, 101–2; TM effects on, 207, 209

insomnia, 184

instruction, in TM, 4–5

insulin, 88

insulin resistance: metabolic syndrome and, 247; from type-2 diabetes, 88–89, 108

insulin sensitivity, 95–96

insurance data. *See* healthcare resource use

Iraq veterans, 126, 128–29

irritable bowel syndrome (IBS): brain and, 51; in children, 101

Israel, 268–69

Jagaret Chetana (waking state of consciousness), 11

James, William, 27, 32

Jeans, James, 260–61

Journal of Conflict Resolution, 264–65

Katha Upanishad, 31

Kearney, D., 29–30, *30*

Keys, Corey, 222–23

King, M. S., 254

Kirp, David, 191

Lagrangian, 260

leaders, 257; managers, 37; rulers, 258–59

learning, *124*, 188–92. *See also* education

Lebanon, 268–69

left ventricular mass (LVM), 70, 77

leisure activity, 26

Levitsky, D., 252

life expectancy, 206. *See also* mortality

Loevinger test of ego development, 252–53

loneliness: from blood glucose, 89, *90*, 91; TM and, 106

loving-kindness research, 30, *30*

Luby, J. L., 26

Lupien, S., 51, 188

LVM. *See* left ventricular mass

magnetoencephalography, 189

Maharishi. *See* Maharishi Mahesh Yogi

Maharishi Ayurveda: depression and, 139–40, 144–45; description of, 17; global effects of, 105; mind-body types in, 18, 93, 145; senses in, 17–18; TM with, 212; type-1 diabetes and, *99*, 99–100. *See also* type-2 diabetes and Maharishi Ayurveda

Maharishi Effect: application of, 269–70; composite index of variables in, 269; natural selection related to, 265–66; One Percent Studies on, 267–68; population size for, 264–65; predictions about, 265–66; research on, 267–69; social indicators on, 266–67; societal change through,

257–60; square root of 1% in, 264–65, 268–69; TM-Sidhi Program for, 264–66, 268–69
Maharishi Mahesh Yogi (Maharishi), 5, 11, 146; on collective consciousness, 257–59, 261; on consciousness, 15; on cosmic consciousness, 35; on higher states of consciousness, 34–35; on problem-focused methods, 8–9; on pure consciousness, 33; on TM, 6
Maharishi Sthapatya-Veda, 17
Maharishi University of Management (MUM), 11–12, 212
Maharishi Vedic Science and Technology, 11; belief and, 8, 12, 18; completely holistic approach of, 15–17; higher Self and lower self in, 31–32, *32*; religion compared to, 12–13; validation in, 12–13
Maharishi Vedic University (MVU), 11
major depression, 142–43
managers, 37
mantra (sound), 4, 32–33
marijuana use, 193
marital satisfaction, 166
Maslow, Abraham, 265–66
Mason, David, 254–55
matched groups, 216
measurement: of collective consciousness, 262–64; of depression, 150; unified field and, 262, 266–69
medical-resource utilization. *See* healthcare resource use
medications, 213–14; for depression, 138, 142–44, 149
meditation comparisons, 216, 219; addictions and, 158–59; alpha EEG coherence in, 245; for effect sizes, 29; for hypertension, 29; meditation procedures in, 28–29; mindfulness meditation in, 6, 29–30, *30*, 57, *124*, 250; problem-focused methods in, 8–9; for PTSD, 29–30, *30*; trait anxiety in, 92, 123–24, *124*

meditation mind-body effects, 29–30, *30*
meditation procedures: in automatic self-transcending meditation, 28–29; in focused attention meditation, 28, 30–31; in meditation comparisons, 28–29; in open monitoring meditation, 28
memory, *124*
mental activity, 7–8
mental control, 5
mental health, 152–53, *207*, *208*. *See also* adolescent mental health; *specific disorders*
Mental Health Inventory (MHI), 57–58
Merikangas, K., 182
meta-analyses, 216; in addictions, 158–59; on anxiety research, 92, 123–24, *124*, 183; of physiological studies, 244, *245*; on trait anxiety, 92, 123–24, *124*
metabolic syndrome, 100; insulin resistance and, 247
MHI. *See* Mental Health Inventory
migraine headaches, 105–6
Millennials, 49
mind, 15
Mind, Matter and Quantum Mechanics (Stapp), 261
mind-body interactions, 51–52
mind-body types, 18, 93, 145
mindfulness meditation: effects of, 28; in meditation comparisons, 6, 29–30, *30*, 57, *124*, 250; research on, 6, 28–30, *30*
Minnesota Multiphasic Personality Inventory (MMPI), 122, 177
minor depression, 144
MMPI. *See* Minnesota Multiphasic Personality Inventory
mood disorders, 183–85. *See also* depression
mood stability, 162
morals, 178
mortality: in aging, 215, 250–51; from breast cancer, 215; from cancer, 75,

215; from CHD, 75–76, 209–10, *210*, 224–25, 251; from CVD, 75–76, 224–25, 251; from suicides, 148–49, 153
mothers: cellular health of, 56–57; pregnancy and, 26, 211, 249, *249*; stress of, 26, 51, 56–57, 185, 194
MUM. *See* Maharishi University of Management
musicians, 37
MVU. *See* Maharishi Vedic University
myocardial ischemia, 209, 247–48

Nader, T., 260
National Association of Mental Illness, 137
National Center on Addiction and Substance Abuse (CASA), 186–87
National Institutes of Health (NIH), 181
National Survey of American Attitudes on Substance Abuse VIII: Teens and Parents, 186–87
Native Americans, 57–58
Native Hawaiians, 139, 215
natural healing, 38; cumulative process of, 8; higher states of consciousness in, 7; imbalances in, 7; mental activity in, 7–8; normalization in, 6–9; rest in, 6–7; transcendental consciousness in, 7
natural selection, 260, 265–66
NE. *See* norepinephrine
negative emotions, 92–93, *124*
neurobiology, 125–26
neuroimaging, 50–51
neurophysiology, 158, *220*, 252
neuroplasticity, 37–38; definition of, 25; habits and, 27; value neutrality of, 25–27. *See also* meditation procedures
neuroticism, *124*
neurovegetative signs, of depression, 137–38
Nidich, S., 73, 184, 191
NIH. *See* National Institutes of Health
nitya-samadhi. See cosmic consciousness

noradrenergic system, 189
norepinephrine (NE), 54, 72, 163
normalization, 6–9
nursing homes, 250

obesity, 100–101
object referral, 147–50
obsessive compulsive disorder, 128
obstetrics. *See* childbirth
One Percent Studies, 267–68
open monitoring meditation, 28, 30–31
Operation Warrior Wellness, 129
order, 259–60
orderliness, 245–46; from inside, 255–56. *See also* brain-wave coherence
Orme-Johnson, David, 92, 124, 184, 187–88, 222. *See also* healthcare resource use
overeating, 92

P300, 248–49
pain, *207*, 209
pain reactivity, 127, 184
panchakarma (body purification therapies), 17
panic attacks, 127–28
parents, 186; adolescents and, 193–94; mothers, 26, 51, 56–57, 185, 194, 211, 249, *249*
Partnership Attitude Tracking Study (PATS Teens), 186–87
Patanjali, 10, 262
PATS Teens. *See* Partnership Attitude Tracking Study
Pauli, Wolfgang, 261
peer support, 192
perception, *124*. *See also* senses
perception-choice experience cycle, 27
personality disorders, 162–63
Personal Orientation Inventory (POI), 162
physicalism, reductive, 15–16
physics: consciousness and, 13–14, 260–61; Lagrangian in, 260; psychophysics, 263–64
physiological mechanisms, 71–72

physiological patterns: of cosmic consciousness, 36; of transcendental consciousness, 33–34
physiological studies, 244, *245*
physiology, 71–72; addictions and, 163–64, 167; wakeful hypometabolic physiologic state, 244–45, *245*
placebo effect, 150, 159
Planck, Max, 14, 261
PMR. *See* progressive muscle relaxation
POI. *See* Personal Orientation Inventory
populations: size for Maharishi Effect, 264–65; for TM, ix–x, 8; vulnerable, 215
post-human era, 16
post-traumatic stress disorder (PTSD): in children, 125; in Congolese refugees, 126–27; meditation comparisons for, 29–30, *30*; neurobiology of, 125–26; prevalence of, 125; research on, 29–30, *30*, 126–27; symptoms of, 126; in veterans, 29–30, *30*, 126
pranayama (breathing exercises), 17
prayer, 165
pregnancy: childbirth, 211, 249, *249*; children and stress related to, 26
prescription medications, 213–14
prevention: CDC for, 137, 185; primary, *218*, 218–20, *220*, 225; secondary, *218*, 218–21, *220*; tertiary, *218*, 218–21, *220*; in U.S., 205. *See also* TM as prevention; *specific topics*
primary prevention, *218*, 218–20, *220*, 225
Principles of Psychology (James), 32
prison inmates, 160–61, 208; behavioral improvements in, 253; psychological improvements in, 252–53; recidivism of, 163, 253–54; in Senegal, 254
probationers, 254–55
problem-focused methods, 8–9
progressive muscle relaxation (PMR), 124

progressive relaxation, 57
psychiatric admissions, 208, 218
psychiatric patients, 122; with bipolar disorder, 151–52
psychological distress, *207*
psychological effects, 161–62
psychological health, 208
psychological improvements, 252–53
psychological integration, 224
psychophysics, 263–64
psychophysiological balance, 17–18
psychosocial stress, 52–57
PTSD. *See* post-traumatic stress disorder
pure consciousness. *See* transcendental consciousness

quality of life, 214–15, 268
Quiet Time program: case study on, 194–95; description of, 190–91; research on, 191–92

race and ethnicity, 191–92; in anxiety research, 57–58, 122–23, 182–83; Hispanics, 57–58; Native Americans, 57–58; Native Hawaiians, 139, 215; trait anxiety in, 122–23, 182–83. *See also* African Americans
Rainforth, M., 74, 254
randomized clinical trials (RCTs), 73–77
randomized controlled trials, 216–17
RCTs. *See* randomized clinical trials
reality, x–xi
recidivism, 163, 253–54
reductive physicalism, 15–16
Rees, B., 29–30, *30*
refined cosmic consciousness (*Bhagavad Chetana*), x–xi, 11, 36
reflux esophagitis, 98–99
refugees, Congolese, 126–27
Rehabilitation Center for Alcoholics, 159–60
relaxation, 57, 250; PMR, 124
religion, 107; TM compared to, 12–13
research, 270; alternative explanations in, 216; blind testing in, 217;

criticism of, 59; dose-response relationship in, 217; evidence strength in, 216–17; extent of, vii, ix; interdisciplinary, xi; matched groups in, 216; placebo effect and, 150, 159; randomized controlled trials in, 216–17; range of, ix–x, 6; RCTs in, 73–77; safety in, 77; time-series analysis for, 268–69. *See also* meta-analyses

resilience, 129; description of, 221; for entrepreneurs, 223; peak levels of, 222–24; relationships related to, 221–22; of soldiers, 57; to stress, 221–24; in TM as prevention, 219–24, *220*

rest, 146; as basis of activity, 6–7

restful alertness, 7, 145–46, 180, 188

resting BP, 76

Rosean, B., 190

Rosenthal, N., 29–30, *30*, 152, 185–86

rulers, 258–59

safety, 77

SAM. *See* sympathetic adrenal medullary (SAM) response

samadhi. See transcendental consciousness

San Francisco, 190–92

SBP. *See* systolic blood pressure

Schneider, Robert, 55, 73, 100, 217

school-based TM programs, 190–92

science, 12–13; social science, 256–57

SDQ. *See* Strengths and Difficulties Questionnaire

secondary prevention, *218*, 218–21, *220*

Sedlmeier, P., 29, 92

selective serotonin reuptake inhibitors (SSRIs), 51

Self: depression and, 146–47; environment and, 10–11; lower self compared to, 31–32, *32*; TM related to, x–xi, 31–32, 37–38, 146–47; transcendental consciousness as, 31–32, 37–38; in Vedic literature, 262

self-actualization, 162, 265–66

self-awareness, 31–32, *32*

self-esteem, 162

self-injury, 187

self-realization, *124*

self referral, 147; in depression, 150–51

Selye, Hans, 91, 105

Senegal, 254

senses, 15; in Maharishi Ayurveda, 17–18; pure consciousness and, 262–64

serotonin: crime related to, 252; 5-HIAA and, 54; SSRIs, 51; stress and, 163–64

seven states of consciousness, 10–11

Shankara, 11

Shankaracharya, 11

Shapiro, S. L., 122

shock treatment. *See* electro-convulsive therapy

side-effects, 16; of medication, 138; of TM, x, 105–6

sidhis. *See* TM-Sidhi Program

Silk, T. J., 189

skin conductance, 222; transcendental consciousness and, 33

sleep, *207*; in ASDs, 185; in cosmic consciousness, 35–36; deprivation of, 97; GH and, 96–97; hormones in, 96; insomnia in, 184; TM effects on, 208; type-2 diabetes and Maharishi Ayurveda and, 97

sleep state of consciousness (*Sushupti Chetana*), 11

SNS. *See* sympathetic nervous system

So, K., 188

social indicators, 266–67

Social Indicators Research, 268

social relationships, 165–66

social science, 256–57

soldiers, 57. *See also* veterans

sound (*mantra*), 4, 32–33

spirituality: in addictions, 165; healthcare professionals and, 107

The Spiritual Recovery Manual: Vedic Knowledge and Yogic Techniques to Accelerate Recovery (Williams), 165

square root of 1%, 264–65, 268–69

SSRIs. *See* selective serotonin reuptake inhibitors
stage-1 hypertension, 29
Stapp, H. P., 261
state anxiety, 122–24, *124*
state effects, 30–31
stitch (*sutra*), 10
Stixrud, William R., 190
St. Louis, Missouri, 254–55
strain, 89
Strengths and Difficulties Questionnaire (SDQ), 57–58
stress: adaptation to, 47; in adolescents, 181; allostatic load of, 50; blood glucose and, 89, 91; brain and, 49–52, 58; cortisol and, 53–54, 163–64, 244–45, *245*; crisis of, 47; CVD and, 55–56, 70–72; definitions of, 52, 70, 89, 91; for depression, 141, 184; diathesis stress model, 50; emotional, 55; environmental, 71–72; healthcare professionals and, 48; hypertension and, 70; learning and, 188; leisure activity related to, 26; of mothers, 26, 51, 56–57, 185, 194; neuroimaging for, 50–51; psychosocial, 52–57; resilience to, 221–24; serotonin and, 163–64; substance abuse related to, 186–87; TM compared to, 53–54; TM's resilience to, 221–22; in U.S., 48–49; of youth, 49. *See also* children and stress; chronic stress; post-traumatic stress disorder
"Stress in America—Missing the Healthcare Connection," 48–49
stress management, 47–49, 58
stressors, 89
stress reactivity, 70–71
stress-reduction: in aging, 244–45, *245*; for EH, 71; techniques for, 56
"Stress Reduction in the Prevention and Treatment of Cardiovascular Disease and African Americans: A Review of Controlled Research" (Schneider), 55
stress-related conditions, 206, *207*, 208; in adolescents, 177–79, 182–87

stroke, 75–76, 209–10, *210*
students: addictions and, 160; anxiety research on, 122–23, 127–28, 182–83. *See also* college students
subclinical inflammation, 101–2
substance abuse, *207*, 208; marijuana in, 193; probationers and, 255; stress related to, 186–87; tobacco use, 74, 159. *See also* alcohol abuse
subsyndromal anxiety, 121–22
sugar, 93
suicide, 148–49, 153
Sushupti Chetana (sleep state of consciousness), 11
sutra (stitch, thread), 10
Swapn Chetana (dreaming state of consciousness), 11
Swedish National Health Board, 208
sympathetic adrenal medullary (SAM) response, 52, 54. *See also* fight or flight response
sympathetic nervous system (SNS), 70, 75
systolic blood pressure (SBP), 72–75, 246–47

teachers: of TM, 4, 255; TM for, 191–92
technology use, 178–79
teens. *See* adolescents; youth
telomerase, 56–57
tertiary prevention, *218*, 218–21, *220*
thoughts, 7–8
thread (*sutra*), 10
thyroid functioning, 103–4, *104*
thyroid stimulating hormone (TSH), 104
time-series analysis, 268–69
TM. *See* Transcendental Meditation
TM as prevention, 152, 187, 225; effectiveness of, 217–21, *218*, *220*; resilience in, 219–24, *220*; understanding of, 219–21, *220*
TM-Sidhi Program, 9–11; for Maharishi Effect, 264–66, 268–69
tobacco use, 74, 159
total knowledge (*Veda*), 3, 11–12
trait anxiety: in anxiety research, 92, 122–24, *124*, 182–83; definition of,

122; in meditation comparisons, 92, 123–24, *124*; meta-analysis on, 92, 123–24, *124*; in race and ethnicity, 122–23, 182–83
transcendental consciousness (Being, pure consciousness, *samadhi*; *Turiya Chetana*), 3–4, 11, 14–15; brain-wave coherence and, 33–34; breath rate and, 33; experience of, 262–63; as holistic active ingredient, 6–7; Maharishi on, 33; nature of, 31–34, *32*; physiological patterns of, 33–34; research on, 6–7; restful alertness as, 7; rest in, 6–7; as Self, 31–32, 37–38; senses and, 262–64; skin conductance and, 33; wakeful hypometabolic physiologic state as, 244–45, *245*; as wakefulness, 33
Transcendental Meditation (TM): belief related to, 107, 255; breathing in, 56; descriptions of, 3–4, 9, 32–33, 129–30, 145–46; effects of, 105–6, 130–31; effortlessness of, 5–6, 13, 16, 255; emphasis in, 8; fight or flight response compared to, 244–45, *245*; global effects of, 105–6; instruction in, 4–5; loneliness and, 106; Maharishi on, 6; origin of, 11; population for, ix–x, 8; religion compared to, 12–13; SAM and, 54; self-referral in, 147, 150–51; Self related to, x–xi, 31–32, 37–38, 146–47; side-effects of, x, 105–6; stress compared to, 53–54; teachers and, 4, 191–92, 255; thoughts in, 7–8; transcendental in, 6. *See also specific topics*
trauma, 26. *See also* post-traumatic stress disorder
Travis, Fred, 184, 190, 224
TSH. *See* thyroid stimulating hormone
Turiya Chetana. See transcendental consciousness
Turyatit Chetana. See cosmic consciousness
type-1 diabetes, *99*, 99–100
type-2 diabetes, *207*; anxiety in, 92–93; blood glucose and, 87–89, 91–92;

cortisol in, 91–92; emotional eating and, 92; HOMA for, 88; insulin in, 88; insulin resistance from, 88–89, *90*, 108; negative emotions in, 92–93; underlying causes of, 89, *90*, 91–93, 106; in U.S., 87
type-2 diabetes and Maharishi Ayurveda: complications and, 100–104, *102*, *104*; daily routine in, 96–100; food for, 93–94; GH and, 96–97; hunger recognition in, 94–95, 98, *99*; insulin sensitivity in, 95–96; sleep and, 97

unified field: as consciousness, 14–15; experience of, 14–15, 262, 265–66; measurement and, 262, 266–69; positive effects from, 265–66
unified field theory, 14; collective consciousness and, 259; completely holistic approach and, 17
unifying ability, 106
United States (U.S.): disease care in, 205; healthcare costs in, 212; prevention in, 205; stress in, 48–49; type-2 diabetes in, 87
unity consciousness (*Brahma Chetana*), x–xi, 11, 36
universal consciousness, 260–61
universal harmony, 107
U.S. *See* United States

Vago, D., 34
vaidya (Ayurvedic physician), 144–45
value neutrality: of neuroplasticity, 25–27; positivity and, 26–27; stress and trauma related to, 26
vasoconstriction, 75
Veda (total knowledge), 3, 11–12
Vedic knowledge, 12–13
Vedic literature, 260; *Katha Upanishad*, 31; Self in, 262; *Yoga Sutras of Patanjali*, 10, 262
Vedic tradition, 34–35
Vermont, 192
veterans, 125, 159–60; Afghanistan, 126, 128–29; Iraq, 126, 128–29; Operation Warrior Wellness for,

129; PTSD in, 29–30, *30*, 126;
    Vietnam War, 92, 126

wakeful hypometabolic physiologic
    state, 244–45, *245*
wakefulness, 33
waking state of consciousness (*Jagaret
    Chetana*), 11
Wallace, R. K., 244–45
Walsh, R., 122
Walton, K. G., 55–56, 252
war, 267–69. *See also* veterans

Wenneberg, S. R., 73
White, S. W., 185
Wigner, Eugene, 14, 261
Williams, Patrick Gresham, 165
women, 26, 211, 249, *249*. *See also*
    mothers

yoga, 10, 262
Yoga Sutras of Patanjali, 10, 262
youth: brain of, 179; stress of, 49;
    technology use by, 178–79. *See also*
    adolescents; college students

The Editors

David F. O'Connell, Ph.D., M.S., CFC, DABPS, is a licensed psychologist with thirty-six years of experience and the author or editor of six books. He has a private practice in forensic and clinical psychology in Pottsville, Pennsylvania. He is a board-certified forensic psychologist with the American College of Forensic Examiners Institute and is listed in the National Register of Health Service Providers in Psychology. He is a member of the American Psychological Association, the American Board of Medical Psychology, and the American Association for the Treatment of Sexual Abusers. He received an M.S. in counseling psychology from Loyola University in 1978, his Ph.D. in psychological studies from Temple University in 1986, and a postdoctoral M.S. in clinical psychopharmacology from Fairleigh Dickinson University in 2009. He has taught in the graduate school of Rosemont College, and he is a conditional prescribing psychologist at St. Christopher in Albuquerque, New Mexico. He has served as the clinical director of Adult and Adolescent Services at Caron Addiction Treatment Center in Pennsylvania and on the editorial board of the *Journal of Adolescent Chemical Dependency*. He is a consulting psychologist at the Reading Health System's Department of Psychiatry. He is a clinical consultant to Lifeworks, an inpatient addictions treatment program in the United Kingdom.

Deborah L. Bevvino, Ph.D., NP, is currently the behavioral medicine faculty associate in the Family Practice and Community Medicine Residency Program at Reading Hospital & Medical Center. She holds adjunct assistant clinical faculty positions at Penn State University School of Medicine and the Sidney Kimmel Family and Community Medicine

College of Jefferson University. She is a practicing psychologist at the Center for Mental Health at Reading Hospital and is also an Adult Nurse Practitioner. She has been practicing Transcendental Meditation and Ayurveda for twenty years.

Contributors

Alarik Arenander, Ph.D.
Director, Brain Research Institute
Fairfield, Iowa

Vernon A. Barnes, Ph.D.
Assistant Professor
Georgia Prevention Center
Institute of Public and Preventive
    Health
Department of Pediatrics
Medical College of Georgia
College of Nursing
The Graduate School
Georgia Regents University
Augusta, Georgia

Deborah L. Bevvino, Ph.D., NP
Adjunct Clinical Assistant
    Professor
Family and Community Medicine
Sidney Kimmel Medical College
    of Thomas Jefferson University
    (SKMC)
Philadelphia, Pennsylvania

Robert W. Boyer, Ph.D.
Certified TM teacher
Applied Developmental
    Psychology
Licensed Psychologist, Iowa
Research Fellow, Institute for
    Advanced Research
Malibu, California

Jim Brooks, M.D.
Certified in Zero Balancing &
Classical Five-Element
    Acupuncture
Ayurvedic Physician
Psychiatrist, Private Practice
Fairfield, Iowa

Sarina Grosswald, Ed.D.
Director of Research
Operation Warrior Wellness
David Lynch Foundation

Robert Herron, Ph.D.
Director
Health Systems Analysis
Fairfield, Iowa

James Krag, M.D.
Distinguished Fellow, American
  Psychiatric Association
Clinical Psychiatrist, Harrisonburg,
  Virginia Community Based
  Outpatient Clinic, Veterans
  Administration
Former Assistant Professor,
  Department of Psychiatry and
  Neurobehavioral Sciences,
  University of Virginia

**David Lovell-Smith, Ph.D., MB,
  Ch.B. FRNZCGP**
Senior Clinical Lecturer
Department of General Practice
University of Otago Christchurch
  School of Medicine
General Practitioner, Private
  Practice
Christchurch, New Zealand

**David F. O'Connell, Ph.D., M.S.,
  DABPS**
Board Certified Forensic
  Psychologist
Medical Psychologist
Private Practice
Pottsville, Pennsylvania

David W. Orme-Johnson, Ph.D.
Research Desk
The Maharishi Foundation

Norman E. Rosenthal, M.D.
Clinical Professor of Psychiatry
Georgetown University School of
  Medicine

Maxwell Rainforth, Ph.D.
Professor, Department of Vedic
  Science
Maharishi University of
  Management
Fairfield, Iowa

William R. Stixrud, Ph.D.
Clinical Neuropsychologist
William Stixrud and Associates
Bethesda, MD

Fred Travis, Ph.D.
Professor, Department of Vedic
  Science
Director, Center for Brain,
  Consciousness and Cognition
Maharishi University of
  Management
Fairfield, Iowa